CBT: Science Into Practice

Series Editor

Nikolaos Kazantzis, Cognitive Behavior Therapy Research Unit
Melbourne, VIC, Australia

This series addresses topics that reflect current thinking in the field of cognitive behavior therapy, the most widely accepted form of therapy across mental health disciplines. Despite the consensus that CBT is an effective treatment modality, much of the existing clinical literature focuses on single facets, such as specific disorders or populations. Mostly it does not take into account the latest evidence for transdiagnostic change mechanisms and processes. This series provides guidance on how the latest evidence can be translated into practice. Volumes focus on enhancing flexibility in both the selection and delivery of techniques tailored to individual clients. Each provides clinical insights enhanced by case studies and vignettes to ensure relevance for the practicing professional.

Kate Wolitzky-Taylor
Editor

Treating Comorbid Substance Use and Emotional Disorders

Springer

CBT Network™

Editor
Kate Wolitzky-Taylor
UCLA Department of Psychiatry and Biobehavioral Sciences
Los Angeles, CA, USA

ISSN 2946-5419 ISSN 2946-5427 (electronic)
CBT: Science Into Practice
ISBN 978-3-031-62970-9 ISBN 978-3-031-62971-6 (eBook)
https://doi.org/10.1007/978-3-031-62971-6

This Springer imprint is published by the registered company Springer Nature Switzerland AG
The registered company address is: Gewerbestrasse 11, 6330 Cham, Switzerland

"It was with high expectations that I greeted the just published volume *Treating Comorbid Substance Use and Emotional Disorders* edited by Dr. Kate Wolitzky-Taylor. Although emotional disorders and substance use disorders are a highly prevalent comorbidity, and their combination results in poorer treatment and life outcomes, the fields of addiction treatment and mental health treatment have been historically bifurcated. Cognitive behavioral therapy (CBT) is the most effective broad-spectrum behavioral intervention available today. Yet clinicians are split on how CBT may be applied to their patients with substance use disorders *or* emotional disorders. This belief is common, despite the fact that CBT shares identical principles and functions agnostic to diagnostic condition or target symptom. This volume assembles the most expert of clinician-scientists who have dedicated their professional careers to developing, delivering, evaluating, and disseminating integrated CBT for co-occurring emotional and substance use disorders. The volume definitely delivered on my high expectations. It is enthusiastically recommended for clinician education and training programs, researchers, and also frontline CBT therapists seeking to provide the best care possible to their complex patients."

—Mark McGovern, *Professor, Department of Psychiatry, Department of Medicine, Stanford University School of Medicine*

"Emotional disorders rarely occur in isolation, but most existing treatment protocols do not account for this. Comorbid substance use problems severely impact interventions that are ordinarily effective for anxiety and mood conditions. Dr. Wolitzky-Taylor tackles this problem head-on in this important book. Leading clinicians and scientists have provided clear and incisive recommendations that will inform beginning-level clinicians as well as experienced mental health professionals."

—N.B. Schmidt, *Distinguished Research Professor and Chair, Department of Psychology, Florida State University; Director, Anxiety and Behavioral Health Clinic*

"*Treating Comorbid Substance Use and Emotional Disorders* is a groundbreaking volume that illuminates a vital shift in mental health care. Authored by leading experts, it confronts the historical divide between treating emotional disorders and substance use disorders (SUD) head-on, offering a comprehensive roadmap for integrated care. Backed by research, this book challenges outdated treatment paradigms, advocating for simultaneous, evidence-based interventions. It's a timely resource, bridging the gap between research and practice, empowering clinicians with actionable strategies to address complex comorbidities effectively. By offering examples of case formulations and therapeutic dialogues, it equips practitioners with practical tools to navigate the clinical scenarios they encounter in practice. This volume is essential reading for anyone committed to delivering the best care for their patients."

—Jasper Smits, Ph.D., *Professor, Department of Psychology, University of Texas at Austin*

To Matt, who was my fiercest and most loyal supporter and partner in all things. Thank you for everything, always.

Foreword

I am delighted that the book *Treating Comorbid Substance Use and Emotional Disorders* is being published in the CBT: Science into Practice book series. As clinicians, we are all too familiar with the complexities that arise when treating individuals with co-occurring emotional disorders and substance use disorders (SUD). The intertwined nature of these conditions presents unique challenges that have long puzzled both researchers and practitioners alike. A primary consideration in the diagnosis of emotional disorders is whether the current presentation occurred in the context of substance use, and if so, there is a need to adapt Cognitive Behavior Therapy (CBT) to take account of this co-occurring use or dependency. Clinicians also have to assess whether the substance use is deemed by the individual to be a goal for therapy, and there are frequent occurrences where the individual is unwilling to consider or act on reduction or abstinence.

The past decades have borne witness to a wealth of research illuminating the intricate relationship between emotional disorders and SUD, highlighting the detrimental impact of their co-occurrence on clinical outcomes and quality of life. Despite this knowledge, effective treatment solutions remained elusive until recent years. This volume stands as a testament to the culmination of this effort, offering a comprehensive exploration of evidence-based interventions that bridge the gap between theory and practice. As a leading researcher in the field, Dr. Wolitzky-Taylor adeptly navigates through the historical context, charting the evolution of treatment paradigms from parallel and sequential interventions to the pivotal emergence of integrated approaches.

Through meticulous synthesis of research findings and practical guidance, Dr. Wolitzky-Taylor and esteemed contributors equip clinicians with the tools to navigate the complexities of integrated care. Following Dr. Wolitzky-Taylor's introduction (Chap. 1), each chapter addresses a frequent comorbidity, including social anxiety disorder and alcohol use (Chap. 2), cannabis use disorder and emotional disorders (Chap. 3), SUD and major depressive disorder (Chap. 4), and posttraumatic stress disorder and SUD (Chap. 5).

Drawing from the rich family of CBTs, this volume transcends traditional diagnostic boundaries, embracing a transdiagnostic framework that addresses underlying processes common to emotional disorders and SUD. By targeting these core constructs, clinicians can effectively dismantle the barriers to recovery and pave the way for lasting change. There are chapters on affect management training (Chap. 6), smoking cessation and anxiety sensitivity (Chap. 7), third-wave treatments for comorbid SUD and emotional disorders (Chap. 8), anxiety and opioid use in those with chronic pain (Chap. 9), and when CBT is applied to benzodiazepines discontinuation (Chap. 10). I applaud all the contributors to this volume for their excellent work.

Dr. Wolitzky-Taylor's comprehensive volume emerges as a landmark resource that offers clarity and innovation in this challenging terrain. Dr. Wolitzky-Taylor's comprehensive exploration in this volume couldn't come at a more crucial time. With decades of research indicating the significant impact of comorbid emotional disorders and SUD on clinical outcomes, the call for effective integrated treatments has never been louder. Importantly, this volume champions a paradigm shift away from siloed approaches toward a more holistic understanding of psychopathology. By embracing a dimensional, transdiagnostic framework, the authors underscore the interconnectedness of emotional disorders and SUD, paving the way for more effective treatment strategies.

The editor brings a wealth of professional experience to this volume. Dr. Kate Wolitzky-Taylor is the Associate Director of the Anxiety and Depression Research Center at UCLA and a Principal Investigator in the Integrated Substance Abuse Programs in the UCLA Semel Institute. Her primary appointment is as an Associate Professor in the UCLA Department of Psychiatry and Biobehavioral Sciences. Dr. Wolitzky-Taylor has published extensively in the areas of CBT for comorbid SUD and emotional disorders, including as a result of being the Principal Investigator for several NIH-funded studies that focus on the development and evaluation of treatments for comorbid emotional disorders and SUD. Dr. Wolitzky-Taylor also treats patients with anxiety and related disorders in the UCLA Faculty Practice Outpatient Clinic and in the Behavioral Health Services. She also directs two clinical practica for clinical psychology doctoral students in UCLA, in which she provides clinical training and supervision in CBT: one that focuses on the treatment of comorbid emotional disorders and SUD, and one that focuses on the treatment of anxiety and depression. Dr. Wolitzky-Taylor is eminently qualified to offer this book, as have produced a book with a rich synthesis of evidence to guide practice.

As we embark on this journey toward integrated care, it is imperative that we heed the call to action articulated within these pages. Dr. Wolitzky-Taylor's important volume serves as a catalyst for change, inspiring clinicians, researchers, and policymakers alike to unite in our collective mission to enhance the well-being of individuals grappling with comorbid emotional disorders and SUD. Dr. Kate Wolitzky-Taylor and her contributors have laid the foundation. It is now up to us, as clinicians and advocates, to build upon it and usher in a new era of integrated care for individuals with comorbid emotional disorders and SUD.

Conflicts of Interest Kazantzis disclosed his royalties from the Guilford Press (Therapeutic Relationship in Cognitive Behavior Therapy; *Cognitive and Behavior*

Theories in Clinical Practice), Routledge (*Using Homework Assignments in Cognitive Behavior Therapy*); SpringerNature publishers (CBT: Science into Practice Book Series; *Handbook of Homework Assignments in Psychotherapy: Research, Practice, and Prevention*). He also disclosed editor stipend from the Association for Behavioral and Cognitive Therapies for his role as Editor-in-Chief for *Cognitive and Behavioral Practice* (Elsevier).

Cognitive Behavior Therapy Research Unit
Melbourne, VIC, Australia
Beck Institute for Cognitive Behavior Therapy
Philadelphia, PA, USA

Nikolaos Kazantzis

Contents

About the Editor

Kate Wolitzky-Taylor, Ph.D., is a licensed clinical psychologist and Associate Professor in the UCLA Department of Psychiatry and Biobehavioral Sciences and Semel Institute for Neuroscience and Human Behavior. With over 100 publications and continuous NIH funding for her research since her predoctoral training, she has extensive experience in the development, evaluation, and implementation of cognitive and behavioral therapies (CBT) for anxiety disorder and comorbid substance use disorders (SUD). Her research expertise was developed during her doctoral training in the Laboratory for the Study of Anxiety Disorders at the University of Texas at Austin, where she was funded by the National Institute of Mental Health (NIMH) on a National Research Service Award (F31) to examine the efficacy of self-administered treatments for pathological worry. She then completed her clinical internship at the Medical University of South Carolina, where she was funded on an NIMH training grant (T32) focusing on the research and treatment of trauma-related problems. She then completed a 3-year postdoctoral research fellowship in the Anxiety and Depression Research Center at UCLA, in which she was Project Director of a 10-year, multi-site, NIMH-funded longitudinal study examining common and specific risk factors for emotional disorders. She developed expertise in the nature and treatment of comorbid anxiety and SUD through her Early Career Development Award (K23) funded by the National Institute on Drug Abuse (NIDA), in which she developed and evaluated a CBT program for anxiety disorders to be delivered in SUD specialty clinics to those with comorbid anxiety and substance use disorders. Since then, she has received continuous funding for several NIH-funded studies aimed at developing and evaluating novel behavioral treatments for comorbid anxiety disorders and SUD. In addition to her innovative program of work in the treatment of comorbid anxiety and SUD, for which she received the Sobell Innovative Addictions Research Award from the Association for Behavioral and Cognitive Therapies, she is the Center co-Director for an NIMH-funded ALACRITY Center that aims to optimize a digitally focused, tiered model of care for anxiety and depression among community college students. In addition to her research, she has an extensive history of providing clinical training and supervision to clinical psychology graduate students, postdoctoral fellows, psychiatry residents, and master's level clinicians in CBT for anxiety disorders, depression, and comorbid emotional disorders and SUD. Dr. Wolitzky-Taylor also treats patients in the UCLA Faculty Practice, specializing in CBT for anxiety, depression, and comorbid emotional disorder/SUD treatment.

Chapter 1
Introduction to the Volume: The Case for Integrating Cognitive Behavioral Therapy for Emotional Disorders and Substance Use Disorders

Kate Wolitzky-Taylor

The high comorbidity of anxiety and depressive disorders (herein referred to as "emotional disorders") and substance use disorders (SUD) has been well documented for several decades (Compton et al., 2007; Grant et al., 2004; Lai et al., 2015; Lee et al., 2022; Leventhal et al., 2010; Savant et al., 2013). This comorbidity has consistently been associated with poorer clinical and functional outcomes in numerous studies over the past several decades as well, including poorer prognosis, greater symptom severity, increased medical utilization, poorer quality of life, poorer engagement in treatment, increased risk of relapse following treatment, and suicide (McKay et al., 2002; Carpentier et al., 2009; Litz & Leslie, 2017; Benningfield et al., 2012; Roy-Byrne et al., 2013; Burns et al., 2005; Glasner-Edwards & Rawson, 2010; Ouimette et al., 2000; Schmitz & Kruse, 2002; Book et al., 2009; Kushner et al., 2005; Schellekens et al., 2015; Smith & Book, 2010). Multiple review articles and even entire books have been written on the nature of emotional disorder and SUD comorbidity (Stewart & Conrod, 2008; Wolitzky-Taylor et al., 2011; McHugh, 2015; Swendsen & Marikangas, 2000; Hesse, 2009).

Despite the knowledge that the comorbidity of emotional disorders and SUD is prevalent and associated with significant consequences, there has been a relative paucity of effective treatment solutions until recently. Early work was limited and primarily evaluated the use of parallel or sequential treatments for each problem/disorder and found limited to no superiority of combined SUD/emotional disorder treatment compared to SUD treatment alone (Bowen et al., 2000; Randall et al., 2001). As the mutual maintenance model of SUD/anxiety comorbidity began to gain traction (Stewart & Conrod, 2008), which also fit well with SUD/emotional

K. Wolitzky-Taylor (✉)
Department of Psychiatry and Biobehavioral Sciences and Semel Institute for Neuroscience and Human Behavior, Integrated Substance Abuse Programs, Los Angeles, CA, USA
e-mail: kbtaylor@mednet.ucla.edu

K. Wolitzky-Taylor (ed.), *Treating Comorbid Substance Use and Emotional Disorders*, CBT: Science Into Practice, https://doi.org/10.1007/978-3-031-62971-6_1

disorder comorbidity more broadly, the importance of developing and evaluating *integrated* treatments for this comorbidity emerged. Indeed, treatments began to emerge that focused directly on breaking the cycle of emotional disorder symptom/substance use by addressing the functional relationships between the two problems and weaving together treatments for both problems in clinically meaningful ways. These integrated interventions, which varied in terms of content, delivery modality, and degree of integration typically demonstrated greater improvements not only in emotional disorders symptoms but in SUD symptom severity compared to SUD treatment alone (e.g., Kushner et al., 2006; Wolitzky-Taylor et al., 2018; Brown et al., 2006; Carpenter et al., 2008; Hien et al., 2010). As a consequence of this growing body of research, the field has reached the point in which the evaluation of the overall effectiveness of these approaches is possible. Indeed, my recent meta-analysis of 11 randomized clinical trials comparing an integrated behavioral treatment for comorbid anxiety disorders/SUD to evidence-based SUD treatment alone demonstrated small to moderate effects favoring the integrated treatment (Wolitzky-Taylor, 2023). Even a small to moderate effect over the gold standard, typically delivered SUD treatment is clinically meaningful. Importantly, the relative superiority of integrated cognitive behavioral therapy (CBT) compared to SUD treatment alone was observed on both anxiety and SUD clinical outcomes, lending support to the mutual maintenance model (Stewart & Conrod, 2008).

In parallel with the development and evaluation of integrated cognitive and behavioral therapy approaches to treating comorbid emotional disorders and SUD, policy calls for addressing this comorbidity have begun to emerge (Barry & Huskamp, 2011; Burnham & Watkins, 2006; SAMHSA, 2022). However, despite an increased awareness of the need for integrated mental health and SUD treatment in community-based settings, SUD treatment and mental health treatment typically remain siloed. This is the consequence of a historical misunderstanding about the nature of emotional disorder/SUD comorbidity which led to the development of two separate pathways for care and the conventional wisdom for decades that one needed to address SUD first, before emotional disorders could be addressed (e.g., Nace, 1988). This misguided division of treatment for problems often so inextricably bound resulted in multiple referrals, problems accessing care, and poorer treatment response (Havassy et al., 2009; McGovern et al., 2006), as well as a system that faces barriers to integrating care for these two problems.

Now that the clinical research and policy recommendations converge around the importance of evidence-based, integrated treatment for comorbid emotional disorders/SUD, it is critical that both the research and clinical communities increase their awareness of what an integrated treatment is,[1] the varied and diverse ways in which cognitive and behavioral treatments for emotional disorder/SUD comorbidity can be effectively delivered, and how to deliver these interventions for a range of emotional disorders. This is a crucial step in bridging the research to community practice gap that is currently leaving a large number of individuals with comorbid

[1] For an operational definition of an integrated treatment and a model for understanding the levels of treatment integration for this population, see Wolitzky-Taylor et al. (2022).

emotional disorders/SUD inadequately treated, making them vulnerable to substance relapse and poor functioning. At present, the majority of research for each of these problems still tends to be siloed, and specialty training in mental health professions tends pigeonhole clinicians into "SUD provider" or "mental health provider". As a consequence, treatment approaches that most clinicians learn and deliver in practice continue to be siloed as well.

This volume attempts to overcome the limitations of training programs and clinical practice paradigms that divide these highly functionally related problems by presenting the first comprehensive overview of integrated treatments for emotional disorders and SUD. As with the other volumes in the *CBT: Science into Practice* series, each chapter in this volume balances the research support for each approach with a practical, step-by-step description of how clinicians can deliver these interventions. Clinical case formulations and client-therapist dialogue are woven throughout to provide concrete tools for clinicians. These chapters do *not*, however, serve as detailed manuals for delivering any given intervention to fidelity.[2] While some chapters describe a specific intervention in detail (e.g., a specific CBT-based intervention targeting comorbid cannabis use disorder and anxiety disorders), others provide a more comprehensive overview of various evidence-based approaches to a particular problem (e.g., PTSD and SUD comorbidity). Further, while some chapters focus on a specific problem (e.g., treating anxiety disorder and opioid use disorder comorbidity among chronic pain patients taking opioids) or specific common comorbidities (e.g., social anxiety disorder and alcohol use disorder), others describe how a particular modality (e.g., third-wave behavioral therapies) can be used to address comorbid emotional disorders and SUD more broadly.

Finally, it is worth noting that, in line with the movement in the field away from traditional diagnoses and towards a dimensional, transdiagnostic framework for understanding and treating psychopathology (NIH, 2008; Insel et al., 2010), and specifically, emotional disorder/SUD comorbidity (Buckner et al., 2007; Wolitzky-Taylor et al., 2015; Bernstein et al., 2009; Buckner et al., 2011a, b; Chawla & Ostafin, 2007; Cougle et al., 2012; Hearon et al., 2011; McHugh & Otto, 2012; Wolitzky-Taylor et al., 2016), this volume includes chapters that focus on targeting relevant transdiagnostic constructs implicated in the onset and maintenance of emotional disorder/SUD comorbidity.[3] For example, chapters discuss how targeting anxiety sensitivity can aid in smoking cessation and how targeting transdiagnostic processes including anxiety sensitivity, distress intolerance, and facets of emotion dysregulation can reduce cannabis use. In sum, the volume begins with chapters focusing on specific comorbidities, then moves into the more transdiagnostic approaches to treating this comorbidity, and concludes with special populations and considerations.

---

[2] For more detailed therapist guides for the treatment approaches, many of the chapter authors would be delighted to share manuals they have developed and evaluated, upon request.

[3] See Wolitzky-Taylor et al. (2022) and Wolitzky-Taylor (2023) for a more detailed discussion.

My hope is that this volume, the first of its kind and written by renowned experts in cognitive and behavioral treatments for comorbid emotional disorders and SUD, will provide a comprehensive overview of the myriad ways that cognitive and behavioral therapies can (and have shown to) be effectively used to address emotional disorder/SUD comorbidity. Although the field faces systemic barriers to effectively integrating care for these commonly comorbid problems, researchers, clinicians, and policymakers are all in agreement that this is the most effective, practical, and parsimonious way to address this comorbidity. One critical step we can take is by providing clinicians with the tools to begin to understand and apply these skills, components, and concepts in their clinical work, and to pique the curiosity of researchers in the hopes they will develop their own programs of work to extend our knowledge of this highly prevalent but sadly understudied population. We are making good headway in the right direction, but there is still significant room for improvement, particularly in bridging the research to practice gap in this area.

References

Barry, C. L., & Huskamp, H. A. (2011). Moving beyond parity — mental health and addiction care under the ACA. *New England Journal of Medicine, 365*(11), 973–975. https://doi.org/10.1056/nejmp1108649

Benningfield, M. M., Dietrich, M. S., Jones, H. E., Kaltenbach, K., Heil, S. H., Stine, S. M., Coyle, M. G., Arria, A. M., O'Grady, K. E., Fischer, G., & Martin, P. R. (2012). Opioid dependence during pregnancy: Relationships of anxiety and depression symptoms to treatment outcomes. *Addiction, 107*, 74–82. https://doi.org/10.1111/j.1360-0443.2012.04041.x

Bernstein, A., Zvolensky, M. J., Vujanovic, A. A., & Moos, R. (2009). Integrating anxiety sensitivity, distress tolerance, and discomfort intolerance: A hierarchical model of affect sensitivity and tolerance. *Behavior Therapy, 40*(3), 291–301. https://doi.org/10.1016/j.beth.2008.08.001

Book, S. W., Thomas, S. E., Dempsey, J. P., Randall, P. K., & Randall, C. L. (2009). Social anxiety impacts willingness to participate in addiction treatment. *Addictive Behaviors, 34*(5), 474–476. https://doi.org/10.1016/j.addbeh.2008.12.011

Bowen, R. C., D'Arcy, C., Keegan, D., & Senthilselvan, A. (2000). A controlled trial of cognitive behavioral treatment of panic in alcoholic inpatients with Comorbid Panic disorder. *Addictive Behaviors, 25*(4), 593–597. https://doi.org/10.1016/s0306-4603(99)00017-9

Brown, S. A., Glasner-Edwards, S. V., Tate, S. R., McQuaid, J. R., Chalekian, J., & Granholm, E. (2006). Integrated cognitive behavioral therapy versus twelve-step facilitation therapy for substance-dependent adults with depressive disorders. *Journal of Psychoactive Drugs, 38*(4), 449–460. https://doi.org/10.1080/02791072.2006.10400584

Buckner, J. D., Bonn-Miller, M. O., Zvolensky, M. J., & Schmidt, N. B. (2007). Marijuana use motives and social anxiety among marijuana-using young adults. *Addictive Behaviors, 32*(10), 2238–2252. https://doi.org/10.1016/j.addbeh.2007.04.004

Buckner, J. D., Heimberg, R. G., & Schmidt, N. B. (2011a). Social anxiety and marijuana-related problems: The role of social avoidance. *Addictive Behaviors, 36*(1–2), 129–132. https://doi.org/10.1016/j.addbeh.2010.08.015

Buckner, J. D., Zvolensky, M. J., Smits, J. A. J., Norton, P. J., Crosby, R. D., Wonderlich, S. A., & Schmidt, N. B. (2011b). Anxiety sensitivity and marijuana use: An analysis from ecological momentary assessment. *Depression and Anxiety, 28*(5), 420–426.

Burnam, M. A., & Watkins, K. E. (2006). Substance abuse with mental disorders: Specialized public systems and integrated care. *Health Affairs, 25*(3), 648–658. https://doi.org/10.1377/hlthaff.25.3.648

Burns, L., Teesson, M., & O'Neill, K. (2005). The impact of comorbid anxiety and depression on alcohol treatment outcomes. *Addiction, 100*(6), 787–796. https://doi.org/10.1111/j.1360-0443.2005.001069.x

Carpenter, K. M., Smith, J. L., Aharonovich, E., & Nunes, E. V. (2008). Developing therapies for depression in drug dependence: Results of a stage 1 therapy study. *The American Journal of Drug and Alcohol Abuse, 34*(5), 642–652. https://doi.org/10.1080/00952990802308171

Carpentier, P. J., Krabbe, P. F., Van Gogh, M. T., Knapen, L. J., Buitelaar, J. K., & De Jong, C. A. (2009). Psychiatric comorbidity reduces quality of life in chronic methadone maintained patients. *American Journal on Addictions, 18*(6), 470–480. https://doi.org/10.3109/10550490903205652

Chawla, N., & Ostafin, B. (2007). Experiential avoidance as a functional dimensional approach to psychopathology: An empirical review. *Journal of Clinical Psychology, 63*(9), 871–890. https://doi.org/10.1002/jclp.20400

Compton, W. M., Thomas, Y. F., Stinson, F. S., & Grant, B. F. (2007). Prevalence, correlates, disability, and comorbidity of DSM-IV drug abuse and dependence in the United States. *Archives of General Psychiatry, 64*(5), 566. https://doi.org/10.1001/archpsyc.64.5.566

Cougle, J. R., Timpano, K. R., & Goetz, A. R. (2012). Exploring the unique and interactive roles of distress tolerance and negative urgency in obsessions. *Personality and Individual Differences, 52*(4), 515–520. https://doi.org/10.1016/j.paid.2011.11.017

Glasner-Edwards, S., & Rawson, R. (2010). Evidence-based practices in addiction treatment: Review and Recommendations for public policy. *Health Policy, 97*(2–3), 93–104. https://doi.org/10.1016/j.healthpol.2010.05.013

Grant, B. F., Stinson, F. S., Dawson, D. A., Chou, S. P., Dufour, M. C., Compton, W., Pickering, R. P., & Kaplan, K. (2004). Prevalence and co-occurrence of substance use disorders and independentmood and anxiety disorders. *Archives of General Psychiatry, 61*(8), 807. https://doi.org/10.1001/archpsyc.61.8.807

Havassy, B. E., Alvidrez, J., & Mericle, A. A. (2009). Disparities in use of mental health and substance abuse services by persons with co-occurring disorders. *Psychiatric Services, 60*(2), 217–223. https://doi.org/10.1176/ps.2009.60.2.217

Hearon, B. A., Calkins, A. W., Halperin, D. M., Kathryn McHugh, R., Murray, H. W., & Otto, M. W. (2011). Anxiety sensitivity and illicit sedative use among opiate-dependent women and men. *The American Journal of Drug and Alcohol Abuse, 37*(1), 43–47. https://doi.org/10.3109/00952990.2010.535581

Hesse, M. (2009). Integrated psychological treatment for substance use and co-morbid anxiety or depression vs. treatment for substance use alone. A systematic review of the published literature. *BMC Psychiatry, 9*(1). https://doi.org/10.1186/1471-244x-9-6

Hien, D. A., Jiang, H., Campbell, A. N., Hu, M. C., Miele, G. M., Cohen, L. R., Brigham, G. S., Capstick, C., Kulaga, A., Robinson, J., Suarez-Morales, L., & Nunes, E. V. (2010). Do treatment improvements in PTSD severity affect substance use outcomes? A secondary analysis from a randomized clinical trial in NIDA's Clinical Trials Network. *American Journal of Psychiatry, 167*(1), 95–101. https://doi.org/10.1176/appi.ajp.2009.09091261

Insel, T., Cuthbert, B., Garvey, M., Heinssen, R., Pine, D. S., Quinn, K., & Wang, P. (2010). Research domain criteria (RDoC): Toward a new classification framework for research on mental disorders. *The American Journal of Psychiatry, 167*(7), 748–751.

Kushner, M. G., Abrams, K., Thuras, P., Hanson, K. L., Brekke, M., & Sletten, S. (2005). Follow-up study of anxiety disorder and alcohol dependence in comorbid alcoholism treatment patients. *Alcoholism: Clinical & Experimental Research, 29*(8), 1432–1443. https://doi.org/10.1097/01.alc.0000175072.17623.f8

Kushner, M. G., Donahue, C., Sletten, S., Thuras, P., Abrams, K., Peterson, J., & Frye, B. (2006). Cognitive behavioral treatment of comorbid anxiety disorder in alcoholism treatment patients:

Presentation of a prototype program and future directions. *Journal of Mental Health, 15*(6), 697–707. https://doi.org/10.1080/09638230600998946

Lai, H. M., Cleary, M., Sitharthan, T., & Hunt, G. E. (2015). Prevalence of comorbid substance use, anxiety and mood disorders in epidemiological surveys, 1990–2014: A systematic review and meta-analysis. *Drug and Alcohol Dependence, 154*, 1–13. https://doi.org/10.1016/j.drugalcdep.2015.05.031

Lee, W.-C., Chang, H.-M., Huang, M.-C., Pan, C.-H., Su, S.-S., Tsai, S.-Y., Chen, C.-C., & Kuo, C.-J. (2022). Healthcare utilization and psychiatric and physical comorbidities before suicide mortality in patients with methamphetamine use disorder: A nationwide case–control study. *Addictive Behaviors, 126*, 107192. https://doi.org/10.1016/j.addbeh.2021.107192

Leventhal, A. M., Mooney, M. E., DeLaune, K. A., & Schmitz, J. M. (2010). Using addiction severity profiles to differentiate cocaine-dependent patients with and without comorbid major depression. *Psychology of Addictive Behaviors, 24*(1), 115–121. https://doi.org/10.1080/10550490600860148

Litz, M., & Leslie, D. (2017). The impact of mental health comorbidities on adherence to buprenorphine: A claims based analysis. *The American Journal on Addictions, 26*(8), 859–863. https://doi.org/10.1111/ajad.12644

McGovern, M. P., Xie, H., Segal, S. R., Siembab, L., & Drake, R. E. (2006). Addiction treatment services and co-occurring disorders: Prevalence estimates, treatment practices, and barriers. *Journal of Substance Abuse Treatment, 31*(3), 267–275. https://doi.org/10.1016/j.jsat.2006.05.003

McHugh, R. K. (2015). Treatment of co-occurring anxiety disorders and substance use disorders. *Harvard Review of Psychiatry, 23*(2), 99–111. https://doi.org/10.1097/hrp.0000000000000058

McHugh, R. K., & Otto, M. W. (2012). Refining the measurement of distress intolerance. *Behavior Therapy, 43*(3), 641–651. https://doi.org/10.1016/j.beth.2011.12.001

McKay, J. R., Pettinati, H. M., Morrison, R., Feeley, M., Mulvaney, F. D., & Gallop, R. (2002). Relation of depression diagnoses to 2-year outcomes in cocaine-dependent patients in a randomized continuing care study. *Psychology of Addictive Behaviors, 16*(3), 225–235.

Nace, E. P. (1988). Posttraumatic stress disorder and substance abuse clinical issues. In M. Galanter et al. (Eds.), Recent developments in alcoholism (pp. 9–26) New York: Plenum Press.

National Institute of Mental Health Strategic Plan (2008). U.S. Department of Health & Human Services, National Institutes of Health. Publication No. 08-6368.

Ouimette, P. C., Moos, R. H., & Finney, J. W. (2000). Two-year mental health service use and course of remission in patients with substance use and posttraumatic stress disorders. *Journal of Studies on Alcohol, 61*(2), 247–253. https://doi.org/10.15288/jsa.2000.61.247

Randall, C. L., Thomas, S., & Thevos, A. K. (2001). Concurrent alcoholism and social anxiety disorder: A first step toward developing effective treatments. *Alcoholism: Clinical and Experimental Research, 25*(2), 210–220. https://doi.org/10.1111/j.1530-0277.2001.tb02201.x

Roy-Byrne, P., Sullivan, M. D., Sherbourne, C. D., Golinelli, D., Craske, M. G., Sullivan, G., & Stein, M. B. (2013). Effects of pain and prescription opioid use on outcomes in a collaborative care intervention for anxiety. *The Clinical Journal of Pain, 29*(9), 800. https://doi.org/10.1097/AJP.0b013e318278d475

Savant, J. D., Barry, D. T., Cutter, C. J., Joy, M. T., Dinh, A., Schottenfeld, R. S., & Fiellin, D. A. (2013). Prevalence of mood and substance use disorders among patients seeking primary care office-based buprenorphine/naloxone treatment. *Drug and Alcohol Dependence, 127*(1–3), 243–247. https://doi.org/10.1016/j.drugalcdep.2012.06.020

Schellekens, A. F. A., de Jong, C. A. J., Buitelaar, J. K., & Verkes, R. J. (2015). Co-morbid anxiety disorders predict early relapse after inpatient alcohol treatment. *European Psychiatry, 30*(1), 128–136. https://doi.org/10.1016/j.eurpsy.2013.08.006

Schmitz, N., & Kruse, J. (2002). The relationship between mental disorders and medical service utilization in a representative community sample. *Social Psychiatry and Psychiatric Epidemiology, 37*(8), 380–386. https://doi.org/10.1007/s00127-002-0567-2

Smith, J. P., & Book, S. W. (2010). Comorbidity of generalized anxiety disorder and alcohol use disorders among individuals seeking outpatient substance abuse treatment. *Addictive Behaviors, 35*(1), 42–45. https://doi.org/10.1016/j.addbeh.2009.07.002

Stewart, S. H., & Conrod, P. (Eds.). (2008). *Anxiety and substance use disorders: The vicious cycle of comorbidity*. Springer.

Substance Abuse and Mental Health Services Administration (SAMHSA) (2022). *The case for screening and treatment of co-occurring disorders*.

Swendsen, J. D., & Merikangas, K. R. (2000). The comorbidity of depression and substance use disorders. *Clinical Psychology Review, 20*(2), 173–189.

Wolitzky-Taylor, K. (2023). Integrated behavioral treatments for comorbid anxiety and substance use disorders: A model for understanding integrated treatment approaches and meta-analysis to evaluate their efficacy. *Drug and Alcohol Dependence, 253*, 110990.

Wolitzky-Taylor, K., Operskalski, J. T., Ries, R., Craske, M. G., & Roy-Byrne, P. (2011). Understanding and treating comorbid anxiety disorders in substance users. *Journal of Addiction Medicine, 5*(4), 233–247. https://doi.org/10.1097/adm.0b013e31823276d7

Wolitzky-Taylor, K., Guillot, C., Pang, R., Kirkpatrick, M., Zvolensky, M., Buckner, J. D., & Leventhal, A. (2015). Examination of anxiety sensitivity and distress tolerance as transdiagnostic mechanisms linking multiple anxiety pathologies to alcohol use problems in adolescents. *Alcoholism: Clinical and Experimental Research, 39*, 532–539.

Wolitzky-Taylor, K., McBeth, J., Guillot, C. R., Stone, M. D., Kirkpatrick, M. G., Zvolensky, M. J., Buckner, J. D., & Leventhal, A. M. (2016). Transdiagnostic processes linking anxiety symptoms and substance use problems among adolescents. *Journal of Addictive Diseases, 35*(4), 266–277. https://doi.org/10.1080/10550887.2016.1207969

Wolitzky-Taylor, K., Krull, J., Rawson, R., Roy-Byrne, P., Ries, R., & Craske, M. G. (2018). Randomized clinical trial evaluating the preliminary effectiveness of an integrated anxiety disorder treatment in substance use disorder specialty clinics. *Journal of Consulting and Clinical Psychology, 86*(1), 81–88. https://doi.org/10.1037/ccp0000276

Wolitzky-Taylor, K., Glasner, S., Tanner, A., Ghahremani, D. G., & London, E. D. (2022). Targeting maladaptive reactivity to negative affect in emerging adults with cannabis use disorder: A preliminary test and proof of concept. *Behaviour Research and Therapy, 150*, 104032. https://doi.org/10.1016/j.brat.2022.104032

Chapter 2
Cognitive Behavioral Therapy for Social Anxiety Disorder and Alcohol Use Disorder

Lexine A. Stapinski, Tara Guckel, Erin Kelly, and Katrina Prior

Co-occurring Social Anxiety Disorder and Alcohol Use Disorder: Prevalence, Correlates, and Associated Harms

Social anxiety disorder (SAD) and alcohol use disorder (AUD) are highly prevalent psychiatric disorders that frequently co-occur. Cross-national epidemiological studies have shown that among people with a lifetime diagnosis of SAD, approximately one in four (25.9%) will experience a lifetime AUD, which is considerably higher than base rates of AUD in the general population (8.6%; range: 0.7–22.7%; Glantz et al., 2020). Conversely, among those with a lifetime AUD, approximately one in eight (12.2%) will meet diagnostic criteria for SAD (Glantz et al., 2020); a rate up to three times higher than those without an AUD (4.0%; range: 0.2–12.1%; Stein et al., 2017). Rates of co-occurrence are even higher among treatment-seeking samples, with up to one in three people receiving AUD or SAD treatment experiencing both disorders (e.g., 21–34%; Bakken et al., 2005; Burns et al., 2005; Terra et al., 2006b).

Several epidemiological and clinical studies have identified sociodemographic factors associated with the co-occurrence of SAD and AUD. Specifically, individuals with co-occurring SAD and AUD tend to be younger (Bakken et al., 2005), female (Kessler et al., 1997; Kushner et al., 2005), less well educated (Terra et al., 2006b; Thevos et al., 1999; Yoshimi et al., 2016), have a family history of alcohol dependence (Terra et al., 2006a), and have a lower occupational status and income (Thevos et al., 1999; Yoshimi et al., 2016) in comparison to those with an AUD but no SAD. Moreover, a recent systematic review identified several risk factors related

L. A. Stapinski (✉) · T. Guckel · E. Kelly · K. Prior
The Matilda Centre for Research in Mental Health and Substance Use,
The University of Sydney, Camperdown, NSW, Australia
e-mail: lexine.stapinski@sydney.edu.au

K. Wolitzky-Taylor (ed.), *Treating Comorbid Substance Use and Emotional Disorders*, CBT: Science Into Practice, https://doi.org/10.1007/978-3-031-62971-6_2

to the association between SAD and alcohol use among adolescents, including being female, seeking approval from peers, affective problems linked to alcohol use, and having secondary comorbidities such as depression and generalized anxiety (Cruz et al., 2017). Nevertheless, some studies have reported no discernible differences between individuals with and without co-occurring SAD and AUD (Book et al., 2009; Schadé et al., 2004; Tonigan et al., 2010).

Although SAD has been estimated to precede the onset of pathological drinking and AUD in approximately 80% of co-occurring cases (Glantz et al., 2020), once both conditions are established, there is an intricate interplay between them that tends to perpetuate or intensify each disorder through a feed-forward cycle (Baillie et al., 2010; Stewart & Conrod, 2008). This mutually reinforcing relationship commonly leads to more severe symptoms and functional impairment, including poorer quality of life, more severe alcohol dependence, increased co-occurrence and severity of disorders such as depression, and heightened risk of suicidal thoughts, plans, and attempts than for either disorder in isolation (Bakken et al., 2005; Marquenie et al., 2006; Schadé et al., 2004; Schneier et al., 2010; Thomas et al., 1999; Yoshimi et al., 2016). Furthermore, alcohol-dependent samples with current SAD have also been shown to experience their first psychiatric disorder at an earlier age and a higher likelihood of past health service utilization (Bakken et al., 2005) than those without this additional diagnosis. Thus, although both SAD and AUD are debilitating in and of themselves, their combination is particularly harmful and requires appropriate treatment.

Efficacy of Psychological Treatment for Co-occurring Social Anxiety Disorder and Alcohol Use Disorder

Empirical evidence suggests that co-occurring SAD-AUD presentations are linked to increased difficulties in treatment and poorer treatment outcomes using conventional psychotherapy approaches (e.g., Cognitive Behavioral Therapy; CBT). Conventional treatments targeting single disorders (i.e., SAD or AUD) may be inadequate for people with co-occurring SAD-AUD because of the interaction between disorders, where each disorder potentially interferes with treatment for the other co-occurring disorder. Given poorer responses to conventional single disorder treatments, the following alternative models of care have been developed and evaluated for co-occurring SAD-AUD:

(a) Dual-focused treatment: where client's SAD and AUD are treated simultaneously, but the treatments are independent of each other, and potentially provided by different therapists.
(b) Integrated treatment: where treatment for the client's SAD and AUD are integrated and provided simultaneously by the same therapist.

This section provides an overview of the existing evidence about the efficacy of single-disorder, dual-focused, and integrated psychological treatment for people with co-occurring SAD and AUD.

Efficacy of AUD-Focused Treatment Among People with Co-occurring SAD-AUD

Evidence from multiple randomized controlled trials (RCTs), spanning the USA, Europe, and Australia, suggests that while people with co-occurring SAD and AUD benefit from AUD-focused treatment, treatment efficacy and sustainability is adversely affected by co-occurring SAD. Two trials identified SAD as the strongest predictor of relapse to drinking (Kushner et al., 2005), especially early relapse (Schellekens et al., 2015), following AUD treatment, compared to other co-occurring anxiety or mental disorders. In a trial of Twelve-Step Facilitation Therapy, females (but not males) with alcohol dependence and co-occurring SAD had a greater likelihood of relapsing to heavy drinking than those without this comorbidity (Tonigan et al., 2010). Similar findings are reported in AUD treatment trials comparing outcomes in individuals with and without co-occurring transdiagnostic anxiety disorders (Burns et al., 2005; Driessen et al., 2001). The poorer AUD treatment outcomes among people with SAD may be due to the detrimental impact of social anxiety on engagement and participation in AUD treatment activities, such as speaking up in group therapy, attending Alcoholics Anonymous meetings, or asking someone to be a sponsor (Book et al., 2009; Tonigan et al., 2010). Additionally, co-occurring phobic anxiety can hinder AUD treatment effects by its association with early treatment drop-out (Haver & Gjestad, 2005). In contrast, a subsequent trial found that men with social anxiety actually stayed longer in treatment (Oakland & McChargue, 2014), while other studies have found that pre-treatment SAD is unrelated to AUD treatment outcomes, such as frequency of drinking (Farris et al., 2012) and alcohol relapse (Marquenie et al., 2006; Terra et al., 2006a). In some cases, these discrepant findings may relate to study-specific factors, such as lower rates of pre-treatment AUD severity among the participants with SAD (Farris et al., 2012) and low overall treatment adherence (Terra et al., 2006a).

Efficacy of SAD-Focused Treatment Among People with Co-occurring SAD-AUD

A co-occurring diagnosis of AUD may complicate and interfere with treatment for SAD, particularly if alcohol is used as a coping mechanism when clients increase their social interactions as part of exposure-based therapy. Drinking alcohol to dampen or cope with anxiety in these social situations is problematic due to the potential for exacerbation of AUD, but also because it may interfere with the benefits of graded exposure (see Harvey et al., 2022). The impact of untreated AUD on SAD treatment has been examined in two trials in Australia and one in the USA. McEvoy and Shand (2008) found that higher pre-treatment alcohol use predicted less improvement in social interaction anxiety (but not performance anxiety) following psychotherapy targeting SAD. Conversely, Subotic-Kerry et al. (2021)

found no evidence that pre-treatment alcohol consumption or AUD diagnosis impacted SAD treatment response in an RCT that included a small number of people with AUD ($n = 7$). Another RCT among individuals receiving anxiety treatment in primary care also found no impact of alcohol use severity on anxiety outcomes across an 18-month period (Wolitzky-Taylor et al., 2015). However, it should be noted that individuals with alcohol dependence (but not abuse) were excluded from this study and treatment was for any anxiety disorder, thus these conclusions may not generalize to treatment of co-occurring SAD-AUD specifically. A significant challenge is that people with AUD are typically excluded from trials of psychotherapy for SAD and other mental disorders (Marel et al., 2022), and therefore there is insufficient evidence about the generalizability of SAD treatment for individuals experiencing both disorders.

Efficacy of Dual-Focused Treatment Among People with Co-occurring SAD-AUD

One trial in the USA and one in the Netherlands have evaluated the efficacy of concurrent (i.e., parallel), dual-focused SAD-AUD treatments. In the earliest trial of a dual-focused treatment approach, Randall et al. (2001) randomly assigned 93 adults with SAD and alcohol dependence into two groups, who both received 12 weeks of individual CBT. For one group, the CBT focused solely on alcohol use, while the dual-focused group spend half of the 90-min session focusing on alcohol, and the other half focused on social anxiety. Contrary to hypotheses, the dual-focused treatment did not provide additional benefits for anxiety, and this group exhibited poorer outcomes at 3 months post-treatment on three of four alcohol indices, including their number of drinks consumed, heavy drinking days, and days abstinent, compared to the alcohol-only condition. A subsequent trial involved 96 alcohol-dependent adults with co-occurring SAD or panic/agoraphobia who attended an intensive 3- to 4-month inpatient program followed by 16 weeks of group-delivered alcohol relapse-prevention (Schadé et al., 2004). Participants were randomized to receive this AUD treatment alone, or in combination with 12 weekly sessions of individual CBT for anxiety at a separate facility and medical management with Fluvoxamine (Schadé et al., 2005). At the 32-week follow-up, the combined group reported significantly greater reductions in anxiety and avoidance behaviors, but no advantage in terms of alcohol relapse or abstinence.

A limitation of dual-focused treatments relates to the cognitive and practical demands of engaging in two disparate, non-integrated treatments for SAD and AUD. With this approach, the onus of integrating the therapeutic principles and strategies falls to the client. The requirement to undergo two intensive treatments simultaneously may weaken otherwise effective treatments by causing confusion, overwhelming clients, and undermining self-efficacy, as indicated by the somewhat higher drop-out rates for dual-focused treatment (Randall et al., 2008). Minimizing complexity may be particularly relevant for this population, as prolonged alcohol use can lead to cognitive impairment and reduced ability to process complex information. Furthermore, exposure to social situations as part of SAD treatment may exacerbate drinking if clients are not provided with guidance to manage the inter-relationship between their SAD and AUD symptoms. Therefore, the unintegrated nature of these treatments may account for the unexpected trial results, and explain the poorer alcohol outcomes observed for dual-focused treatment in the Randall et al. (2001) study.

Efficacy of Integrated Treatment Among People with Co-occurring SAD-AUD

Addressing the potential limitations of dual-focused treatments, integrated treatments have been developed that synthesize effective treatment protocols for SAD and AUD, and offer explicit guidance for managing the inter-relationship between these disorders (Stapinski et al., 2021d; Wolitzky-Taylor et al., 2022). To date, two RCTs have examined the effectiveness of integrated SAD-AUD psychotherapy among adults in Australia and the USA. The first compared individually delivered CBT focused on alcohol only, to integrated CBT targeting SAD, AUD, and the connections between these disorders (n = 117; Stapinski et al., 2021d). With the same number of treatment sessions (i.e., 10 × 90-minute sessions of individual CBT), the integrated group showed greater improvements in SAD symptoms, depression, and quality of life, while the two treatments were equally effective in reducing alcohol consumption and severity of alcohol dependence over a 6-month period. Similar results were observed by Wolitzky-Taylor et al. (2022) who evaluated an integrated, intensive group program for co-occurring SAD and AUD among adults receiving treatment in a community-based substance use disorder (SUD) specialty clinic. Participants (n = 56) were randomized to receive three, 3-h group CBT sessions per week, for 12 weeks of either: the integrated treatment, which combined group-based CBT exposure protocols for SAD and specific anxiety-related exposures relevant to the treatment of AUD, or usual care, which consisted of the CBT-based Matrix Model of Addiction Intensive Outpatient Program (Obert et al., 2000). At post-intervention, the integrated group showed significantly greater decreases in avoidance of social situations when alcohol is unavailable, and at 6-month follow-up, the integrated treatment outperformed usual care on reductions in the severity of social anxiety and avoidance, and the number of drinking days in the past month. Taken together, the findings of these two trials support the clinical utility of integrated treatments in differing contexts as a comprehensive approach for individuals with co-occurring SAD and AUD, achieving additional benefits compared to isolated management of AUD.

In addition to integrated treatments specific to co-occurring SAD-AUD, several studies have investigated the efficacy of integrated treatments for comorbid AUD and transdiagnostic anxiety disorders, yielding mixed results. Stapinski et al. (2019) adapted their integrated SAD-AUD treatment (Stapinski et al., 2015) for brief intervention among youth, delivered via five web-based modules combined with psychologist support via email/phone targeting transdiagnostic anxiety and hazardous alcohol use. The program was evaluated in an RCT among 123 young adults (aged 17–24 years) presenting with symptoms of both anxiety (SAD, generalized anxiety disorder, or panic disorder) and AUD, ranging in severity from subclinical to disorder (60% probable alcohol dependence and 81% probable SAD based on symptom scores). Results showed that the integrated program resulted in significantly greater reductions in SAD symptoms and hazardous alcohol use compared to alcohol psychoeducation at both the post-intervention and 6-month follow-up (Stapinski et al., 2021c). Superior outcomes for generalized anxiety and depression symptoms compared to control were observed at post-intervention only. Additionally, while both groups reduced their alcohol consumption and binge-drinking (≥5 standard drinks on one occasion) at post-intervention, significant between-group differences emerged at 6-month follow-up, suggesting a rebound in the control group but sustained improvements for the integrated group.

Two further studies among adults with an AUD and co-occurring anxiety disorder found beneficial treatment effects from six to ten integrated anxiety and AUD-focused CBT sessions on most alcohol outcomes (e.g., rates of relapse, days of abstinence, total drinks, drinking days, and binge days) but not anxiety outcomes (e.g., diagnosis severity, anxiety severity), compared to routine outpatient AUD treatment (Kushner et al., 2013; Morley et al., 2016) or community-based residential AUD treatment plus Progressive Muscle Relaxation Training program (Kushner et al., 2013). Changes in anxiety did not account for the group differences in alcohol outcomes over time in either study; suggesting the superior outcomes instead reflect benefits of CBT compared to alternative counselling or twelve-step focused AUD treatments.

In summary, evaluation of integrated treatments specifically developed for co-occurring SAD and AUD suggest they offer unique benefits for ameliorating anxiety symptoms and other mental health indicators, in addition to improving alcohol-related outcomes. However, integrated treatments for AUD and transdiagnostic anxiety disorders have demonstrated less pronounced effects on anxiety symptoms, which suggests there are advantages to protocols tailored to the particular cognitive and behavioral processes underpinning distinct anxiety disorders. Further research is needed to identify the essential therapeutic components and psychological mechanisms that contribute to treatment efficacy for co-occurring SAD-AUD presentations.

Summary and Recommendations

Research evidence to date suggests that people with co-occurring SAD and AUD can benefit from conventional single-disorder treatments; however, treatment efficacy and long-term outcomes are negatively impacted by the co-occurring disorders. The evidence for detrimental impacts of co-occurring SAD-AUD on AUD-focused treatment is more substantial, due to the limited number of evaluations of SAD treatment among people with co-occurring AUD. In general, evidence for the efficacy of conventional treatments in this population is sparse, as it is common for RCTs to exclude participants with co-occurring diagnoses.

Dual-focused and integrated treatments for co-occurring SAD and AUD have been developed in an effort to improve outcomes for this population. Only one trial of dual-focused treatment found greater anxiety symptom reduction compared to routine AUD treatment, while the other found that dual-focused CBT resulted in worse alcohol outcomes, potentially due to the demands of simultaneously engaging in two separate treatments. Integrated SAD-AUD treatment addresses this concern by offering a coherent, synthesized therapeutic rationale and set of techniques that can be applied to address the cognitive behavioral processes underlying each disorder, and their interconnections. Two trials found that with the same number of treatment sessions, integrated CBT for co-occurring SAD-AUD improved outcomes over and above AUD-focused treatment, reducing anxiety symptoms and improving quality of life, without jeopardizing efficacy for alcohol outcomes.

Additional research efforts are needed to strengthen the evidence base regarding the efficacy of treatment for co-occurring SAD and AUD, and to identify the underlying mechanisms of change. In addition, a significant limitation of the research to date has been the predominance of studies conducted in the USA, Australia, and Europe. Further research is needed to understand how these findings generalize to people from diverse cultural backgrounds, as well any considerations about how treatment might need to be adapted to align with a person's age, gender, sexual, or racial identity, or to accommodate past experiences of marginalization, stigma, and discrimination.

Overall, the available evidence suggests that where no integrated treatment is available, people with co-occurring SAD-AUD should be offered evidence-based single-disorder treatments, which will likely achieve some symptom reduction. However, there are significant advantages to providing integrated SAD-AUD treatment. In a study of the lived experience of co-occurring AUD and mental disorders, participants commonly viewed their problems to be inter-related, and expressed a preference for integrated treatment (Barrett et al., 2019). Often, people with co-occurring AUD and mental disorders experience "wrong door syndrome", where they struggle to find appropriate treatment services, and can be moved on from service to service. Integration of treatments for mental and substance use disorders is a key recommendation of the World Health Organization and United Nations Office on Drugs and Crime for improving access to services, enhancing treatment outcomes, and preventing people from falling through the gaps (Volkow et al., 2020). Lack of therapist training and confidence is one of the primary barriers to delivering integrated treatment, and thus, the next section provides a detailed overview and case example of integrated CBT for co-occurring SAD and AUD.

Integrated CBT for Co-occurring Social Anxiety Disorder and Alcohol Use Disorder

In this section we describe the strategies and clinical application of an integrated cognitive behavioral treatment for co-occurring SAD and AUD. The integrated approach we describe has been evaluated in two RCTs described in detail earlier in this chapter, and found to achieve benefits above and beyond routine care for alcohol use when delivered to Australian adults with SAD and AUD (Stapinski et al., 2021d), and when adapted for brief web-based and telehealth delivery among young adults with transdiagnostic anxiety symptoms and hazardous alcohol use (Stapinski et al., 2021c). The integrated treatment we describe is similar in focus and clinical components to the only other integrated SAD-AUD treatment that has been evaluated in a RCT (Wolitzky-Taylor et al., 2022), which similarly demonstrated benefits over usual care. In these RCTs, treatment was delivered by clinical psychologists and masters' level clinicians who ranged in experience level from recent graduate to experienced clinician. Detailed therapist guides and accompanying client workbooks are available to support delivery by non-specialist psychologists (Stapinski et al., 2021a, b, 2015).

Theoretical Framework for Integrated SAD-AUD Treatment

The overarching theoretical framework for treatment integrates evidence-based CBT models for SAD (Heimberg et al., 2014; Rapee et al., 2009), AUD (Beck et al., 1993; Miller, 2004; Monti et al., 2002), and comorbidity (Baillie & Sannibale, 2007). In addition, we recognize the critical role of client motivation for treatment engagement, retention, and maintenance of changes to drinking in the long-term (Miller et al., 2019; Westra & Dozois, 2008). Integrating these frameworks, the aim of treatment is to assist clients to build an integrated SAD-AUD problem formulation and repertoire of skills (see Table 2.1) to manage the cognitions, distorted negative self-image, attentional processes, and behaviors that maintain and mutually reinforce these disorders (Stapinski et al., 2015). These CBT skills are offered within the context of an empowering therapeutic style that acknowledges the client's agency and enhances their intrinsic motivation to make changes.

In contrast to earlier programs which offered dual-focused treatment for SAD and AUD delivered in parallel (see section "Efficacy of Psychological Treatment for Co-occurring SAD and AUD"), integrated treatment reduces complexity by explicitly synthesizing the problem formulation, treatment rationale and strategies, such that clients are supported to develop a repertoire of techniques that can be applied to target the cognitions, behaviors, and attentional processes that underlie both disorders. Critically, the therapist and client also develop a shared understanding of the inter-relationship between the client's social anxiety and alcohol use. This integrated problem formulation draws from current theoretical frameworks and research

Table 2.1 Overview of integrated treatment components and suggested structure

Session	Treatment component	Description
All	Motivational interviewing therapeutic style	Non-confrontational style to explore ambivalence and enhance motivation to change "Elicit-Provide-Elicit" approach to skill development
1–2	Motivation enhancement	Provide structured personalized feedback about drinking Explore patterns of drinking and motivation to reduce consumption Client determines initial goals (to be reviewed as treatment progresses)
	Integrated problem formulation & treatment plan	Therapist and client collaboratively develop an initial problem formulation Develop shared understanding of expectations, rules, and model for treatment
2–4	Development of alternative reinforcers	Identify interests and activities other than drinking Collaboratively develop an action plan, adopting a hierarchy approach beginning with manageable goals to enhance self-efficacy Introduce "emotion surfing" to manage anxiety that may be elicited as activities are attempted
	Develop coping alternatives for high-risk situations	Identify high-risk triggers for drinking and current coping strategies; review past successes to enhance self-efficacy Suggest and practice additional coping strategies Introduce weekly routine of identifying and planning for upcoming triggers
4–6	Cognitive therapy	Identify social threat cognitions Identify expectancies about positive effects of alcohol (e.g., anxiety reduction, improved social performance and enjoyment) Introduce cognitive therapy rationale and technique; practice in and out of session
5–8	Behavioral experiments	Identify overt social avoidance and "safety behaviors" (including alcohol consumption) and related cognitions Formulate avoidance-anxiety relationship and rationale for behavioral experiments Develop hierarchy of behavioral experiments, explicitly link to the cognitions that will be tested
	Attention training	Introduce distinction between task and self-focused attention Establish rationale and technique to assist disengagement from self-focused attention and "sticky thoughts" Practice task-focused attention during behavioral experiments
7	Social support session	Assist client to provide brief overview of the problem formulation, treatment plan and progress to date Identify interpersonal dynamics that may contribute exacerbate anxiety/drinking Acknowledge support person's role; elicit current helpful behaviors and form long-term support plan
9	Skill review and advanced practice	Review skills and refine/trouble-shoot skill integration Advanced behavioral experiments accompanied by therapist to consolidate skill integration
9–10	Relapse prevention and continuing change	Reflect on progress, prepare for termination Identify long- and short-term goals for post-treatment Psychoeducation and planning for potential setbacks

Note. Table 2.1 reproduced with permission from Stapinski et al. (2015)

evidence suggesting important bidirectional connections between anxiety and AUD (Anker & Kushner, 2019; Smith & Randall, 2012; Stewart et al., 2016). Anxiety disorders are consistently associated with self-reported use of alcohol to self-medicate or cope with their anxiety (Cooper et al., 2014; Morris et al., 2005). For people with social anxiety, alcohol can be conceptualized as one of many "safety behaviors" (avoidance strategies) used in an attempt to prevent feared social outcomes (Piccirillo et al., 2016; Wong & Rapee, 2016). Use of alcohol in this way is influenced by positive expectancies about the relaxant and social lubrication effects of alcohol (Moss & Albery, 2009), and may be reinforced by the impact of alcohol on attention and memory, resulting in perceptual narrowing, decreased self-awareness, and less self-evaluation during and after the event (Goodwin & Sayette, 2022). While these short-term effects may contribute to the perception that alcohol alleviates anxiety; evidence suggests that over the longer-term, social anxiety and alcohol use are mutually exacerbating because (a) alcohol can have neurobiological effects during intoxication and withdrawal that exacerbate anxiety symptoms (Koob et al., 2014); (b) relying on alcohol in social contexts prevent disconfirmation of unrealistic social fears, and erodes confidence to manage these situations unaided (Baillie & Sannibale, 2007; Tran & Haaga, 2002); and (c) increasing alcohol tolerance and consumption leads to increases in negative social outcomes, alcohol-related problems (e.g., work, relationship, legal or financial problems), and negative affect (e.g., embarrassment, shame, anxiety, low mood). In this way, a feed-forward cycle can emerge, whereby the experience or perception of alcohol as a mood enhancer reinforces alcohol consumption, which in turn increases negative affect and triggers further drinking (Anker & Kushner, 2019; Smith & Randall, 2012; Stewart et al., 2016). By developing an individualized formulation and functional analysis of a client's anxiety and alcohol, relevant treatment strategies can be identified to align with the specific cognitive, motivational, attentional, and behavioral processes that maintain and mutually exacerbate these disorders.

Target Population and Setting

This treatment was developed for individuals who have symptoms consistent with a *Diagnostic and Statistical Manual of Mental Disorders* (*DSM-5*) diagnosis of SAD, and who also meet criteria for an AUD or are consuming alcohol at a hazardous and/or harmful level as determined by the Alcohol Use Disorders Identification Test (scores of 8 or above indicate hazardous use, while scores of 16 or above indicate high level alcohol problems; Babor et al., 2001). Evidence from young adult samples suggests this integrated approach is also beneficial for individuals presenting with subclinical symptoms (Stapinski et al., 2021c), where treatment can prevent exacerbation of the anxiety-alcohol cycle. Even in cases when alcohol use is at lower levels of severity, there is good reason to consider integrated anxiety-alcohol treatment, given the potential that alcohol use may disrupt or reduce the benefits of graded exposure, particularly if it is used as a safety behavior to prevent anxiety in social-evaluative situations (see Harvey et al., 2022). Assessment of alcohol and other substance use among individuals presenting with social anxiety should form part of the initial problem formulation and be reviewed regularly over the course of treatment. A combination of informal and standardized assessment tools can be used to gain an understanding of the person's alcohol use, alcohol-related problems, dependence level, and inter-relationship with social anxiety. An accessible toolkit of potential assessment instruments is provided by Marel et al. (2022).

The treatment outlined in this chapter was developed for individual administration over 10 sessions of 90 min' duration each, which allowed for a basic structure of 20 min to review motivation and progress, with the remainder of the session to focus on new content and skill development. However, treatment format and duration could be adapted in accordance with individual needs, for example, clients with alcohol-related cognitive deficits may require additional time for skill development. Alternatively, Wolitzky-Taylor et al. (2022) have demonstrated beneficial outcomes when integrated SAD-AUD treatment is delivered in a group format. Although individual customization is limited by group delivery, this format offers other advantages due to the beneficial effects for clients with SAD of exposure to group discussions, and the opportunity to use the group for exposure tasks (e.g., giving a speech, sharing an opinion with a small group), provided their anxiety does not prevent them from joining the group at all. The use of evidence-informed technological tools (e.g., interactive apps or online forms) may assist with client engagement and retention (Muroff & Robinson, 2022), with some tools available that have been specifically designed for co-occurring anxiety and AUD (Stapinski et al., 2019).

Safety Considerations and Medical Management

It is common for clients with SAD and AUD to present with additional psychosocial concerns, such as childhood sexual or physical abuse, suicidal ideation and past suicide attempts, and additional psychiatric diagnoses. In particular, mood disorders are commonly comorbid with both social anxiety and alcohol use disorders (Glantz et al., 2020; McGrath et al., 2023) and likely to be comparatively over-represented in this group. Additional disorders are not necessarily contraindications for integrated treatment; indeed there is evidence that some emotional disorders (e.g., depression and generalized anxiety disorder) tend to remit following a period of abstinence from alcohol (Kushner et al., 2005). When additional psychosocial issues are present, it is important to consider on a case-by-case basis their potential impact and modify the treatment plan accordingly or refer to alternate services. Particular attention should be given to assessing, monitoring, and managing any safety concerns for the client or those around them, including risk of suicide or violence, accidental injury, and safety of any children in the client's care (Saunders et al., 2021). In many cases, supporting the client to abstain from alcohol will significantly reduce these psychosocial risks.

It is ideal for psychological treatment to be conducted in collaboration with an appropriate medical practitioner who can assist with assessment and management of any alcohol-related health complications (e.g., alcohol-related liver disease, gastrointestinal disorders). Pharmacotherapy may be considered as an adjunct to the psychological therapy: there is evidence that selective serotonin reuptake inhibitors reduce anxiety symptoms among individuals with co-occurring and alcohol use (Baillie et al., 2021), and acamprosate or naltrexone are recommended to prevent relapse among clients with moderate to severe AUD (Knox et al., 2019; Morley et al., 2021). For clients with more severe alcohol use, it is important to consider and plan for potential risks associated with withdrawal from alcohol. While some clients may be able to manage withdrawal symptoms at home with the support of relatives or friends, others may require referral for supervised inpatient or outpatient withdrawal management. Home-based withdrawal is unlikely to be suitable for clients at risk of severe alcohol withdrawal, such as severe tremor, severe tachycardia, seizures, delirium, or hallucinations; nor for clients who have a history of severe withdrawal symptoms (Haber & Lintzeris, 2021). The Clinical Institute Withdrawal Assessment for Alcohol Revised (CIWA-AR; Sullivan et al., 1989) is useful for assessment and to guide decision-making regarding management of alcohol withdrawal.

Core Treatment Components and Approach

Table 2.1 provides an overview of the integrated components and suggested session structure. While we recommend routine implementation of all components, specific strategies may be prioritized (in terms of time allocated or session order) according to the client's presentation and needs. Furthermore, the treatment integrates CBT skills within a motivational interviewing framework and therapeutic style, recognizing the client's personal agency in the therapeutic process and their recovery. The first treatment session (described below) is dedicated to clarifying the clients' intrinsic motivation and goals for change, and thereafter motivation and self-efficacy for change are revisited each session. Motivation and commitment to change will likely fluctuate across the course of treatment, so additional time may be needed in some sessions to explore and resolve ambivalence. When cognitive behavioral skills are introduced to assist with change, it is optimal for this to also be approached in a collaborative manner that enhances the client's autonomy and self-efficacy. Westra and Dozois (2008) suggest an "Elicit-Provide-Elicit" approach, whereby the therapist first asks permission to suggest a potential strategy for change, then offers information, and asks for the client's response.

Within a motivational framework for treatment, clients are expected and encouraged to take an active role in therapy and agenda setting, and overarching goals for treatment are determined collaboratively. As such, goals for alcohol reduction are not stipulated, and clients may arrive at a goal of abstinence or moderated drinking. We recommend providing psychoeducation about the benefits of an initial period of abstinence, which serves to create some momentum, boost self-efficacy, and achieve some initial symptom reduction (e.g., improved mood, decreased lethargy, and agitation). However, an abstinence-focused approach is not imposed, and thus clients may select a goal of reducing their alcohol consumption. While abstinence is typically recommended as the optimal goal for more severely dependent drinkers (Berglund et al., 2019), a recent meta-analysis found no evidence that abstinence compared to moderated drinking treatment goals achieve superior outcomes, nor was there evidence that alcohol use severity was related to success at moderated drinking (Henssler et al., 2021). From a harm-minimization perspective, it is clear that reductions in alcohol consumption significantly reduce the risk of negative outcomes (Mann et al., 2017). Offering a choice of treatment goals is important for decreasing the risk of early treatment drop-out and encouraging a greater number of people to seek treatment. National surveys conducted in the USA found that among people with untreated AUD, nearly half reported they were not ready to commit to alcohol abstinence (SAMHSA, 2014). In some cases, clients who trial a goal of moderated drinking initially will subsequently reconsider and shift to an alcohol abstinence goal, and therefore we view goal setting and treatment planning to be an evolving discussion, with time allocated for review and re-evaluation over the course of treatment.

Motivation Enhancement

During initial treatment sessions, it is important to build a shared understanding of the client's personal treatment goals and enhance their intrinsic motivations for change. Our procedure follows the Motivation Enhancement Therapy (MET) approach described and updated by Miller and colleagues (Miller, 2004; Miller & Rollnick, 2012; Miller et al., 1992). The primary objectives are (a) to develop an empathic understanding of the client's relationship with alcohol; (b) to explore the discrepancy between the client's values and current drinking; (c) to provide personalized feedback about current problem severity; and (d) to enhance the client's self-efficacy for change. It is essential that the therapist's style is non-confrontational and affirming, incorporating micro-skills such as reflective listening, exploring the consequences of action and inaction, summarizing, and reframing. By avoiding arguments or persuasion, and emphasizing the client's autonomy, this therapeutic style avoids evoking "sustain talk"—the person's own arguments for not changing their alcohol use (Miller & Rollnick, 2012). The way the therapist responds to any sustain talk or ambivalence expressed by the client is critically important. Micro-skills such as listening with empathy, reflection, and exploring goals and values are less likely to exacerbate resistance, and more likely to elicit the client's intrinsic reasons for change. If the client is receptive, it can be beneficial to provide structured personalized feedback derived from standardized assessment instruments regarding the severity of the client's alcohol consumption and related problems (Miller et al., 2019). This could include presenting alcohol consumption patterns in comparison with normative population data, information about severity of dependence or identified risk factors for chronic problems (e.g., familial risk, age of onset). It is ideal for treatment to be conducted in collaboration with a medical practitioner who review and provide feedback about any alcohol-related health consequences (e.g., results of liver function tests). As per the "Elicit-Provide-Elicit" approach described above (Westra & Dozois, 2008), any feedback should be provided in a non-confrontational manner, with the therapist first confirming the client's willingness to receive feedback, and listening reflectively to understand how the client understands and responds to the feedback.

While the above provides suggested objectives for the initial treatment sessions, a therapist attitude that emphasizes the client's autonomy and promotes a trusting, mutually respectful working relationship is more important than adhering to a predetermined session structure. In a helpful clarification of the essence of motivational interviewing, Miller and Rollnick (2009) emphasize the importance of adapting session content in accordance with the client's motivational state and readiness for change. For some clients, this may mean that a plan for change is not developed until later sessions. To promote therapeutic engagement and positively affirm clients' participation, we follow the Miller (2004) approach of e-mailing or mailing a brief, personalized letter immediately following the initial therapy session. This letter incorporates a summary of the reasons for change and goals identified by the client, and most importantly, expresses optimism and enthusiasm about working with the client towards these goals (for an example letter, see Stapinski et al., 2021a).

Coping Alternatives for High-Risk Situations

Craving and urges to drink alcohol are a common and normal component of alcohol use disorder, and may be triggered by particular thoughts, emotions, physical sensations, people, places, situations, and times of the day. It is important that clients identify and plan for their personal drinking triggers, through functional analysis of current and past alcohol use patterns. Once alcohol triggers are identified, the therapist and client can work collaboratively to develop a repertoire of coping alternatives tailored to the client's individual needs. Helpful strategies may include (a) distraction with alternative activities, (b) constructive self-talk, (c) talking cravings through, (d) substitution with alternate behaviors or drinks, (e) limiting the amount of money that can be accessed, or modifying transit routes to avoid high-risk encounters, (f) problem-solving skills training, (g) use of flashcards with reminders of intrinsic motivation and/or coping statements, and (h) assertive drink refusal to assist coping with real or perceived pressure from others (Miller, 2004; Monti et al., 2002). In addition, "emotion surfing" is a strategy that can be applied to urges to drink (e.g., "urge surfing") as well as uncomfortable emotional states more broadly (e.g., anxiety, frustration, boredom, low mood). This approach encourages clients to observe uncomfortable feelings from a non-reactive and accepting stance, and "surf" or ride out these feelings rather than fighting against or exacerbating them (Baillie & Rapee, 2003; Miller, 2004).

In-session practice exercises and role plays are recommended to refine and consolidate skill development. Imaginal or actual cue exposure may be beneficial to reduce reactivity to alcohol cues and consolidate alternate coping responses (Monti et al., 2002). For example, clients can be guided in session to imagine the sights, sounds, tastes, and situations that act as triggers for drinking. Imaginal or actual cue exposure can be incorporated as part of a graded exposure hierarchy, with clients prompted to use (or imagine themselves using) an identified coping strategy until the urge to drink decreases in intensity.

During each session, clients are encouraged to identify and plan for management of high-risk situations in the upcoming week/s. This includes explicit planning of strategies to manage any anxiety symptoms or craving for alcohol may be elicited by the behavioral experiments or activity scheduling conducted as part of treatment. Review and debriefing of past efforts to manage triggers is vital to crystallize learning, inform future planning, and enhance self-efficacy.

Development of Alternate Reinforcers

Clients may have few activities or interests other than drinking. Reliance on alcohol to manage social anxiety may mean that most, if not all, social interactions have also come to involve alcohol. Thus, it is essential that clients are assisted to develop or re-establish interests, activities and a lifestyle that is more rewarding than drinking. From the outset of treatment, we recommend setting weekly goals around identifying and sampling potentially rewarding activities that have been avoided or neglected due to drinking or anxiety (for ideas see p. 215, Miller et al., 2019). Give particular emphasis to activities that are incompatible with drinking (e.g., sports and fitness, outdoor activities, sober relationships, or support groups). Activity scheduling is also advantageous in terms of commencing exposure to and re-engagement with previously avoided social situations. Although anxiety-provoking for this population, socializing and building relationships are important steps towards establishing a fulfilling life in the longer-term. We recommend a hierarchical approach to activity scheduling beginning with manageable goals to enhance self-efficacy.

Cognitive Therapy

This component draws from established protocols for cognitive therapy applied to the treatment of social anxiety (McEvoy et al., 2018; Rapee et al., 2009) and substance use disorders (Beck et al., 1993; Epstein & McCrady, 2009). The therapist and client work together to uncover idiosyncratic beliefs that underlie these disorders. In the case of social anxiety disorder, underlying cognitions tend to incorporate inflated appraisals of the likelihood and consequences of negative evaluation. That is, individuals with social anxiety disorder tend to underestimate how well they perform socially, expect to be embarrassed or negatively judged by others, and consider the social cost of any perceived negative evaluation to be high. There is also evidence that individuals with social anxiety disorder overestimate the extent to which their anxiety is evident to others, and anticipate that others expect a higher standard of performance than they will be able to deliver (Heimberg et al., 2014). This underestimation of social performance and overestimation of the salience of their anxiety symptoms can often manifest in a negative mental representation of how they appear to others. Cognitive therapy therefore aims to facilitate identification and reappraisal of the threat cognitions and negative self-imagery that occur during anticipatory, concurrent, and post-event processing of social stressors (McEvoy et al., 2018; Rapee et al., 2009).

Cognitions that maintain alcohol use, also known as "Drinking Thinking", encompass overly positive expectancies regarding the benefits of drinking, as well as underestimates of the negative consequences of drinking. Empirical data indicate that heavy drinkers are more likely to expect alcohol will transform experiences in a positive way, improve social and sexual performance/experiences, improve mood, and decrease tension and anxiety (Boness et al., 2021; Hamonniere & Varescon, 2018). Other cognitions that contribute to drinking may include permission-giving thoughts, and meta-cognitive belief about the uncontrollable, persistent, and irresistible nature of craving (Beck et al., 1993; Hamonniere & Varescon, 2018). For example, cognitions such as "I'm not strong enough to resist this craving" may result in surrendering to the urge to drink. Entitlement beliefs, such as "I've been having a hard time, I deserve some relief" may seem to justify drinking. Alcohol-related cognitions are thought to play a causal role in the maintenance of alcohol use disorders (see Goldman et al., 1999; Halvorson et al., 2023), and are an important target for intervention with cognitive therapy. Identification of relevant cognitions may be assisted by administration of the Tension Reduction Subscale of the Alcohol Expectancies Questionnaire (Kushner et al., 1994).

Specific cognitive therapy techniques to assist reappraisal include: (a) evaluating the evidence to determine the realistic probability and cost of negative evaluation; (b) considering the realistic outcomes associated with drinking (see Table 2.4: Cognitive therapy for drinking thinking: Example for "Anna"); (c) considering alternative perspectives and the helpfulness or value of current thinking patterns; and (d) obtaining objective feedback about social performance and consequences of drinking (e.g., video feedback, feedback from supportive person). In addition, individualized behavioral experiments are designed to test out target expectancies and provide corrective evidence to inform cognitive therapy.

Behavioral Experiments

We encourage introduction of behavioral experiments early in treatment, potentially aligned with activity scheduling, with more comprehensive hierarchies developed as treatment progresses. The benefits of behavioral experiments are twofold. Firstly, they provide exposure to previously avoided situations, and the opportunity for a corrective learning experience (Jacquart et al., 2022). This may include increasing tolerance and acceptance of the resulting anxious arousal, and the opportunity to practice and refine coping strategies. Secondly, behavioral experiments are designed to test out the automatic expectancies and cognitions underlying anxiety and drinking. Clients are encouraged to explicitly identify expected outcomes for each experiment, and then compare this with the reality of what actually occurs. To optimize benefits and corrective learning, we recommended that the therapist initially accompany the client to complete some behavioral experiments. Guided sessions help motivate the client to get started on anxiety-provoking hierarchies, and the opportunity to model the optimal procedure and prompt use of cognitive therapy, task-focused attention, and coping skills before, during and after completing behavioral experiments.

For integrated SAD-AUD treatment, the primary targets for behavioral experiments are (a) experiments designed to test inflated social threat expectancies, (b) experiments designed to elicit realistic objective feedback about social performance and appearance to others, (c) experiments to challenge perceived reliance on safety behaviors, and (d) experiments designed to evaluate alcohol outcome expectancies. Design of behavioral experiments begins with a comprehensive analysis to identify idiosyncratic expectancies, avoidance patterns, and safety behaviors relevant to anxiety and drinking. The therapist and client then work collaboratively to develop a graded hierarchy of experiments to test the underlying expectancies. For example, consider a client who avoids being the center of attention, and identifies the underlying fears: "I will say something stupid and everyone will laugh", and "I will look nervous and everyone will notice and think I am weird". The first step for this client might be to tell an anecdote in front of a small group. With this behavioral experiment, they will be able to collect evidence as to both the *probability* and the *cost* of the outcomes they fear. They may discover that it is likely that they will stumble over their words at some point, but much less likely that others will notice and laugh. Subsequent behavioral experiments may incorporate the dropping of common safety behaviors, such as rehearsal or over-preparation, to test out the perception that these behaviors are necessary in order to prevent feared outcomes (Clark, 2005; McEvoy et al., 2018). Debriefing after behavioral experiments is critical to minimize the extent that the client's interpretation biases the observed outcomes. Clients should be discouraged from inferring the reactions of others and instead instructed to focus on directly observable evidence.

It is common for behavioral experiments to elicit craving for alcohol, and it is important that this is discussed explicitly, and an alternate coping plan developed. Furthermore, we suggest that behavioral experiments are designed to explicitly target the inter-connectedness between drinking and social anxiety. Experimental data suggest expectancies about the positive effects of alcohol can be manipulated, and this shift is associated with decreased drinking in non-clinical populations (Darkes & Goldman, 1998; Scott-Sheldon et al., 2012). Thus, we recommended that clients are supported to identify and challenge the alcohol-related cognitions linked to drinking in social and/or anxiety provoking contexts. For example, a client may hold the belief "alcohol makes me more interesting", and consequently fears "others will find me boring and dull if I socialize without drinking". To challenge these beliefs, behavioral experiments might initially focus on attending social activities that do not involve alcohol, and eventually build up to events where others might be drinking (see case example and Table 2.3 for an illustration of this approach). Through these experiments, clients have the opportunity to explore the actual outcomes of attending events sober, and realistically evaluate predictions about the feared consequences of not drinking. This approach represents a deviation from traditional protocols for alcohol treatment that typically advocate avoidance of situations that may be high risk for drinking. Our integrated treatment framework is more consistent with the approach-coping framework of anxiety treatment protocols and alcohol treatments incorporating cue exposure (Kushner et al., 2006; Monti et al., 2002). That is, whilst clients may be encouraged to avoid high-risk triggers for drinking initially, this is considered impractical in the longer-term, and thus they are supported to gradually encounter triggers and practice alternate coping strategies as they gain confidence to do so. This approach may be particularly important for helping clients overcome AUD, given the abundance of alcohol-related cues they are likely to encounter in everyday life (Byrne et al., 2019). Clients may feel more secure to begin with experiments accompanied by the therapist, for example, going together to an establishment that serves alcohol to practicing urge surfing and ordering a non-alcoholic beverage. In some cases, imaginal exposure techniques may be beneficial when identified behavioral experiments are deemed impractical or not clinically advisable.

Attention Training

Drawing from Rapee and colleagues (McEvoy et al., 2018; Rapee et al., 2009), this component encompasses two aspects of attention training: attention strengthening and applied task-focused attention. These components are important given mounting evidence that individuals with social anxiety preferentially attend to, and find it difficult to disengage from, threatening social information such as signs of disapproval from others and internal anxiety symptoms (Heimberg et al., 2014; Morrison & Heimberg, 2013). Strengthening clients' ability (and self-efficacy) to manipulate their focus of attention is also likely to have additional benefits in terms of improving their capacity to refocus from "sticky" (i.e., persistent) thoughts that may contribute to drinking or anxiety. Attention strengthening is achieved through regular practice of a 10-min meditation during which attention is focused on developing a full awareness of each breath. It is expected that during this practice a variety of thoughts, sensations and feelings will arise, and the client is encouraged to acknowledge these experiences but refocus attention on the breath. While frustration is a common response to wandering thoughts, clients should instead be encouraged to view these as the opportunity for further practice and strengthening of the ability to refocus attention. Alternative attention strengthening exercises (e.g., actively focusing on and switching attention between specific sounds in an array of competing sounds) may be used in cases where breath meditation is unsuitable (Wells, 2011).

Applied task-focused attention builds on the increased flexibility and control gained through attention strengthening practice. Clients are encouraged to become aware of the focus of their attention during social situations, and differentiate between "self-focused" and "task-focused" attention. Self-focused attention encompasses attention directed towards internal experiences such as physical symptoms, recollections of past negative social experiences, or hypotheses about how one appears to or is being evaluated by others (McEvoy et al., 2018; Rapee et al., 2009). Applied attention training refers to the practice of consciously re-directing attention towards more adaptive task-related foci. In the context of social interactions, this often involves redirecting the focus of attention to the conversation topic, being curious about what the other person is saying and noticing common interests or experiences. Prior to practicing task-focused attention in a given situation, it is beneficial to apply cognitive therapy techniques to critically evaluate social threat appraisals, as the ability to refocus attention on the task at hand will improve as the salience of potential threat cues decreases. Clients are also encouraged to apply attention re-focus where relevant to assist with disengaging and refocusing away from alcohol-related thoughts, cravings, or cues in the environment (e.g., walking past a pub). Over time, deliberate modification of attention in this manner may deactivate maladaptive cognitive processing routines and promote more flexible control over these processes and the subsequent behavioral response. In addition, reduced self-focus likely results in a greater capacity to attend to and integrate information that disconfirms anxiety-related threat appraisals. For this reason, we recommend that clients incorporate task-focused attention during behavioral experiments to maximize the potential for corrective learning experiences and cognitive reappraisal.

Social Support

AUD and SAD are both associated with impoverished social networks and support (Dobkin et al., 2002; Teo et al., 2013). Existing friendships may tend to revolve around drinking. It is important that clients are encouraged to develop positive social networks, and/or access appropriate support from existing relationships, as social support is a robust predictor of sustained recovery (Sliedrecht et al., 2019). Enhancing social networks may involve development of (a) communication skills to enhance the client's ability to ask for support, (b) interpersonal and listening skills to improve reciprocity in relationships, and (c) identifying and planning ways to form new sober friendships. We recommend that these objectives be pursued in conjunction with cognitive therapy to target social threat cognitions that emerge as barriers to healthy relationships.

Where possible, it is beneficial for clients to attend at least one therapy session together with an identified support person. Involving significant others in treatment has been found to improve treatment adherence and reduce relapse rates (see Miller et al., 2019). The support person should be someone the client identifies within their existing network who is willing to support their goals and involvement in treatment. Aims of the session include providing the support person with psychoeducation about SAD and AUD, and clarifying any misconceptions about these problems or the treatment approach. The session is an opportunity to acknowledge and affirm the support person's role and form a collaborative plan for continued support. It is useful to review and discuss the effectiveness of current support behaviors, to reinforce helpful behaviors and highlight counter-productive behaviors such as nagging or enabling anxiety and drinking (e.g., offering drinks, facilitating avoidance, or protecting the client from the natural consequences). By supporting the client's efforts to change and increasing engagement with positive activities that do not involve alcohol, the support person can play an important role in recovery and maintenance. However, it is important to emphasize that the support person is not expected to act as co-therapist or enforcer, and assistance should not be offered at the expense of the support person's own well-being (Miller, 2004).

Continuing Change and Coping with Setbacks

Towards the end of treatment, staggered sessions help to prepare the client for termination. We suggest the therapist and client work together to develop a long-term action plan for continued change post-termination. This plan can incorporate (a) long-term goals for a fulfilling post-recovery lifestyle, with a focus on alcohol-free activities, (b) advanced behavioral experiments, and (c) identification and planning for potential high-risk situations and setbacks. It is critical to provide clients with psychoeducation about the gradual, uneven nature of progress and recovery, and prepare them to form realistic, non-catastrophic interpretation of any future setbacks. Therapists need to find a balance between communicating that setbacks and/or lapses to drinking are common, without conveying that relapse is inevitable (DiClemente & Crisafulli, 2022). Most important, is the way that clients respond to and move forward from any lapses or setbacks. Throughout therapy and when preparing for termination, clients should be encouraged to respond with self-compassion, and view setbacks as important learning opportunities. It is valuable to identify the environmental, emotional, interpersonal, cognitive, and behavioral factors that contributed to the lapse or setback, and consider how these could be managed and planned for in the future (DiClemente & Crisafulli, 2022; Witkiewitz & Marlatt, 2004). The final sessions should also focus on exploring the client's feelings and any concerns about termination and reflect on the progress that has been made. It is important that these therapeutic interactions enhance the client's sense of self-efficacy, and that credit for positive changes is attributed to the client rather than the therapist, medication, or external factors.

Common Challenges

People with co-occurring SAD-AUD often present with a wide range of complex and severe problems. Co-occurring substance use dependence other than alcohol may require referral or management in collaboration with specialist services. Suicide and child protection risk assessment and management may be required and we recommend that therapists are well acquainted with the local procedures to address these concerns.

With some clients, therapeutic progress may be hindered due to a pattern of recurrent situational stressors, which may be related to the person's anxiety or alcohol use, social networks, experiences of marginalization, or just due to chance. A first consideration in these situations is assessing and responding to any risk to the immediate safety of the client or their networks. Reflective listening is important to help the client make sense of what has happened, including understanding the contributing cognitive, attentional and/or behavioral processes. While it is important that clients are given the opportunity to explore these issues, it is equally important that these conversations do not occur at the expense of the skill development necessary for amelioration of problems in the longer-term (Linehan, 1993). When supporting the client to identify possible practical actions, look for opportunities to apply or develop cognitive behavioral skills as a way of responding to immediate crises or stressors. In this way, crises need not obstruct skill development, but can be used as an opportunity to practice or refine application of the skills the client has been working to develop.

It is important to consider how the client's unique social, cultural, gender, sexual, racial, and sexual identity affects their perspective and engagement with treatment. AUD is more prevalent and difficult to overcome among marginalized populations, who do not have the same opportunities to seek, access or engage with treatment consistently (Lavalley et al., 2020). These disparities can be amplified by the stigma and prejudice that is commonly experienced by people with AUD. Given these individual differences, it is important that treatment is adapted to the client's individual needs and circumstances. The motivational interviewing framework and flexible session structure allow for tailoring of treatment in line with clients' needs. For example, it may be beneficial to schedule a social support session earlier in treatment for clients who identify their partners' alcohol consumption and/or enabling behaviors as key drinking triggers. Clients who present with alcohol-related cognitive deficits or memory impairment may require simplification of the components and/or additional time for comprehension and skill development. Co-occurring depression and low self-efficacy add to the motivational challenges of treatment. Additional time may be needed to enhance motivation and rebuild momentum in response to a lapse or fluctuating motivation. Miller et al. (2019) provide a useful discussion of additional challenges and professional issues that commonly arise in AUD treatment. Regular clinical supervision is important to ensure that therapists are adequately supported through the complex psychosocial issues, suicidal ideation, and fluctuating motivation that are common in this population.

Clinical Case and Treatment Vignette

The following vignette describes the clinical presentation and application of integrated CBT for co-occurring SAD and AUD. To ensure client anonymity, the vignette has been drawn from file notes of several clients and potentially identifying information has been changed. For additional examples, we refer readers to previous case vignettes described in our earlier work (Stapinski et al., 2015).

Clinical Characteristics and Treatment Overview

"Anna" was a 29-year-old queer woman (pronouns: she/her) who emigrated with her family from South America to Australia when she was 9. She was in stable full-time employment in retail and lived with her partner. Anna met criteria for a diagnosis of SAD (severe) and alcohol dependence (moderate); she also described subclinical symptoms and a history of major depressive disorder and disordered eating. Initial treatment sessions focused on developing a shared problem formulation (see Fig. 2.1), exploring Anna's motivations and goals for change (see example dialogue), and beginning to implement strategies to reduce her drinking. Anna's primary motivation for changing her alcohol consumption was to reduce the negative impact on her relationship with her partner due to arguments when intoxicated. In addition, Anna's alcohol use had led to some gastrointestinal complications, and she was concerned about the impact on her work performance. Anna's long-term goal was to be able to drink in moderation; however, she set an initial goal of abstinence for the first month to build momentum and shift her current patterns prior to re-introducing moderated drinking. Another important treatment goal was to reduce her social avoidance and cultivate friendships and interests outside of her relationship with her partner. Treatment proceeded in collaboration with Anna's general practitioner, who was managing her alcohol-related gastrointestinal issues, and provided ongoing medical monitoring. Anna declined the option of adjunct pharmacotherapy.

Initially, Anna found it challenging to abstain from drinking, and sessions focused on enhancing her motivation, and detailed planning of strategies to manage her cravings and triggers for drinking. The strategies she found most effective were modifying her route home from work to avoid passing the liquor store, and replacing her "wind-down" drink with an evening walk or yoga class. Abstaining from drinking alcohol before/during social events was more difficult for her, but she found it helped to tell her partner in advance that she would not be drinking and offer to be the designated driver. Initially she avoided events that centered around drinking and instead opted for alternative social activities (e.g., going to the theatre, beach day). Anna appreciated the approach of "emotion surfing" and applied this to wait out feelings of anxiety and alcohol craving that she experienced, noticing that her intense cravings typically subsided after 30 min. During weekly debriefing, Anna reflected on the benefits associated with her reduced alcohol consumption: including more energy, improved work performance, less irritability, and less wasted time from hangovers. Working towards her longer-term goal of moderated alcohol use involved identifying what "healthy" vs unhealthy alcohol use looked like for her and articulating some guidelines to follow for the remainder of the treatment and beyond (see Table 2.2).

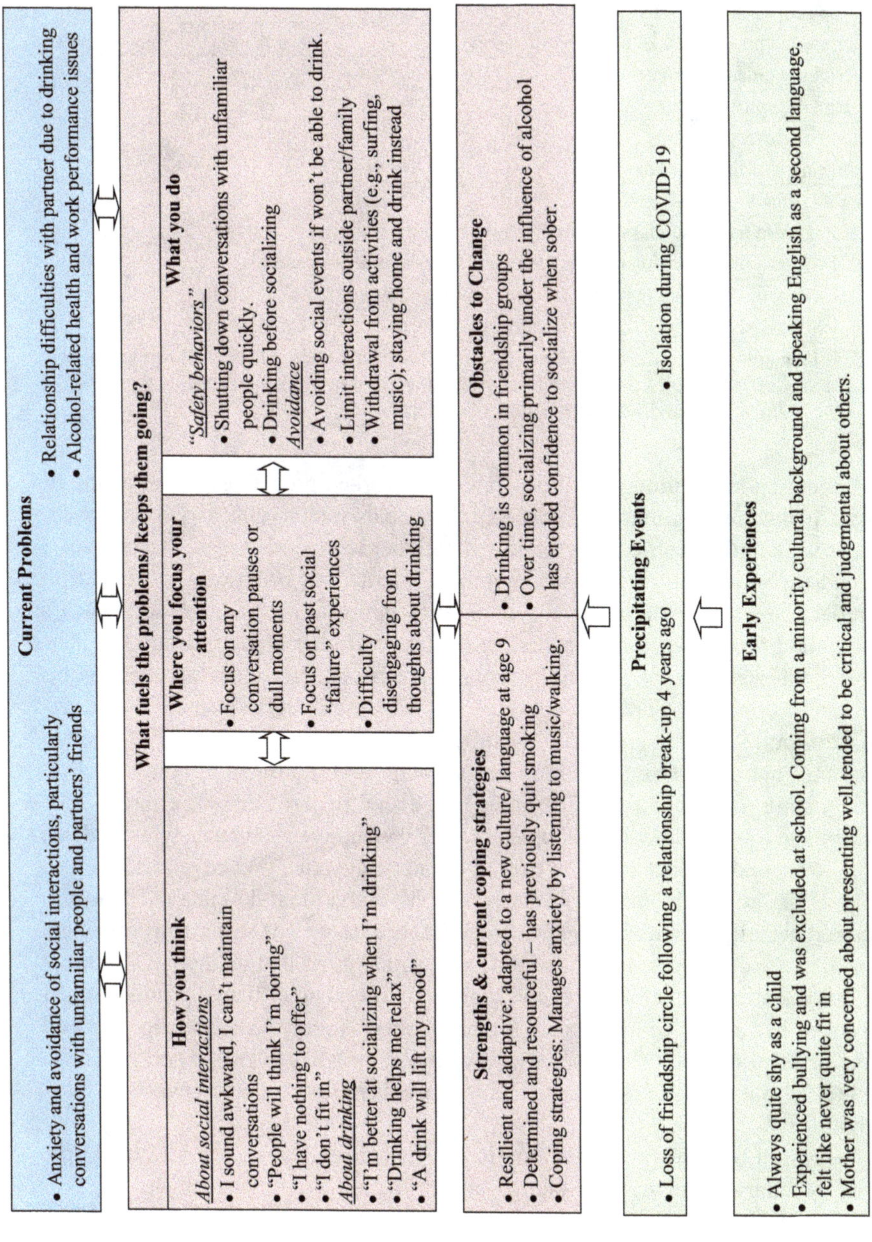

Fig. 2.1 Problem formulation worksheet for "Anna"

Table 2.2 Developing safe drinking guidelines: Example for "Anna"

What does unsafe or unhealthy drinking look like for me?
Drinking because I feel anxious, stressed or depressed
Drinking alone
Drinking "pre-drink/s" before a social event
Drinking quickly or to get drunk
Drinking spirits or shots
Drinking everyday
Starting to drink at midday
My safe drinking guidelines:
1. It is ok to have one glass of wine with dinner or on a special occasion
2. I will avoid drinking more than 2 standard drinks on one occasion
3. I will avoid drinking regularly (i.e., maximum once per month)
4. I will avoid drinking to cope with anxiety or stress
5. If I am going to drink alcohol, I will plan in advance and make use the following coping strategies: decide on a drinks limit in advance, eat prior to drinking, drink slowly (savor the taste), space out drinks with non-alcoholic options

Beginning in the initial sessions, Anna also worked proactively on reducing her social avoidance, beginning with less difficult goals such as chatting to dog owners on her walk and agreeing to go for coffee with her work colleagues. She noticed an immediate boost to her confidence and these interactions provided useful evidence to reflect on when reappraising social threat cognitions in subsequent sessions. For Anna, the primary targets for cognitive therapy were her cognitions around being boring, awkward, or inadequate in social interactions. Her concerns that she had nothing to offer and didn't "fit in" were longstanding beliefs since childhood, and most difficult to shift. Anna found it helpful to learn about the role that biased attention and memory processes play in shaping and entrenching these beliefs. Recognizing that memories of negative past social experiences were most salient for her, she found it helpful to supplement her own counter-evidence with feedback about her social abilities from her trusted friends/colleagues. When reflecting on the focus of her attention during social interactions, Anna identified that she tended to focus on herself, scrutinizing her own performance, as well as scanning for potential signs that the other person was disinterested. Anna found that deliberately redirecting her attention to the conversation topic (i.e., the content being communicated) improved her ability to maintain and enjoy conversations. As therapy progressed, Anna planned for and progressed to more challenging behavioral experiments (see Table 2.3) to gain further evidence and increase her confidence to engage in social activities while sober.

At session 6, Anna presented reporting a lapse to heavy drinking, initially triggered by an argument with her partner about whether and how much she had been drinking. Anna identified thoughts such as "stuff it" and "nothing I do helps anyway" that contributed to her return to drinking. The session focused on positively affirming Anna's continued commitment to attending therapy, normalizing the experience of setbacks, and revisiting Anna's own motivations for wanting to change

Table 2.3 Behavioral experiment hierarchy: Example for "Anna". In collaboration with her therapist, Anna developed the following behavioral experiment hierarchy to collect evidence and critically evaluate the cognitions "People find me boring" and "I need a few drinks to be able to socialize". Where possible, Anna repeated each step multiple times. Anna was reminded to practice task-focused attention when completing each step. Following each interaction, she recorded what she had learned from the experiment (limited to observable, objective evidence) to debrief and discuss in the subsequent therapy session

Steps	Predicted difficulty (0–8)
Attend the women's surfing academy group course.	8
Attend a birthday dinner with partner's friends; non-alcoholic drinks only. Make an effort to chat with at least two new people.	8
Go for 1 h to after-work drinks with colleagues at the pub. Order a non-alcoholic drink and chat with at least two people.	7
Chat with at least two people while at the song-writing course.	7
Go to dinner with partner and their friends. Tell partner in advance that I won't be drinking and ask if her to do the same.	6
Join the 8-week song-writing course at local arts center.	6
Ask trusted colleague for feedback about my social abilities with customers at work.	6
Go to a pub accompanied by therapist, practice ordering a non-alcoholic drink.	5
Visit the women's surfing academy and ask for information about the next course.	5
Invite an old friend to catch up over dinner. Tell her in advance that I'm taking a break from drinking and practice assertive drink if she offers me a drink.	5
Strike up a conversation with another dog owner when out for a walk.	4
Agree to go for coffee at lunch with work colleague.	4
Chat for 5–10 min with colleague at work.	4
Say hello to other dog owners when out walking the dog.	3

as distinct from her partner's desire that she change. Critically evaluating the cognitions that contributed to her choosing to drink (i.e., drinking thinking; see Table 2.4) helped to strengthen her resolve and prepare for urges to drink in the future. The subsequent support session, which Anna attended together with her partner Sam, was an opportunity to clarify Sam's role as a support but not an enforcer, and collaboratively develop a plan for how Sam could most effectively support Anna's goals for treatment. Sam acknowledged there had been fewer arguments since Anna started treatment but was frustrated that Anna had not made more progress in addressing her anxiety and alcohol use. Sam described feeling "left in the dark", which made her suspicious and worried about Anna sneaking drinks. Anna set a goal of trying to communicate her feelings, goals, and achievements more openly, acknowledging that this was something that she found difficult but could build up to using the behavioral stepladder approach. With affirmation and encouragement from the therapist, Anna was able to make a start in session, by reflecting on the achievements that she felt most proud of, and her long-term goals for the future.

Table 2.4 Cognitive therapy for drinking thinking: Example for "Anna"

Situation	Drinking thinking	What do I hope alcohol will do for me?	What is the reality? (Consider immediate & delayed outcome)	Helpful alternative thought
Meeting partner and her friends for dinner.	"I'm awkward and have nothing to contribute to conversations" "I'll be more sociable and interesting if I drink"	Help me to feel more sociable and less worried about others judging me.	Drank two drinks quickly because I was nervous. Had some pretty good conversations early in the night but kept drinking. Have some memory gaps for later conversations so worry I might have said something stupid or inappropriate. Felt criticized in a conversation with partner and became defensive. Felt embarrassed that Sam's friends will think I over-reacted and might judge me for how much I was drinking.	Drinking more than one or two drinks has a negative effect on me socially and I become over-sensitive and reactive. I know from past experience that I can be sociable and interesting without drinking.
Argument with partner about whether I had been drinking. Felt let down, angry and hopeless.	"Stuff it" "Nothing I do helps anyway—may as well drink"	Show my partner how angry I am. Make me feel good, squash the angry/hopeless thoughts.	Felt a bit better after the first few drinks but continued to drink. Had another argument with partner. Felt terrible the next day: vomiting, anxious, and ashamed. Worried all day about the future and my relationship. For the next few days, fell back into a pattern of drinking when I got home from work.	Drinking damages my relationship. There are better ways to communicate that I felt let down. I'm reducing my drinking for me, not just for Sam (partner). I feel better when I'm not drinking. Drinking makes me feel ashamed and physically unwell. Going for a surf or listening to music is a better way to lift my mood.

In the remaining sessions, Anna focused on progressing and extending her behavioral experiment hierarchies, working towards her longer-term goals of broadening her activities and social networks outside of those shared with her partner. For example, Anna built up to joining an 8-week surfing course, which provided her with important social experiences and counterevidence to her anxious predictions that people found her boring and she needed alcohol to socialize. Anna also explored a podcast series about evidence-based strategies for managing conflict and promoting healthy communication in relationships. Anna described the experience of persevering with her alcohol reduction goals following her mid-treatment lapse as giving her the confidence to stay focused on her personal reasons for not drinking when navigating relationship conflict and other potential setbacks in the future. Although Anna continued to experience anxiety at social events, particularly when socializing with her partner's friends, she found these events less difficult and no longer felt that she needed to drink to socialize. Re-engagement with activities she had come to avoid, particularly surfing and making music, had enriched her day-to-day life and she reported feeling more content and fulfilled.

Example of Therapeutic Dialogue: Exploring the Anxiety-Alcohol Inter-Relationship

The following dialogue between the therapist and Anna took place in the initial therapy sessions. This part of the session focused on building an understanding of Anna's reasons for using alcohol, the relationship between her anxiety and alcohol use, and enhancing her intrinsic motivation to make some changes.

Therapist	Now I'd like to hear some more about what you're hoping to get out of treatment and understand what drinking and anxiety are like for you at the moment. Let's start by getting a bit more detail about your alcohol use—does that sound ok?
Anna	Yeah, okay.
Therapist	In our assessment you told me that your typical pattern is drinking 4 or 5 glasses of wine or beer on the weekdays, generally when you get home from work or before an event. And then on weekends, you'll start drinking earlier and have more like 1 or sometimes 2 bottles of wine each day. Have I got that right? [Clarification]
Anna	Yeah, that's usually how it is… and then often on a Monday I'll feel really bad and decide I'm not going to drink—so those days I won't have any.
Therapist	Okay, so you have been able to have some alcohol-free days, about once a week? [Highlight self-efficacy to control drinking]
Anna	Yep, and sometimes Tuesday as well.. if I feel really guilty after the weekend and decide I need to cut back. But then by Wednesday… I feel like a drink again.
Therapist	So the after-effects of a weekend of drinking motivate you to avoid drinking at first, but after a couple of days the urges to drink get strong again… Is that right?

[Introducing the idea of cravings].

Anna	Yeah… I know my drinking is a problem, but it's hard to stop.
Therapist	What are some of the things that tell you that your drinking is a problem? [Elicit reasons for change].
Anna	Well… feeling bad physically and then there have been a few occasions when I have been late to work—I'm on my second notice and our rent is a lot so I can't afford to lose my job. But, … the thing is, drinking is one of the few things that makes me feel good and that I can look forward to..
Therapist	So it's hard to think about making changes because you see drinking alcohol as something you can look forward to. [Reflective listening, avoid persuasion]
Anna	Yes.. and it helps me to relax. I mean at work I have to talk with people all day. I find that really stressful and so I'm just so tense by the time I go home. Or the other thing is, sometimes my partner will want me to come and meet her and her friends somewhere—and then I'll definitely need a drink. As soon as I get there, or before if I can.
Therapist	So when you're going to a social event with others—that's a time when you really feel like having a drink. What do you hope that drinking will do for you in those situations? [Explore function of drinking].
Anna	Make it easier to talk with people… After a few drinks I don't care as much what they are thinking about me—drinking helps to squash all the thoughts running through my head..
Therapist	Ok, I'm understanding that drinking alcohol is one of the ways that you cope with worries about what others think of you. And are you saying that your social interactions go better if you've drunk alcohol? [Explore discrepancy between perceived benefits and negative social consequences reported during assessment].
Anna	Ummm… well there's definitely a tipping point, after a few drinks I can get ultra-sensitive and just take things the wrong way… or get angry—react to things and get into arguments with my partner. Or if I have had a really bad day—nothing helps. On those days, drinking takes me to a pretty dark place.. where I'm just thinking how awkward I am socially and that I can't make friends..
Therapist	Ok so drinking leads to some pretty dark thoughts sometimes.. and means that you are sensitive and react strongly to things.
Anna	Yeah it's not been great with my partner the last few months. We've just been having too many arguments and it's one of the reasons that she doesn't like me drinking..
Therapist	It sounds like you've noticed that drinking has affected your relationship?
Anna	Yeh, like last week at dinner we ended up arguing in front of her friends and I stormed out… the next day I woke up and just felt so guilty and so embarrassed—that I'd acted insecure and irrational like that in front of her friends.. it's just not me to act that way and I feel so ashamed that it keeps happening.

Therapist	That's so hard—I can see that going to social events has been tough, and using alcohol has been your way of coping with the nervousness and worries. But at the same time, drinking can mean that you do or say things that are out of character, and then you feel even worse. [Summarizing; Highlight anxiety-alcohol inter-relationship and discrepancy between goals and current behavior].
Anna	Yep.. pretty much, that's why I'm here.. I need to do something.
Therapist	I hear how important it is for you to make some changes—it's so great that you have taken the first steps by coming here—I'm sure that wasn't easy. What is it that you are hoping to get out of our work together—what would you like to be different? [Positive affirmation, explore goals, emphasizing autonomy]
Anna	I want to be able to have a drink occasionally, but without feeling like I *need* to drink or that I am using alcohol as a crutch…. I feel like I have gotten so used to drinking to socialize that I don't know how to do it sober anymore.
Therapist	Ok so it is important to feel that you have control over your alcohol use. And to be able to socialize without relying on alcohol. You're not alone—it's common for people to experience that over time, using alcohol to cope with anxiety in social situations can reduce their confidence to socialize without alcohol. So, to make it easier to cut back on your drinking, we can work on some really practical strategies to help you manage your anxiety—instead of drinking. Would you find that useful? [Affirm change talk, provide information about how treatment will help]
Anna	That's what I want—to not feel so stressed all the time about worrying about what other people think of me. And to reduce the pressure on my relationship... by having my own life outside my partner—and not getting into those silly arguments 'cos I'm drinking. I really want things to be good between us.
Therapist	Those are some really important goals then for us to work on in our time together. What if we start by making a plan together for some things you can do in the next week, to begin to make some positive changes? [Collaborative, encourage small changes to build momentum]

Acknowledgments The authors gratefully acknowledge Andrew Baillie, Ron Rapee, Claudia Sannibale, Maree Teesson, Mirjana Subotic-Kerry, and Paul Haber, who contributed to the development and/or trial of the integrated cognitive behavioral treatment for co-occurring social anxiety disorder and alcohol use disorder described in this chapter.

References

Anker, J. J., & Kushner, M. G. (2019). Co-occurring alcohol use disorder and anxiety: Bridging psychiatric, psychological, and neurobiological perspectives. *Alcohol Research: Current Reviews, 40*(1), arcr.v40.41.03. https://doi.org/10.35946/arcr.v40.1.03

Babor, T. F., Higgins-Biddle, J. C., Saunders, J. B., & Monteiro, M. G. (2001). *The alcohol use disorders identification test: Guidelines for use in primary care* (Vol. 2). World Health Organization.

Baillie, A. J., & Rapee, R. M. (2003). *Panic surfing: Early intervention treatment manual for panic disorder*. Macquarie Lighthouse Press.

Baillie, A. J., & Sannibale, C. (2007). Anxiety and drug and alcohol problems. In A. Baker & R. Velleman (Eds.), *Clinical handbook of co-existing mental health and drug and alcohol problems* (pp. 195–214). Brunner-Routledge.

Baillie, A. J., Stapinski, L., Crome, E., Morley, K., Sannibale, C., Haber, P., & Teesson, M. (2010). Some new directions for research on psychological interventions for comorbid anxiety and substance use disorders. *Drug and Alcohol Review, 29*(5), 518–524.

Baillie, A., Pham, J., Morley, K., Stapinski, L., Mills, K., Marel, C., Kay-Lambkin, F., & Teesson, M. (2021). Comorbidities: Co-occurring mental and alcohol use disorders. In *Guidelines for the treatment of alcohol problems*. Specialty of Addiction Medicine, Faculty of Medicine and Health, The University of Sydney.

Bakken, K., Landheim, A. S., & Vaglum, P. (2005). Substance-dependent patients with and without social anxiety disorder: Occurrence and clinical differences. *Drug and Alcohol Dependence, 80*(3), 321–328. https://doi.org/10.1016/j.drugalcdep.2005.04.011

Barrett, E., Mills, K., Dudley, L., Holmes, D., Conroy, C., Teesson, M., & Kay-Lambkin, F. (2019). Lived experiences of Australians with mental health and AOD comorbidity and their perspectives on integrated treatment. *newparadigm*, Summer 2018-2019.

Beck, A. T., Wright, F. D., Newman, C. F., & Liese, B. S. (1993). *Cognitive therapy of substance abuse*. Guilford Press.

Berglund, K. J., Rauwolf, K. K., Berggren, U., Balldin, J., & Fahlke, C. (2019). Outcome in relation to drinking goals in alcohol-dependent individuals: A follow-up study 2.5 and 5 years after treatment entry. *Alcohol and Alcoholism, 54*(4), 439–445. https://doi.org/10.1093/alcalc/agz042

Boness, C. L., Watts, A. L., Moeller, K. N., & Sher, K. J. (2021). The etiologic, theory-based, ontogenetic hierarchical framework of alcohol use disorder: A translational systematic review of reviews. *Psychological Bulletin, 147*(10), 1075–1123. https://doi.org/10.1037/bul0000333

Book, S., Thomas, S., Dempsey, J., Randall, P., & Randall, C. (2009). Social anxiety impacts willingness to participate in addiction treatment. *Addictive Behaviors, 34*(5), 474–476. https://doi.org/10.1016/j.addbeh.2008.12.011

Burns, L., Teesson, M., & O'Neill, K. (2005). The impact of comorbid anxiety and depression on alcohol treatment outcomes. *Addiction, 100*(6), 787–796. https://doi.org/10.1111/j.1360-0443.2005.001069.x

Byrne, S. P., Haber, P., Baillie, A., Giannopolous, V., & Morley, K. (2019). Cue exposure therapy for alcohol use disorders: What can be learned from exposure therapy for anxiety disorders? *Substance Use & Misuse, 54*(12), 2053–2063. https://doi.org/10.1080/10826084.2019.1618328

Clark, D. M. (2005). A cognitive perspective on social phobia. In *The essential handbook of social anxiety for clinicians* (pp. 193–218). Wiley.

Cooper, R., Hildebrandt, S., & Gerlach, A. (2014). Drinking motives in alcohol use disorder patients with and without social anxiety disorder. *Anxiety, Stress & Coping, 27*(1), 113–122. https://doi.org/10.1080/10615806.2013.823482

Cruz, E., Martins, P. D. C., & Diniz, P. R. B. (2017). Factors related to the association of social anxiety disorder and alcohol use among adolescents: A systematic review. *Jornal de Pediatria, 93*(5), 442–451. https://doi.org/10.1016/j.jped.2017.05.001

Darkes, J., & Goldman, M. S. (1998). Expectancy challenge and drinking reduction: Process and structure in the alcohol expectancy network. *Experimental and Clinical Psychopharmacology, 6*(1), 64–76. https://doi.org/10.1037/1064-1297.6.1.64

DiClemente, C. C., & Crisafulli, M. A. (2022). Relapse on the road to recovery: Learning the lessons of failure on the way to successful behavior change. *Journal of Health Service Psychology, 48*(2), 59–68.

Dobkin, P. L., Civita, M. D., Paraherakis, A., & Gill, K. (2002). The role of functional social support in treatment retention and outcomes among outpatient adult substance abusers. *Addiction, 97*(3), 347–356. https://doi.org/10.1046/j.1360-0443.2002.00083.x

Driessen, M., Meier, S., Hill, A., Wetterling, T., Lange, W., & Junghanns, K. (2001). The course of anxiety, depression and drinking behaviours after completed detoxification in alcoholics with and without comorbid anxiety and depressive disorders. *Alcohol and Alcoholism, 36*, 249–255. https://doi.org/10.1093/alcalc/36.3.249

Epstein, E. E., & McCrady, B. S. (2009). *Overcoming alcohol use problems: Therapist guide: A cognitive-behavioural treatment program*. Oxford University Press. https://doi.org/10.1093/med:psych/9780195322811.001.0001

Farris, S. G., Epstein, E. E., McCrady, B. S., & Hunter-Reel, D. (2012). Do co-morbid anxiety disorders predict drinking outcomes in women with alcohol use disorders? *Alcohol and Alcoholism, 47*(2), 143–148.

Glantz, M. D., Bharat, C., Degenhardt, L., Sampson, N. A., Scott, K. M., Lim, C. C. W., Al-Hamzawi, A., Alonso, J., Andrade, L. H., Cardoso, G., De Girolamo, G., Gureje, O., He, Y., Hinkov, H., Karam, E. G., Karam, G., Kovess-Masfety, V., Lasebikan, V., Lee, S., Levinson, D., McGrath, J., Medina-Mora, M. E., Mihaescu-Pintia, C., Mneimneh, Z., Moskalewicz, J., Navarro-Mateu, F., Posada-Villa, J., Rapsey, C., Stagnaro, J. C., Tachimori, H., Ten Have, M., Tintle, N., Torres, Y., Williams, D. R., Ziv, Y., & Kessler, R. C. (2020). The epidemiology of alcohol use disorders cross-nationally: Findings from the World Mental Health Surveys. *Addictive Behaviors, 102*, 106128. https://doi.org/10.1016/j.addbeh.2019.106128

Goldman, M. S., Del Boca, F. K., & Darkes, J. (1999). Alcohol expectancy theory: The application of cognitive neuroscience. *Psychological Theories of Drinking and Alcoholism, 2*, 203–246.

Goodwin, M. E., & Sayette, M. A. (2022). A social contextual review of the effects of alcohol on emotion. *Pharmacology Biochemistry and Behavior, 221*, 173486. https://doi.org/10.1016/j.pbb.2022.173486

Haber, P. S., & Lintzeris, N. (2021). Alcohol withdrawal. In P. S. Haber & B. C. Riordan (Eds.), *Guidelines for the treatment of alcohol problems*. Specialty of Addiction Medicine, Faculty of Medicine and Health, The University of Sydney.

Halvorson, M. A., Lengua, L. J., Smith, G. T., & King, K. M. (2023). Pathways of personality and learning risk for addictive behaviors: A systematic review of mediational research on the acquired preparedness model. *Journal of Personality, 91*(3), 613–637. https://doi.org/10.1111/jopy.12761

Hamonniere, T., & Varescon, I. (2018). Metacognitive beliefs in addictive behaviours: A systematic review. *Addictive Behaviors, 85*, 51–63. https://doi.org/10.1016/j.addbeh.2018.05.018

Harvey, L. R., Saraiya, T. C., Mills, K. L., Brown, D. G., Jarnecke, A. M., Back, S. E., & Stapinski, L. A. (2022). Exposure therapy when patients present with comorbid substance use disorders. In *Clinical guide to exposure therapy: Beyond phobias* (pp. 87–107). Springer.

Haver, B., & Gjestad, R. (2005). Phobic anxiety and depression as predictor variables for treatment outcome. A LISREL analysis on treated female alcoholics. *Nordic Journal of Psychiatry, 59*(1), 25–30. https://doi.org/10.1080/08039480510018797

Heimberg, R. G., Brozovich, F. A., & Rapee, R. M. (2014). A cognitive-behavioral model of social anxiety disorder. *Social Anxiety*, 705–728.

Henssler, J., Müller, M., Carreira, H., Bschor, T., Heinz, A., & Baethge, C. (2021). Controlled drinking—non-abstinent versus abstinent treatment goals in alcohol use disorder: A systematic review, meta-analysis and meta-regression. *Addiction, 116*(8), 1973–1987. https://doi.org/10.1111/add.15329

Jacquart, J., Abramowitz, J., Arch, J., Margraf, J., & Smits, J. A. (2022). The basics of exposure therapy. In *Clinical guide to exposure therapy: Beyond phobias* (pp. 1–31). Springer.

Kessler, R. C., Crum, R. M., Warner, L. A., Nelson, C. B., Schulenberg, J., & Anthony, J. C. (1997). Lifetime co-occurrence of DSM-III-R alcohol abuse and dependence with other psychiatric disorders in the National Comorbidity Survey. *Archives of General Psychiatry, 54*(4), 313–321. https://doi.org/10.1001/archpsyc.1997.01830160031005

Knox, J., Hasin, D. S., Larson, F. R., & Kranzler, H. R. (2019). Prevention, screening, and treatment for heavy drinking and alcohol use disorder. *The Lancet Psychiatry, 6*(12), 1054–1067.

Koob, G. F., Buck, C. L., Cohen, A., Edwards, S., Park, P. E., Schlosburg, J. E., Schmeichel, B., Vendruscolo, L. F., Wade, C. L., Whitfield, T. W., Jr., & George, O. (2014). Addiction as a stress surfeit disorder. *Neuropharmacology, 76*, 370–382. https://doi.org/10.1016/j.neuropharm.2013.05.024

Kushner, M. G., Sher, K. J., Wood, M. D., & Wood, P. K. (1994). Anxiety and drinking behavior: Moderating effects of tension-reduction alcohol outcome expectancies. *Alcoholism: Clinical & Experimental Research, 18*(4), 852–860.

Kushner, M. G., Abrams, K., Thuras, P., Hanson, K. L., Brekke, M., & Sletten, S. (2005). Follow-up study of anxiety disorder and alcohol dependence in comorbid alcoholism treatment patients. *Alcoholism, Clinical and Experimental Research, 29*(8), 1432–1443. https://doi.org/10.1097/01.alc.0000175072.17623.f8

Kushner, M. G., Donahue, C., Sletten, S., Thuras, P., Abrams, K., Peterson, J., & Frye, B. (2006). Cognitive behavioral treatment of comorbid anxiety disorder in alcoholism treatment patients: Presentation of a prototype program and future directions. *Journal of Mental Health, 15*(6), 697–707. http://www.informaworld.com/10.1080/09638230600998946

Kushner, M. G., Maurer, E. W., Thuras, P., Donahue, C., Frye, B., Menary, K. R., Hobbs, J., Haeny, A. M., & Van Demark, J. (2013). Hybrid cognitive behavioral therapy versus relaxation training for co-occurring anxiety and alcohol disorder: A randomized clinical trial. *Journal of Consulting and Clinical Psychology, 81*(3), 429. https://www.ncbi.nlm.nih.gov/pmc/articles/PMC3756682/pdf/nihms503814.pdf

Lavalley, J., Kastor, S., Tourangeau, M., Goodman, A., Kerr, T., & Western Aboriginal Harm Reduction, S. (2020). You just have to have other models, our DNA is different: The experiences of indigenous people who use illicit drugs and/or alcohol accessing substance use treatment. *Harm Reduction Journal, 17*(1), 19. https://doi.org/10.1186/s12954-020-00366-3

Linehan, M. M. (1993). *Cognitive-behavioral treatment of borderline personality disorder*. Guilford.

Mann, K., Aubin, H. J., & Witkiewitz, K. (2017). Reduced drinking in alcohol dependence treatment, what is the evidence? *European Addiction Research, 23*(5), 219–230. https://doi.org/10.1159/000481348

Marel, C., Siedlecka, E., Fisher, A., Gournay, K., Deady, M., Baker, A., Kay-Lambkin, F., Teesson, M., Baillie, A., & Mills, K. (2022). *Guidelines on the management of co-occurring alcohol and other drug and mental health conditions in alcohol and other drug treatment settings* (3rd ed.). Matilda Centre for Research in Mental Health and Substance Use, The University of Sydney.

Marquenie, L. A., Schadé, A., Van Balkom, A. J. L. M., Koeter, M., Frenken, S., Van Den Brink, W., & Van Dyck, R. (2006). Comorbid phobic disorders do not influence outcome of alcohol dependence treatment. Results of a naturalistic follow-up study. *Alcohol and Alcoholism, 41*(2), 168–173. https://doi.org/10.1093/alcalc/agh252

McEvoy, P. M., & Shand, F. (2008). The effect of comorbid substance use disorders on treatment outcome for anxiety disorders. *Journal of Anxiety Disorders, 22*(6), 1087–1098. https://doi.org/10.1016/j.janxdis.2007.11.007

McEvoy, P. M., Saulsman, L. M., & Rapee, R. M. (2018). *Imagery-enhanced CBT for social anxiety disorder*. The Guilford Press.

McGrath, J. J., Al-Hamzawi, A., Alonso, J., Altwaijri, Y., Andrade, L. H., Bromet, E. J., Bruffaerts, R., de Almeida, J. M. C., Chardoul, S., Chiu, W. T., Degenhardt, L., Demler, O. V., Ferry, F., Gureje, O., Haro, J. M., Karam, E. G., Karam, G., Khaled, S. M., Kovess-Masfety, V., Magno,

M., Medina-Mora, M. E., Moskalewicz, J., Navarro-Mateu, F., Nishi, D., Plana-Ripoll, O., Posada-Villa, J., Rapsey, C., Sampson, N. A., Stagnaro, J. C., Stein, D. J., ten Have, M., Torres, Y., Vladescu, C., Woodruff, P. W., Zarkov, Z., Kessler, R. C., Aguilar-Gaxiola, S., Al-Hamzawi, A., Alonso, J., Altwaijri, Y. A., Andrade, L. H., Atwoli, L., Benjet, C., Bromet, E. J., Bruffaerts, R., Bunting, B., Caldas-de-Almeida, J. M., Cardoso, G., Chardoul, S., Cía, A. H., Degenhardt, L., De Girolamo, G., Gureje, O., Haro, J. M., Harris, M. G., Hinkov, H., Hu, C.-Y., De Jonge, P., Karam, A. N., Karam, E. G., Karam, G., Kazdin, A. E., Kawakami, N., Kessler, R. C., Kiejna, A., Kovess-Masfety, V., McGrath, J. J., Medina-Mora, M. E., Moskalewicz, J., Navarro-Mateu, F., Nishi, D., Piazza, M., Posada-Villa, J., Scott, K. M., Stagnaro, J. C., Stein, D. J., Ten Have, M., Torres, Y., Viana, M. C., Vigo, D. V., Vladescu, C., Williams, D. R., Woodruff, P., Wojtyniak, B., Xavier, M., & Zaslavsky, A. M. (2023). Age of onset and cumulative risk of mental disorders: A cross-national analysis of population surveys from 29 countries. *The Lancet Psychiatry*. https://doi.org/10.1016/S2215-0366(23)00193-1

Miller, W. R. (2004). *Combined behavioral intervention manual: A clinical research guide for therapists treating people with alcohol abuse and dependence*. US Department of Health and Human Services, National Institutes of Health.

Miller, W. R., & Rollnick, S. (2009). Ten things that motivational interviewing is not. *Behavioural and Cognitive Psychotherapy, 37*(2), 129–140. https://doi.org/10.1017/S1352465809005128

Miller, W. R., & Rollnick, S. (2012). *Motivational interviewing: Helping people change* (3rd ed.). Guilford Publications.

Miller, W. R., Zweben, A., DiClemente, C. C., & Rychatrik, R. G. (1992). *Motivational enhancement therapy manual* (Vol. 2). National Institute on Alcohol Abuse and Alcoholism.

Miller, W. R., Forcehimes, A. A., & Zweben, A. (2019). *Treating addiction: A guide for professionals* (2nd ed.). The Guilford Press.

Monti, P. E., Kadden, R. M., Rohsenow, D. J., Abrams, D. B., & Cooney, N. L. (2002). *Treating alcohol dependence: A coping skills training guide* (2nd ed.). Guilford Press.

Morley, K. C., Baillie, A., Leung, S., Sannibale, C., Teesson, M., & Haber, P. S. (2016). Is specialized integrated treatment for comorbid anxiety, depression and alcohol dependence better than treatment as usual in a public hospital setting? *Alcohol and Alcoholism, 51*(4), 402–409. https://doi.org/10.1093/alcalc/agv131

Morley, K., Rombouts, S., Jamshidi, N., & Haber, P. (2021). Pharmacotherapies. In P. S. Haber & B. C. Riordan (Eds.), *Guidelines for the treatment of alcohol problems* (4th ed., pp. 37–68). Specialty of Addiction Medicine, Faculty of Medicine and Health, The University of Sydney.

Morris, E. P., Stewart, S. H., & Ham, L. S. (2005). The relationship between social anxiety disorder and alcohol use disorders: A critical review. *Clinical Psychology Review, 25*(6), 734–760. https://doi.org/10.1016/j.cpr.2005.05.004

Morrison, A. S., & Heimberg, R. G. (2013). Social anxiety and social anxiety disorder. *Annual Review of Clinical Psychology, 9*(1), 249–274. https://doi.org/10.1146/annurev-clinpsy-050212-185631

Moss, A. C., & Albery, I. P. (2009). A dual-process model of the alcohol-behavior link for social drinking. [References]. *Psychological Bulletin, 135*(4), 516–530. https://doi.org/10.1037/a0015991

Muroff, J., & Robinson, W. (2022). Tools of engagement: Practical considerations for utilizing technology-based tools in CBT practice. *Cognitive and Behavioral Practice, 29*(1), 81–96.

Oakland, A., & McChargue, D. (2014). Polysubstance use, social anxiety, and length of treatment for alcohol use disorders. *Journal of Dual Diagnosis, 10*(1), 3–8. https://doi.org/10.1080/15504263.2013.866799

Obert, J. L., McCann, M. J., Marinelli-Casey, P., Weiner, A., Minsky, S., Brethen, P., & Rawson, R. (2000). The matrix model of outpatient stimulant abuse treatment: History and description. *Journal of Psychoactive Drugs, 32*(2), 157–164. https://doi.org/10.1080/02791072.2000.10400224

Piccirillo, M. L., Taylor Dryman, M., & Heimberg, R. G. (2016). Safety behaviors in adults with social anxiety: Review and future directions. *Behavior Therapy, 47*(5), 675–687. https://doi.org/10.1016/j.beth.2015.11.005

Randall, C. L., Thomas, S., & Thevos, A. K. (2001). Concurrent alcoholism and social anxiety disorder: A first step toward developing effective treatments. *Alcoholism, Clinical and Experimental Research, 25*(2), 210–220. https://doi.org/10.1111/j.1530-0277.2001.tb02201.x

Randall, C. L., Book, S. W., Carrigan, M. H., & Thomas, S. (2008). Treatment of co-occurring alcoholism and social anxiety disorder. In S. H. Stewart & P. J. Conrod (Eds.), *Anxiety and substance use disorders: The vicious cycle of comorbidity* (pp. 139–155). Springer Science & Business Media; US.

Rapee, R. M., Gaston, J. E., & Abbott, M. J. (2009). Testing the efficacy of theoretically derived improvements in the treatment of social phobia. *Journal of Consulting and Clinical Psychology, 77*, 317–327.

SAMHSA. (2014). *Results from the 2013 National Survey on Drug Use and Health: Summary of National Findings, NSDUH Series H-48, HHS Publication No. (SMA) 14–4863.* Substance Abuse and Mental Health Services Administration.

Saunders, J. B., Stjepanovic, D., & Connor, J. P. (2021). Screening and assessment. In P. S. Haber & B. C. Riordan (Eds.), *Guidelines for the treatment of alcohol problems* (4th ed., pp. 37–68). Specialty of Addiction Medicine, Faculty of Medicine and Health, The University of Sydney.

Schadé, A., Marquenie, L. A., Van Balkom, A. J., Koeter, M. W., De Beurs, E., Van Den Brink, W., & Van Dyck, R. (2004). Alcohol-dependent patients with comorbid phobic disorders: A comparison between comorbid patients, pure alcohol-dependent and pure phobic patients. *Alcohol & Alcoholism, 39*(3), 241–246. https://doi.org/10.1093/alcalc/agh039

Schadé, A., Marquenie, L. A., van Balkom, A. J. L. M., Koeter, M. W. J., de Beurs, E., van den Brink, W., & van Dyck, R. (2005). The effectiveness of anxiety treatment on alcohol-dependent patients with a comorbid phobic disorder: A randomized controlled trial. *Alcoholism: Clinical and Experimental Research, 29*(5), 794–800. https://doi.org/10.1097/01.ALC.0000163511.24583.33

Schellekens, A., de Jong, C., Buitelaar, J., & Verkes, R. (2015). Co-morbid anxiety disorders predict early relapse after inpatient alcohol treatment. *European Psychiatry, 30*(1), 128–136.

Schneier, F. R., Foose, T. E., Hasin, D. S., Heimberg, R. G., Liu, S. M., Grant, B. F., & Blanco, C. (2010). Social anxiety disorder and alcohol use disorder co-morbidity in the National Epidemiologic Survey on alcohol and related conditions. *Psychological Medicine, 40*(6), 977–988. https://doi.org/10.1017/S0033291709991231

Scott-Sheldon, L. A. J., Terry, D. L., Carey, K. B., Garey, L., & Carey, M. P. (2012). Efficacy of expectancy challenge interventions to reduce college student drinking: A meta-analytic review. *Psychology of Addictive Behaviors, 26*(3), 393–405. https://doi.org/10.1037/a0027565

Sliedrecht, W., de Waart, R., Witkiewitz, K., & Roozen, H. G. (2019). Alcohol use disorder relapse factors: A systematic review. *Psychiatry Research, 278*, 97–115. https://doi.org/10.1016/j.psychres.2019.05.038

Smith, J. P., & Randall, C. L. (2012). Anxiety and alcohol use disorders comorbidity and treatment considerations. *Alcohol Research-Current Reviews, 34*(4), 414–431.

Stapinski, L. A., Rapee, R. M., Sannibale, C., Teesson, M., Haber, P., & Baillie, A. J. (2015). The clinical and theoretical basis for integrated cognitive behavioral treatment of comorbid social anxiety and alcohol use disorders. *Cognitive and Behavioral Practice, 22*(4), 504–521. https://doi.org/10.1016/j.cbpra.2014.05.004

Stapinski, L. A., Prior, K., Newton, N. C., Deady, M., Kelly, E., Lees, B., Teesson, M., & Baillie, A. J. (2019). Protocol for the Inroads Study: A randomized controlled trial of an internet-delivered, cognitive behavioral therapy–based early intervention to reduce anxiety and hazardous alcohol use among young people. *People, 8*(4), e12370.

Stapinski, L., Rapee, R., Haggman, S., Sannibale, C., & Baillie, A. J. (2021a). *Combined cognitive behavioural therapy for social phobia & harmful drinking: Client workbook (revised edition).* Available from: https://osf.io/9zwfn

Stapinski, L., Rapee, R., Haggman, S., Sannibale, C., Winkler, C., & Baillie, A. J. (2021b). *Combined cognitive behavioural therapy for social phobia & harmful drinking: Therapist guide, revised version*. Available from: https://osf.io/76fau

Stapinski, L. A., Prior, K., Newton, N. C., Biswas, R. K., Kelly, E., Deady, M., Lees, B., Teesson, M., & Baillie, A. J. (2021c). Are we making inroads? A randomized controlled trial of a psychologist-supported, web-based, cognitive behavioral therapy intervention to reduce anxiety and hazardous alcohol use among emerging adults. *EClinicalMedicine, 39*(101048). https://doi.org/10.1016/j.eclinm.2021.101048

Stapinski, L. A., Sannibale, C., Subotic, M., Rapee, R. M., Teesson, M., Haber, P. S., & Baillie, A. J. (2021d). Randomised controlled trial of integrated cognitive behavioural treatment and motivational enhancement for comorbid social anxiety and alcohol use disorders. *Australian & New Zealand Journal of Psychiatry, 55*(2), 207–220. https://doi.org/10.1177/0004867420952539

Stein, D. J., Lim, C. C. W., Roest, A. M., de Jonge, P., Aguilar-Gaxiola, S., Al-Hamzawi, A., Alonso, J., Benjet, C., Bromet, E. J., Bruffaerts, R., de Girolamo, G., Florescu, S., Gureje, O., Haro, J. M., Harris, M. G., He, Y., Hinkov, H., Horiguchi, I., Hu, C., Karam, A., Karam, E. G., Lee, S., Lepine, J. P., Navarro-Mateu, F., Pennell, B. E., Piazza, M., Posada-Villa, J., Ten Have, M., Torres, Y., Viana, M. C., Wojtyniak, B., Xavier, M., Kessler, R. C., & Scott, K. M. (2017). The cross-national epidemiology of social anxiety disorder: Data from the World Mental Health Survey Initiative. *BMC Medicine, 15*(1), 143. https://doi.org/10.1186/s12916-017-0889-2

Stewart, S. H., & Conrod, P. J. (2008). Anxiety disorder and substance use disorder co-morbidity: Common themes and future directions. In S. H. Stewart & P. J. Conrod (Eds.), *Anxiety and substance use disorders: The vicious cycle of comorbidity* (pp. 239–257). Springer. https://doi.org/10.1007/978-0-387-74290-8_13

Stewart, S. H., Grant, V. V., Mackie, C. J., & Conrod, P. J. (2016). Comorbidity of anxiety and depression with substance use disorders. In K. J. Sher (Ed.), *The Oxford handbook of substance use and substance use disorders* (Vol. 2, pp. 149–186). Oxford University Press.

Subotic-Kerry, M., Baillie, A. J., Stapinski, L. A., Abbott, M. J., MacDonald, J., Gaston, J. E., & Rapee, R. M. (2021). The impact of alcohol use disorders and alcohol consumption on treatment-seeking individuals with social anxiety disorder. *Bulletin of the Menninger Clinic, 85*(2), 100–122. https://doi.org/10.1521/bumc.2021.85.2.100

Sullivan, J., Sykora, K., Schneiderman, J., Naranjo, C., & Sellers, E. (1989). Assessment of alcohol withdrawal: The revised clinical institute withdrawal assessment for alcohol scale (CIWA-Ar). *British Journal of Addiction, 84*, 1353–1357. https://doi.org/10.1111/j.1360-0443.1989.tb00737.x

Teo, A. R., Lerrigo, R., & Rogers, M. A. M. (2013). The role of social isolation in social anxiety disorder: A systematic review and meta-analysis. *Journal of Anxiety Disorders, 27*(4), 353–364. https://doi.org/10.1016/j.janxdis.2013.03.010

Terra, M. B., Barros, H. M., Stein, A. T., Figueira, I., Athayde, L. D., Spanemberg, L., de Aguiar Possa, M., Filho, L. D., & da Silveira, D. X. (2006a). Does co-occurring social phobia interfere with alcoholism treatment adherence and relapse? *Journal of Substance Abuse Treatment, 31*(4), 403–409. https://doi.org/10.1016/j.jsat.2006.05.013

Terra, M. B., Barros, H. M., Stein, A. T., Figueira, I., Jorge, M. R., Palermo, L. H., Athayde, L. D., Goncalves, M. S., Spanemberg, L., Possa, M. A., Daruy Filho, L., & Da Silveira, D. X. (2006b). Social anxiety disorder in 300 patients hospitalized for alcoholism in Brazil: High prevalence and undertreatment. *Comprehensive Psychiatry, 47*(6), 463–467. https://doi.org/10.1016/j.comppsych.2006.02.004

Thevos, A. K., Thomas, S. E., & Randall, C. L. (1999). Baseline differences in social support among treatment-seeking alcoholics with and without social phobia. *Substance Abuse, 20*(2), 107–118. https://doi.org/10.1080/08897079909511399

Thomas, S. E., Thevos, A. K., & Randall, C. L. (1999). Alcoholics with and without social phobia: A comparison of substance use and psychiatric variables. *Journal of Studies on Alcohol, 60*(4), 472–479.

Tonigan, J. S., Book, S. W., Pagano, M. E., Randall, P. K., Smith, J. P., & Randall, C. L. (2010). 12-Step therapy and women with and without social phobia: A study of the effectiveness of 12-Step therapy to facilitate AA engagement. *Alcoholism Treatment Quarterly, 28*(2), 151–162. https://doi.org/10.1080/07347321003648596

Tran, G. Q., & Haaga, D. A. F. (2002). Coping responses and alcohol outcome expectancies in alcohol abusing and nonabusing social phobics. *Cognitive Therapy and Research, 26*(1), 1–17. https://doi.org/10.1023/A:1013803803192

Volkow, N. D., Torrens, M., Poznyak, V., Sáenz, E., Busse, A., Kashino, W., Krupchanka, D., Kestel, D., Campello, G., & Gerra, G. (2020). Managing dual disorders: A statement by the informal scientific network, UN Commission on narcotic drugs. *World Psychiatry, 19*(3), 396–397. https://doi.org/10.1002/wps.20796

Wells, A. (2011). *Metacognitive therapy for anxiety and depression*. Guilford press.

Westra, H. A., & Dozois, D. J. A. (2008). Integrating motivational interviewing in the treatment of anxiety. In H. Arkowitz, H. A. Westra, W. R. Miller, & S. Rollnick (Eds.), *Motivational interviewing in the treatment of psychological problems* (pp. 26–56). Guilford.

Witkiewitz, K., & Marlatt, G. A. (2004). Relapse prevention for alcohol and drug problems: That was Zen, this is Tao. *American Psychologist, 59*(4), 224–35. https://doi.org/10.1037/0003-066X.59.4.224.

Wolitzky-Taylor, K., Brown, L. A., Roy-Byrne, P., Sherbourne, C., Stein, M. B., Sullivan, G., Bystritsky, A., & Craske, M. G. (2015). The impact of alcohol use severity on anxiety treatment outcomes in a large effectiveness trial in primary care. *Journal of Anxiety Disorders, 30*, 88–93. https://doi.org/10.1016/j.janxdis.2014.12.011

Wolitzky-Taylor, K., Sewart, A., Karno, M., Ries, R., & Stimson, J. (2022). Development and initial pilot testing of a fully integrated treatment for comorbid social anxiety disorder and alcohol use disorder in a community-based SUD clinic setting. *Behaviour Research and Therapy, 148*, 103999. https://doi.org/10.1016/j.brat.2021.103999

Wong, Q. J. J., & Rapee, R. M. (2016). The aetiology and maintenance of social anxiety disorder: A synthesis of complementary theoretical models and formulation of a new integrated model. *Journal of Affective Disorders, 203*, 84–100. https://doi.org/10.1016/j.jad.2016.05.069

Yoshimi, N. T., Campos, L. M., Simão, M. O., Torresan, R. C., & Torres, A. R. (2016). Social anxiety symptoms in alcohol-dependent outpatients: Prevalence, severity and predictors. *Jornal Brasileiro de Psiquiatria, 65*(2), 117–126. https://doi.org/10.1590/0047-2085000000112

Chapter 3
Cognitive Behavioral Therapy for Comorbid Cannabis Use Disorder and Emotional Disorders

Julia D. Buckner, Paige E. Morris, Caroline R. Scherzer, Anthony H. Ecker, and Jennifer S. Beighley

Rates of cannabis use and related problems are at an all-time high. To illustrate, nearly half (42.6%) of young adults have used cannabis in the past year and over one-fourth (28.5%) have used in the past month (National Institute on Drug Abuse, 2022). Further, rates of daily use continue to increase (National Institute on Drug Abuse, 2022). Corresponding to the increase in cannabis use rates, rates of cannabis use disorder (CUD) are also increasing. To illustrate, epidemiological data estimate that 16.3 million Americans met diagnostic criteria for a current CUD in 2021, and rates of CUD are over three times that of opioid use disorder and are greater than the rates of cocaine, methamphetamine, stimulant, and opioid use disorders combined (Substance Abuse and Mental Health Services Administration, 2021). As rates of CUD continue to rise, there is an increased demand for CUD treatment, with an increasing proportion of substance use disorder (SUD) treatment being provided for patients with CUD (United Nations Office on Drugs and Crime, 2020).

J. D. Buckner (✉) · P. E. Morris · C. R. Scherzer
Department of Psychology, Louisiana State University, Baton Rouge, LA, USA
e-mail: jbuckner@lsu.edu

A. H. Ecker
Houston Center for Innovations in Qualify, Effectiveness and Safety, Michael E. DeBakey VA Medical Center, Houston, TX, USA

South Central Mental Illness Research, Education and Clinical Center, Menninger Department of Psychiatry and Behavioral Sciences, Baylor College of Medicine, Houston, TX, USA

J. S. Beighley
Providence Boyden Family Autism Center, Providence Regional Medical Center, Everett, WA, USA

K. Wolitzky-Taylor (ed.), *Treating Comorbid Substance Use and Emotional Disorders*, CBT: Science Into Practice, https://doi.org/10.1007/978-3-031-62971-6_3

Comorbidity of CUD with Emotional Disorders

Accumulating data indicate that CUD is related to especially high rates of emotional disorders (ED), such as anxiety and depressive disorders and their symptoms. In fact, nearly 50% of individuals with CUD meet criteria for a comorbid anxiety disorder (Guillem et al., 2015). Further, anxiety is related to more cannabis problems and perceived barriers to quitting (e.g., Schmidt et al., 2007; Zvolensky et al., 2018). These high rates are evident across specific types of anxiety—for example, individuals with CUD are three times more likely to meet criteria for comorbid generalized anxiety disorder (GAD) than individuals without CUD (Onaemo et al., 2021). Depressive disorders are also highly prevalent among individuals with CUD compared to the general population (8.4%; Substance Abuse and Mental Health Services Administration, 2021), ranging from 18.25% to 32.4% for major depressive disorder (MDD) in epidemiological samples (Arias et al., 2013; Lai & Sitharthan, 2012; Teesson et al., 2012; Wu et al., 2017) and up to 66.6% among high-risk samples such as U.S. veterans with CUD (Ecker et al., 2020). Notably, the increase in rates of cannabis use in the U.S.A. from 2005 to 2017 was greater among individuals with (10.19% in 2005 vs. 18.84% in 2017) versus without (5.65% in 2005 vs. 8.67% in 2017) depression (Pacek et al., 2020).

Theories of Etiology/Maintenance of Comorbidity

Consistent with affect regulation models of substance use (Baker et al., 2004), individuals with emotional disorders or sub-clinically elevated emotional disorders symptoms may use cannabis to manage subjective and/or physiological symptoms associated with chronically elevated negative affect. In support of this conceptualization, social anxiety is related to more cannabis problems and coping (to decrease negative affect generally) and social anxiety (to manage negative affect in social situations) cannabis use motives; and the relation between social anxiety and cannabis problems occurs indirectly via these coping motives (Morris & Buckner, 2023). Relatedly, greater social anxiety was related to more cannabis problems indirectly via the singular effect of use to decrease negative affect in social situations and the sequential effects of use to decrease negative affect in social situations and more frequent cannabis use (Walukevich-Dienst et al., 2020). Similarly, the positive association between depressive symptoms and cannabis use, use-related problems, and CUD symptoms occurs via the indirect effect of coping motives (Livingston et al., 2023). Notably, recent data from a nationally representative sample indicate that the perceived risk of cannabis use is lower and decreased more rapidly from 2005 to 2017 among individuals with depression compared to those without depression (Pacek et al., 2020).

Temporal Relations

There is some variability in the temporal sequencing of CUD with emotional disorders. Consistent with self-medication (Khantzian, 1997) and affect regulation models (Baker et al., 2004), some types of emotional disorders appear to be risk factors for CUD. Social anxiety is one such type of emotional disorder. To illustrate, social anxiety is associated with an increased risk of transitioning from cannabis use to CUD (e.g., Marel et al., 2019) and SAD in adolescence predicted greater rates of CUD by age 30 (Buckner et al., 2008). Further, although some individuals report that their SAD onset after their CUD, over 80% indicate that SAD onset occurred prior to onset of CUD (Buckner et al., 2012b). Similarly, cross-sectional and epidemiological data indicate that a diagnosis of panic disorder (PD), but not GAD, appears to be a risk factor for the onset of cannabis use initiation (Feingold et al., 2016). It is also unclear whether using cannabis actually decreases state anxiety. Data collected using ecological momentary assessment (also known as experiential sampling) suggests that although anxiety was somewhat higher prior to cannabis use, cannabis use did not significantly decrease state anxiety (Buckner et al., 2012a).

However, some data indicate that some types of anxiety may be the result of cannabis use. To illustrate, cannabis use and CUD may predict the development of GAD and GAD symptoms (e.g., Kedzior & Laeber, 2014; Onaemo et al., 2021); however, this relation is not maintained in studies after controlling for confound variables such as education and other illicit drug use (Danielsson et al., 2016). In sum, it appears that panic and social anxiety may predict subsequent cannabis use and related problems, but that cannabis use may increase risk of generalized anxiety.

The relationship between depressive disorders and cannabis use is complex and existing evidence on the directionality of the association is mixed. Some studies suggest that cannabis use, particularly during adolescence, leads to the development of depression; however, other studies suggest that depression serves as a risk factor for initiating or increasing cannabis use frequency (for review see Feingold & Weinstein, 2021). To illustrate, cross-sectional data indicate that although the acute effects of cannabis may include a temporary reduction in perceived depressive symptoms (Cuttler et al., 2018) and data from ecological momentary assessment indicates that cannabis use results in subsequent decreases in negative affect generally (Buckner et al., 2015). Yet, longitudinal studies suggest that initiation of cannabis use during adolescence (specifically before age 18) and continued regular cannabis use may contribute to the maintenance and/or worsening of depressive symptoms over time (Gobbi et al., 2019).

In sum, the relationships between emotional disorders and their symptoms and cannabis use/CUD may be complex, with state anxiety predicting cannabis use and some types of anxiety (e.g., social anxiety) serving as a risk factor for continuing to use cannabis despite cannabis-related problems. On other hand, some types of emotional disorder conditions (e.g., depression, GAD) may develop as a result of chronic cannabis use. These differential relations may play important roles in treatment of comorbid emotional disorders and CUD in some patients use cannabis to manage pre-existing emotional disorder conditions whereas other patients may experience emotional disorder symptoms as a negative consequence of their cannabis misuse.

Public Health Significance of the Comorbidity

The co-occurrence of CUD with emotional disorders (as well as the co-occurrence of subclinical symptoms) is associated with greater impairment than either condition alone. To illustrate, epidemiological data indicate that individuals with comorbid CUD-SAD report worse physical health and more psychiatric comorbidity than those with CUD without SAD or SAD without CUD (Buckner et al., 2012b). Further, comorbid CUD-SAD was related to greater use of other illicit drugs and more functional impairment (e.g., less likely to graduate from high school or be married) than those with CUD without SAD. Similarly, compared to those with SAD without CUD, those with CUD-SAD reported more avoidance of social situations. Notably, individuals with comorbid anxiety disorders and CUD engaged in CUD treatment report greater cannabis withdrawal severity and less efficacy to refrain from using cannabis in emotionally distressing situations (Buckner et al., 2017a). Among patients presenting for CUD treatment, anxiety was positively significantly related to more severe CUD, more cannabis-related problems, and greater number of cannabis joints smoked per day (Buckner & Carroll, 2010).

Similarly, both elevated subclinical depression (e.g., Crane et al., 2015; Horwood et al., 2012; Troup et al., 2016) and MDD (e.g., Fairman & Anthony, 2012; Gage et al., 2015) are related to greater cannabis use, including heavy use (e.g., Rasic et al., 2013) and cannabis dependence (Dierker et al., 2018; Mathews et al., 2011). Moreover, longitudinal data indicate that reductions in cannabis use are associated with improvements in depression symptoms over time (Hser et al., 2017). Compared to individuals with MDD that do not use cannabis, those with MDD that use cannabis have greater negative symptoms (Bersani et al., 2016) and greater symptom severity (Bahorik et al., 2013). The detrimental impact of cannabis use on emotional disorder symptoms such as depression has been identified as a primary reason for treatment seeking among individuals with CUD (van der Pol et al., 2013) and MDD increases risk of relapse among individuals with CUD in remission (Flórez-Salamanca et al., 2013).

Impact of Emotional Disorders on CBT for CUD and the Impact of Cannabis Use on CBT for Emotional Disorders

Patients with emotional disorder or elevated emotional disorder symptoms evince worse CUD treatment outcomes. To illustrate, female patients with elevated baseline anxiety report more cannabis use and related problems following treatment

(Buckner & Carroll, 2010). Greater anxiety at discharge was related to greater risk of cannabis relapse on year later (Bonn-Miller & Moos, 2009). Further, frequent cannabis use (using at least twice per week) was related to worse anxiety-related outcomes following cognitive behavioral therapy (CBT) for anxiety disorders (Ouellette et al., 2022).

Notably, MET-CBT for CUD was associated with less anxiety at follow-up compared to MET for CUD alone and reductions in anxiety during the course of treatment among patients in both the MET-CBT and MET alone conditions were related to better cannabis-related outcomes (less cannabis use, fewer cannabis-related problems) at 9-month follow-up, whereas reduction in cannabis use did not predict subsequent anxiety (Buckner & Carroll, 2010). These data suggest that targeting anxiety in the context of MET-CBT for CUD may improve treatment outcomes and this may be especially the case among patients with elevated anxiety symptoms.

The co-occurrence of depression and depressive disorders with CUD also appears related to poorer CUD and depression treatment outcomes. Regarding depression treatment, contrary to notions that cannabis can be used to self-medicate depressive symptoms, accumulating evidence indicates that cannabis use has deleterious effects on the course and treatment of depression. For example, recent meta-analytic data indicates that cannabis use is associated with poorer course, symptoms, and functioning for major depressive disorder (Tourjman et al., 2023). Further, among individuals receiving outpatient treatment for depression, patients that used cannabis at baseline had greater suicidal ideation, less improvement in depressive symptoms, less treatment utilization, worse mental health functioning, and greater suicidal ideation at 12-month follow-up compared to those without baseline cannabis use (Bahorik et al., 2018). Further, frequent (at least monthly) cannabis use among clinical samples has been linked to decreased efficacy of pharmacological treatment of depression (Bricker et al., 2007). Regarding CUD treatment, among individuals receiving pharmacological treatment for CUD plus abstinence-based contingency management, greater baseline depressive symptoms were related to decreased likelihood of cannabis abstinence during treatment (Tomko et al., 2020). Further, at 4, 8, and 12 weeks into treatment, depressive symptoms were related to greater cannabis use quantities concurrently (i.e., at each time point) and subsequently (i.e., depression related to greater cannabis use quantities at the next time point), suggesting that depression is associated with worse CUD outcomes. Similarly, depressive symptoms moderated outcomes for a text message-based treatment for CUD, such that patients with clinically elevated depression had greater cannabis use post-treatment compared to those with less depression (Mason, 2020).

CBT for CUD and Emotional Disorders

In response to calls for the development of personalized treatments for dually diagnosed patients that treat anxiety and substance use disorders in an integrated fashion that addresses the reciprocal nature of these disorders (e.g., Stewart & Conrod,

2008), we developed an integrated cannabis and anxiety reduction treatment (ICART) to simultaneously treat comorbid anxiety and cannabis use disorders in an integrated manner (Buckner et al., 2016a, 2014). ICART integrates an MET-CBT for CUD (Steinberg et al., 2005) with a transdiagnostic CBT that addresses *false safety behaviors*, or behaviors that help one avoid or alleviate false threats (i.e., phobic stimuli) (Schmidt et al., 2012). False safety behaviors are commonly used among individuals with a variety of across anxiety disorders because these behaviors may temporarily alleviate anxiety (e.g., by avoiding a phobic stimulus); however, research indicates that repeated use of these behaviors can contribute to the maintenance of anxiety disorders (Salkovskis et al., 1991). Thus, a transdiagnostic CBT, False Safety behavior Elimination Therapy (FSET), was developed to identify and eliminate use of false safety behaviors, resulting in decreased anxiety and depression and improve quality of life (e.g., Riccardi et al., 2017; Schmidt et al., 2012).

During ICART, we conceptualize at least some cannabis use as a false safety behavior that can be used to temporarily alleviate anxiety (i.e., coping motivated cannabis use; e.g., Schmidt et al., 2007) but that can maintain or even exacerbate anxiety in the long-term. We designed ICART using a translational approach based on data indicating that the majority of individuals who use cannabis (regardless of level of anxiety) report using cannabis to cope with negative affect (Buckner et al., 2015, 2016b) and that non-cannabis-related false safety behaviors and use of these behaviors is robustly related to more frequent cannabis use and as well as more cannabis-related problems (Buckner et al., 2018, 2017b). Further, false safety behaviors mediated the relation between anxiety severity and cannabis problems (Buckner et al., 2017b). Thus, ICART was designed to target both cannabis use as a false safety behavior and the use of non-cannabis-related false safety behaviors that may maintain anxiety and cannabis use, while teaching CBT skills to help manage high-risk cannabis use situations (regardless of whether cannabis is used for anxiety management) and using MET techniques to attend to motivation to change cannabis use.

In a pilot randomized controlled trial, patients in the ICART condition attended significantly more treatment sessions than those in the MET-CBT for CUD only condition and ICART produced decreases in cannabis-related problems; in fact, patients in the ICART condition were more likely to be abstinent post-treatment than those in MET-CBT (Buckner et al., 2019). Baseline severity of cannabis use and use-related problems moderated the relation between condition and post-treatment outcomes, such that among patients with the greatest baseline cannabis use, ICART was associated with less post-treatment cannabis use than MET-CBT alone (Buckner et al., 2021). Similarly, among those with the greatest number of cannabis-related problems, patients in the ICART condition reported fewer post-treatment problems than those in the MET-CBT alone condition.

Table 3.1 outlines the MET-CBT for CUD and FSET skills taught in each of the 12 sessions of ICART. Additionally, motivational interviewing (MI) skills are incorporated throughout the treatment when necessary, especially to explore and resolve ambivalence about substance use and treatment adherence. ICART skills have also

Table 3.1 Integrated cannabis and anxiety reduction treatment (ICART) session topics

Session #	Session topic
1	Psychoeducation regarding anxiety disorders & CUD Psychoeducation regarding the reciprocal relation between anxiety & cannabis Reasons for quitting Personalized feedback report Change plan Barriers to quitting
2	Psychoeducation regarding types of anxiety Psychoeducation regarding the emotional processing model of anxiety & how it relates to cannabis use New cannabis coping strategies
3	Psychoeducation regarding false safety behaviors & strategies to eliminate them
4	Cannabis & other substance use as false safety behaviors Function analysis of cannabis use Cannabis coping strategies
5	Antiphobic attitude Coping with cannabis cravings (including urge surfing)
6	Other false safety behaviors (checking, reassurance seeking, companions, avoidance of bodily sensations) Managing thoughts related to cannabis use
7	Avoidance as a false safety behavior Managing negative moods & depression as triggers for cannabis Increasing pleasant activities
8	Other false safety behaviors (cognitive avoidance, idiosyncratic behaviors) Seemingly irrelevant decisions
9	Problem-solving
10	Cannabis refusal skills Assertiveness training
11	Planning for emergencies & coping with a lapse
12	Prevention of relapse of anxiety disorders and CUD

Note. Topics were adapted from MET-CBT for CUD (Steinberg et al., 2005) and False Safety Behavior Elimination Therapy (Schmidt et al., 2012). Motivational interviewing techniques (Miller & Rollnick, 2013) were used to explore and resolve ambivalence about changing cannabis use and to address motivation to change cannabis use throughout treatment as clinically appropriate

been described in prior work (Buckner et al., 2016a) and are presented here to provide illustrative examples of how to apply these skills with patients with comorbid CUD and anxiety disorders. Sessions 1 and 2 include the MET technique of provision of personalized feedback related to the patient's cannabis use to explore and resolve ambivalence about quitting or reducing cannabis and to strengthen commitment to change problematic cannabis use. Diagnostic feedback and psychoeducation on the relationships between CUD and anxiety disorders are also included in the initial sessions. Psychoeducation includes describing the prevalence of the comorbidity of anxiety disorders and CUD as well as a discussion of the mutual maintenance model of anxiety and substance misuse (e.g., Stewart & Conrod, 2008), highlighting that coping motivated cannabis use increases reliance on cannabis, which in turn can exacerbate anxiety symptoms, to provide rationale for fading cannabis use as a false safety behavior to help patients better manage anxiety and meet their cannabis-related goals of reduction or abstinence.

In the remaining sessions, aspects of both MET-CBT for CUD and FSET for anxiety disorders are presented each week to facilitate integrated, simultaneous attention to patients' dual goals of managing anxiety and changing cannabis use, given that patients' anxiety and cannabis use are often related—for example, exposure to anxiety-provoking situations may increase craving to use cannabis to cope with increased anxiety symptoms, decreased cannabis use may result in increased anxiety as a symptom of withdrawal. Specifically, Session 3 introduces the notion of false safety behaviors as strategies patients use in an attempt to reduce their anxiety but that these behaviors actually maintain and possibly exacerbate their anxiety long-term. Patients are also taught FSET techniques to begin to eliminate false safety behaviors, including delaying use, decreasing degree of use, and decreasing frequency of false safety behaviors. One of our patients (who was diagnosed with CUD and SAD) identified several false safety behaviors in which she engaged, including avoiding eye contact with others and using her phone as a distraction when in public places. The therapist explained how engaging in such false safety behaviors maintains her anxiety disorder, and that by gradually decreasing the use of these behaviors, the patient would begin to change the associations between feared stimuli and the anxiety response. The patient agreed to fade these false safety behaviors for homework. To discourage the use of cannabis as a false safety behavior to replace the behaviors the patient agreed to fade, the therapist worked with the patient to identify identified alternative coping strategies the patient could use instead of using cannabis, including exercise and engaging in distracting activities (e.g., reading).

Session 4 focuses on substance use (including cannabis use) as a false safety behavior. To further examine the relationship of patients' cannabis use to their anxiety, Session 4 also includes functional analysis of cannabis use to begin to identify triggers of cannabis use, thoughts related to use, and consequences of use. Conceptualizing cannabis use as a false safety behavior allows for integration of the key FSET anxiety treatment components (e.g., exposure to feared stimuli when not under influence) and CBT for CUD treatment components (i.e., understanding triggers, related thoughts/feelings, and consequences of cannabis use) in one integrated session. A major goal of this session is helping patients understand their particular cannabis use patterns, both coping and non-coping motivated use, as not all cannabis use will be for anxiety management. For example, a patient with comorbid CUD-SAD-GAD reported that she learned that she used cannabis to manage anxiety approximately half the time and the other half was because she wanted to rather than for anxiety or other negative affect management. She stated that in the past week, she used cannabis when friends offered to her because she found it to be enjoyable to use cannabis with her friends. The therapist used the functional analysis to identify pros and cons of using with friends and assessed whether this was cannabis use the patient wanted to reduce. The patient stated that she would like to reduce use with her friends, so she and the therapist identified alternative ways to spend time with friends that did not include cannabis use (e.g., go to a movie theater or meet at a restaurant, places where cannabis cannot be used).

In Session 5, antiphobic exercises are introduced. These are activities that intentionally bring about an anxiety-provoking situation. In the case of fear of negative evaluation (a hallmark feature of social anxiety), antiphobic exercises may include intentionally wearing non-matching clothes or earrings, or intentionally misspeaking or calling someone by the wrong name—behaviors that could elicit negative evaluation from others. Given that increased anxiety as a result of engaging in antiphobic exercises can be a trigger for cannabis use, alternative strategies for coping with cannabis craving (e.g., *urge surfing*, *delaying decisions to use*, *using self-talk*) from the MET-CBT for CUD manual (Steinberg et al., 2005) are also presented in this session to help patients mange increases in urges to use cannabis that may accompany increases in anxiety. When she returned for therapy during Session 6, our patient with CUD-SAD reported that she found self-talk (e.g., reviewing reasons for quitting, reviewing positive consequences of abstinence, reviewing negative consequences of use) especially helpful in managing the increased anxiety she experienced from doing her antiphobic exercise, as well as cravings she experienced in response to non-anxiety triggers, such as being around other people when they were using cannabis and during the time of day she typically used cannabis prior to quitting. Our patient with CUD-SAD-GAD was more reluctant to begin antiphobic exercise, so she initially made small antiphobic gestures (e.g., wearing suspenders rather than a belt to increase the likelihood that others may notice her), and she engaged in more challenging antiphobic behaviors over the next few weeks—for example, she went to a store while wearing clothes with stains on them, without her hair done, and without shaving her legs.

Sessions 6 through 8 include discussions of specific categories of false safety behaviors (e.g., situational avoidance, cognitive avoidance) that are integrated with discussions of CBT skills for reducing cannabis use to provide the patient with coping strategies other than cannabis use to cope with increased anxiety experienced during fading of additional false safety behaviors. To illustrate, during Session 6, the CBT for CUD skill *challenging thoughts about cannabis use*, is presented after discussing fading the false safety behaviors, given that patients may experience thoughts about using cannabis to cope with increased anxiety as response to fading and eliminating these safety behaviors. Our patient with CUD-SAD reported that although she was initially reluctant to fade her false safety behaviors, after several weeks of having done so, she found that situations she would normally avoid (e.g., making eye contact with strangers, social interactions with coworkers) were not as threatening as she believed they were. In other words, she learned that eliminating her false safety behaviors allowed her the opportunity to learn that her feared situations were not actually threatening, which reduced her anxiety in these situations. Our patient with CUD-SAD-GAD reported that engaging in antiphobic activities combined with fading false safety behaviors (e.g., only going in public with her partner present) resulted in her feeling very proud of herself. Session 7 consisted of skills to manage negative moods including depression, which was a strong, recurring trigger for cannabis use for our patient with CUD-SAD-GAD. Although the patient did not meet criteria for a depressive disorder, she reported that she struggled with feelings of sadness related to a family member's death several years prior. She reported that she found it very helpful to challenge maladaptive depression-inducing automatic thoughts as an alternative to using cannabis to cope with negative moods.

Sessions 9 through 11 are dedicated to continued identification and fading of false safety behaviors and engaging in antiphobic exercises. Decreases in social avoidance could result in risk for cannabis use for a variety of reasons including increased anxiety in previously avoided situations along with greater exposure to cannabis-using other people. Thus, to help patients manage new challenges that accompany engagement in more and/or novel social interactions, the CBT for CUD skill of *problem-solving* training is introduced in Session 9. Our patient with CUD-SAD-GAD wanted to address her family relationships within the framework of problem-solving. Problem-solving steps were introduced and included recognition of a problem, elaboration of the problem, consideration of multiple options followed by selection of the most promising approach, and implementation and evaluation of effectiveness. Our patient had a greater deal of difficulty coming up with possible options given the strong negative emotions the patient experienced when thinking about her family relationships. However, she stuck with it and with the therapist's help, came up with a plan for managing her family relationships. Following the session, the patient reported improved perceptions of her family relationships as a result.

In Session 10, the CBT for CUD skills of *refusal skills* and *assertiveness* are introduced given that at this point in treatment, patients are ideally engaging in less social avoidance and may potentially be experiencing social pressure to use cannabis. Patients have also ideally learned to manage their anxiety to the point that they are able to practice refusal and assertiveness skills by Session 10.

In Session 11, *planning for emergencies and cannabis use lapse* is introduced to prepare patients for termination and to help generalization of cannabis reduction techniques to new, anticipated situations. Session 12 focuses on relapse prevention for both anxiety and cannabis use disorders. High-risk situations are identified and discussed as opportunities for each patient to become their own therapist, implement problem-solving techniques, and cope with high-risk situations related to anxiety/depression and cannabis use. Our patient with CUD-SAD-GAD reported feeling confident to challenge thoughts related to use and negative emotions as well as problem-solving during her high-risk cannabis use situations.

In sum, targeting CUD and pathological anxiety in an integrated manner shows promising for reducing cannabis use, use-related problems, anxiety, and depression. Our conversations with our patients highlight that although a good deal of cannabis use occurred in an attempt to manage negative affect (i.e., cannabis use as a false safety behavior), not all of it did and thus it is important to assess for non-coping motivated cannabis use to teach patients skills such as refusal skills, avoiding triggers, self-talk, and distraction to managing those other high-risk situations.

Case Example

Here we present a case of a patient from our clinic to illustrate the use of ICART to treat comorbid CUD and anxiety disorders. This patient was a 30-something-year-old Black woman who presented for the treatment of and a desire to quit using cannabis, which she reported she used primarily to manage her anxiety. She stated that she was seeking treatment for SAD because she experienced clinically elevated social anxiety in most social situations that was interfering with several domains of her life—for example, she wanted to finish college and make more friends, but she avoided these things due to fears others would negatively judge her. She reported that she was highly motivated to quit using cannabis because she wanted to set a better example for her children and she wanted to change jobs and be able to pass a drug test if one was required. The patient had over 10 years of pharmacotherapy for anxiety that she discontinued several years prior because she believed that the medications did not improve her symptoms.

This patient completed 12 sessions of ICART. As described above, Session 1 included diagnostic feedback and psychoeducation on the relationships between CUD and anxiety disorders. The following clinical exchange from Session 1 demonstrates the patient's realization of the link between her cannabis use and anxiety:

Therapist	"What situations are you concerned are going to be most difficult for to not use cannabis?"
Patient	"It's more like I worry just going through these things. Just coming here and talking about my anxiety, just having to deal with stuff like that, and I'm just turning to that [cannabis use] every time, like, I get an inkling about anything or just going into restaurants or, you know, stuff like that, I feel nervous and then I start thinking about smoking. It's just like a vicious cycle."
Therapist	"So, this information is making you realize..."
Patient	"How big of a problem it is! How hard I deal with everything. How much it [cannabis use] makes things worse. Yeah, it's definitely a hard slap in the face. And, you know, I don't know how to deal with these feelings without smoking. That makes me very nervous and anxious in itself."

The patient then stated that her main reasons for using cannabis were to stop worrying, help her relax, and to cope with stress, including stress related to social fears. The patient agreed that she used cannabis to decrease her anxiety but that it actually made her anxiety worse, per the mutual maintenance model of anxiety.

Session 3 introduced the notion of false safety behaviors. The patient identified safety behaviors in which she engaged, including only going in public if her spouse was with her. The therapist explained how engaging in such false safety behaviors maintains anxiety disorders, and that by gradually decreasing their use, she would begin to change the associations between feared stimuli and her anxiety response. The patient began to fade these false safety behaviors for homework. The below exchange occurred at the beginning of the next session when discussing homework on fading the use of companions when shopping as a false safety behavior:

Patient "I went to the mall and tried on clothes by myself."
Therapist "Awesome!"
Patient "I didn't enjoy it, though."
Therapist "That's ok. Remember you're doing this to face your fears and learn that you can go to the mall without your spouse and that over time you'll learn that going to the mall by yourself is a 'false threat' and that there is nothing actually threatening about being in the mall without your spouse."
Patient "The lady was extremely nice, and she helped me pick out some things. But I didn't feel comfortable purchasing anything without getting my spouse's opinion."
Therapist "You did it! You went in and did it! So, buying something by yourself is the next step."
Patient "Yep! I feel like I came a good way this week! … I feel like I'm doing well with not using [cannabis] to cope."

Session 4 focused on substance use as a false safety behavior. Session 4 integrated functional analysis of cannabis use with discussions of cannabis use as a false safety behavior, facilitating the patient's understanding of her particular cannabis use patterns (both coping and non-coping motivated use) as well as positive/negative consequences of using cannabis.

In Session 5, the patient's cannabis use had reduced from daily use to two occasions in the past week. The following exchange reflects her first steps reducing cannabis use as a false safety behavior:

Patient "As far as smoking marijuana, I did have my day to stop, and I have smoked but it's not the same. Any other time I would use it like a crutch, like, 'Oh my son's getting into trouble, let me smoke,' but it hasn't been like that. It did work out that I smoked when I looked at all the things I had to do, but I felt bad about it. I didn't have to do it. I thought, 'I don't have to be high to get this done.'"
Therapist "Wow!"
Patient "I felt like, wow, you have to be high to handle this? I felt stupid, like, ugh, I used to ride around and smoke in my car, but now that feels stupid. I was like, 'you've been doing good all these days, why mess that up?'"
Therapist "Sounds like you've been able to go a few days without smoking."
Patient "Yeah, I used to smoke every day, but now when I think about that paper I signed [referring to Cannabis Change Plan] I think about that date [cannabis quit day], I said I was going to stop. I don't know, I've just really been waking up to some stuff lately."

The patient went on to describe that in addition to fading cannabis use as a false safety behavior, she reduced her cannabis use by avoiding cannabis cues (e.g., paraphernalia) and using alternative coping strategies when she wanted to use (e.g., reading a book).

Also in Session 5, antiphobic exercises were introduced, and the patient gave several examples antiphobic exercises she could do (e.g., seeking out conversations with her superiors at work). To help her cope with increases in cannabis craving that may occur as a result of antiphobic exercises, the CBT for CUD skill of *coping with craving* was presented during this session. Skills the patient chose to use to help her cope with craving included using distractions and using self-talk (e.g., reviewing reasons for quitting, reviewing positive consequences of abstinence, reviewing negative consequences of use).

In Session 10, our patient reported that she had completely stopped using cannabis as a false safety behavior, nearly eliminating her cannabis use. She reported several additional improvements related to SAD symptoms, such as applying for a new job. Yet, she continued to use cannabis for reasons unrelated to her anxiety and thus had not yet met her goal of abstinence from cannabis. She was therefore eager to try these additional MET-CBT skills to help manage her remaining cannabis use and meet her goals. The following exchange from Session 10 illustrates how CBT for CUD skills were integrated into the FSET treatment and reflects this patient's decrease in cannabis use to cope with her SAD symptoms:

Therapist	"What situations this week brought on marijuana use?"
Patient	"Just this weekend, I hit it then put it down…it was just social, and not knowing how to tell somebody, like 'Hey, I thought I was going to come here and not have to smoke, and y'all smoking over here.'"
Therapist	"So not really knowing how to say no."
Patient	"Exactly"
Therapist	"Well, that's exactly what we're going to cover today, how to effectively say no to people when they offer to smoke. What situations this week brought on marijuana use in response to anxiety?"
Patient	"To be honest, you know, during the week, not really. I'm realizing that it only makes me feel worse."
Therapist	"That's huge that you're not smoking during the week to cope with anxiety, because that's where we started—smoking almost all day every day because you were feeling anxious."
Patient	"It was. I really want to be honest when I tell people that I don't smoke."

This exchange highlights that ceasing cannabis as a false safety behavior was not sufficient to attain the patient's goal of abstinence. Rather, she benefited from additional MET-CBT skills to manage her cannabis use (in this case, learning effective refusal skills).

The final session consisted of relapse prevention. High-risk situations were identified and discussed as opportunities to become her own therapist, implement problem-solving techniques, and cope with high-risk situations related to anxiety/depression and cannabis use. The patient reported feeling more confident to deal with using thought challenges and problem-solving during these high-risk cannabis use situations.

Throughout treatment, the patient completed all weekly homework assignments (including self-monitoring daily, practicing anxiety management skills including fading of safety behaviors and antiphobic exercises, and using MET-CBT for CUD skills to manage craving and high-risk cannabis use situations). By the termination session (Session 12), she no longer met diagnostic criteria for CUD or for SAD and she had only used cannabis twice in the month prior to termination, both times because she "wanted to" not because she was trying to "fix something" (i.e., her anxiety). This is a significant decrease from her use at intake, which was daily. Further, the patient denied any problems related to her cannabis use.

Other Approaches

According to a recent review, ICART is the only investigated psychosocial treatment designed to treat co-occurring CUD and anxiety disorders (Lees et al., 2021). Although other studies have investigated similar treatment approaches for specific anxiety disorders and substance use broadly (e.g., 10 weeks of weekly group CBT for co-occurring SAD and SUD [38% with CUD]; Courbasson & Nishikawa, 2010), there is a paucity of treatment studies examining co-occurring CUD and anxiety disorders specifically. Further, pharmacological treatments have been investigated for CUD and have demonstrated initial efficacy in reducing cannabis use (e.g., 400 mg oral cannabidiol; Freeman et al., 2020); yet, no studies have investigated pharmacological treatment methods to treat co-occurring CUD and anxiety disorders.

CBT for CUD and Depression or Mixed Emotional Disorder Symptoms

Although empirical attention has been limited, psychosocial treatments targeting both CUD and depression have demonstrated promising initial outcomes. To illustrate, among young adults with co-occurring MDD and SUD (53.3% of the whom had CUD) or risky substance use (defined as past-month alcohol use exceeding national guidelines or at least weekly illicit substance use), 10 individual sessions of integrated CBT for both depression and risky substance use delivered with case management over 20 weeks was effective at reducing depression and cannabis use quantities at mid-treatment, post-treatment, and follow-up compared to baseline (Hides et al., 2010). However, the lack of a control group, small sample size, and focus on risky substance use/SUD broadly (rather than cannabis use/CUD specifically) in this study indicates that additional research is needed to confirm the efficacy of CBT for comorbid MDD and CUD. Several studies have also investigated pharmacological treatments (e.g., venlafaxine, fluoxetine) for co-occurring CUD and depressive disorders and found that patients that received active medications did not have more favorable cannabis (e.g., rates of abstinence or cannabis use frequency) or depressive outcomes (e.g., less depression) compared to those in the placebo conditions (e.g., Cornelius et al., 2010; Levin et al., 2013).

Future Directions

Computerized Interventions

Although ICART is a promising approach to treating comorbid CUD and anxiety disorders, the majority of patients do not seek treatment for CUD (Hasin et al., 2016; Wu et al., 2017). Thus, online interventions can be one method to intervene with patients. We therefore developed an online intervention designed to specifically target risky cannabis use and elevated negative affect, a personalized feedback intervention (PFI) that integrates personalized normative feedback regarding cannabis with strategies to manage negative affect (PFI-NAC). In a pilot test of PFI-NAC, undergraduates who endorsed past-month cannabis use (who used cannabis weekly, on average) were randomly assigned to the 1-session PFI-NAC or an assessment-only control and completed a 2-week follow-up assessment (Buckner et al., 2020). Participants were unselected for baseline severity of negative affect. After controlling for baseline negative affect and cannabis use frequency, social anxiety interacted with condition to predict follow-up cannabis use frequency, such that among those with moderate or high (but not lower) levels of social anxiety, those in PFI-NAC reported cannabis less use at follow-up than those in the control. Results of this pilot study suggest that a 1-session online intervention that teaches simultaneously teaching skills to manage negative affect and cannabis may benefit those cannabis users with moderate to high social anxiety.

There is similarly a paucity of research on the efficacy of computer-based interventions for co-occurring CUD and depression. One study compared a brief intervention control condition to nine sessions of MI/CBT targeting both depression and substance misuse, delivered either in-person or via computer, to individuals with clinically elevated depression and either alcohol or cannabis misuse (defined as at least weekly cannabis use; Kay-Lambkin et al., 2009). They found that although participants in both in-person and computerized MI/CBT conditions reported reductions in depression and cannabis use.

The Need to Attend to Sex Differences and Psycho-Sociocultural Factors

Little attention has been paid to the role of demographic and thus sociocultural factors that may impact the relation of CUD to emotional disorders and the treatment implications of such relations. However, emerging data indicate that there may be important differences in the experience of the CUD-emotional disorders comorbidity based on psycho-sociocultural factors that may impact treatment. Sex is one such factor that appears to impact the relation of emotional disorder symptoms and CUD outcomes. To illustrate, among patients undergoing either MET or MET-CBT for CUD, there was a significant effect of anxiety on post-treatment cannabis problems such that after controlling for baseline cannabis problems, treatment site, and treatment condition, baseline anxiety was related to more cannabis problems at 4- and 9-month follow-up assessments among women, but not among men (Buckner & Carroll, 2010). Although the mechanisms underlying sex differences related to the impact of anxiety on CUD treatment outcomes have not yet been identified, it may be due to differences in cannabis use motives. To illustrate, although social anxiety was related to more cannabis problems and coping (to decrease NA generally) and social anxiety (to manage NA in social situations) cannabis use motives among both men and women, there were sex differences in the relation of social anxiety to other high-risk motives such that among men (not women) social anxiety was related to less frequent cannabis use and more conformity motives, whereas among women (not men), social anxiety was related to more enjoyment, experimentation, boredom alleviation, altered perceptions (to modulate perceptual experiences), and relatively low risk (perceived low risk) motives (Morris & Buckner, 2023). Data such as these suggest that clinicians may consider different cognitive restructuring techniques that address these different reasons for use among men versus women.

Similarly, rates of MDD are higher among women with CUD than men with CUD (Kerridge et al., 2018) and accumulating evidence suggests that women with co-occurring depressive disorders and CUD may have poorer treatment outcomes than men. To illustrate, a randomized placebo-controlled trial examining the effectiveness of 12-week N-Acetylcysteine (NAC) plus abstinence-based contingency management in reducing depressive symptoms and promoting cannabis abstinence among individuals with CUD found that higher levels of depressive symptoms were more strongly associated with a lower likelihood of achieving cannabis abstinence among women compared to men (Tomko et al., 2020). Given that women are more likely to use cannabis to cope than men, mental health professionals may consider teaching these patients alternative methods to cope with negative affect (e.g., behavior activation) as a strategy to improve outcomes for female patients.

Race/ethnicity may also impact the relation of emotional disorder symptoms to cannabis outcomes, although this hypothesis has been understudied. We recently found that Black adults use more false safety behaviors than White adults, and that use of false safety behaviors among Black adults was related to more anxiety, depression, and suicidal thoughts and behaviors (Buckner et al., 2023). Thus, future work is necessary to test whether ICART, which targets false safety behaviors to improve anxiety and cannabis outcomes, is efficacious with Black patients, as these data indicate that ICART may be especially useful to help these patients learn more adaptive ways to cope with negative affect. However, it is important to test the role of psycho-sociocultural factors that may account for any observed racial/ethnic differences, as those factors could also be important therapeutic targets. For example, we recently found that the experience of microaggressions (common, everyday instances of race-based discrimination; e.g., locking car doors when a Black person walks by) is related to more emotional disorder symptoms (anxiety, depression, stress) as well as more cannabis problems and coping and conformity motivated cannabis use and Black young adults (Buckner et al., in press). Importantly, the relation of microaggressions with cannabis problems occurred serially via emotional disorder symptoms and coping motives, suggesting that Black individuals may use cannabis despite cannabis-related problems in an attempt to cope with negative affect associated with all-too-common experiences of race-based microaggressions. Thus, clinicians are encouraged to strive to create an inclusive, culturally sensitive environment when working with Black patients (American Psychological Association Task Force on Race and Ethnicity Guidelines in Psychology, 2019) and assess for and address emotional disorder symptoms associated with race-based discrimination and trauma. Further, future work is necessary to test whether incorporation of skills to help patients better manage emotional disorder symptoms resulting from race-based discrimination result in better cannabis-related outcomes.

Medical Cannabis to Manage Emotional Disorder Symptoms

Another area of future work is the utility of cannabis to manage emotional disorder symptoms. Although patients in several countries and in several U.S. states can receive medical cannabis to help them manage their emotional disorder symptoms, there is a paucity of research on whether cannabis is efficacious for alleviating these symptoms. To illustrate, among patients who use cannabis for medicinal purposes in Canada, nearly half (43.7%) indicated that they used medicinal cannabis to treat their anxiety (Turna et al., 2019). Anxiety disorders included GAD (45.6%), SAD (45.6%), and panic disorder (25.7%), with the majority (63.4%) meeting criteria for more than one anxiety disorder. Further, 25.7% met for MDD. Of note, nearly all (92%) indicated that they believed their cannabis use improved their anxiety symptoms and 56.9% indicated it helped with "low mood"; yet they continued to exhibit moderate levels of anxiety. Further, these patients used cannabis daily, with more frequent use associated with more severe emotional disorder symptoms, making it unclear whether patients with more severe anxiety used more cannabis to manage it or whether more cannabis use was resulted in greater anxiety. Patients reported that some strains of cannabis were anxiolytic (e.g., *Cannabis indica* was endorsed as anxiolytic by 52% of those with anxiety disorders), whereas others were anxiogenic (e.g., *Cannabis sativa*). Thus, it also remains unclear the extent to which the medicinal cannabis did in fact help with their anxiety symptoms. This is consistent with other work indicating that it remains unclear whether medicinal cannabis is useful for managing anxiety (for review see Walukevich-Dienst et al., 2019). Taken together, these data indicate that additional work is necessary to determine whether medicinal cannabis is useful for managing emotional disorder symptoms and if so, which stains of cannabis at which doses are most efficacious in helping these patients. Additional work is also necessary to determine whether combined treatment of medical cannabis plus psychotherapy such as ICART or other MET-CBT for anxiety and/or CUD improves treatment outcomes over singular cannabis-based medical intervention or CBT-based psychotherapy. Future research is also necessary to determine whether the use of medical cannabis serves as a false safety behavior that actually maintains pathological anxiety among patients with CUD with comorbid anxiety disorders, including but not limited to when medical cannabis is used among patients undergoing ICART for CUD-anxiety disorders.

Summary of Key Findings and Concluding Remarks

Cannabis misuse and CUD are highly prevalent and rates continue to rise with the increased access and decreased risk perceptions that accompany increases in legalization of cannabis. Further, cannabis misuse and CUD are associated with especially high rates of anxiety and depressive disorders, and the co-occurrence of these conditions are associated with worse CUD treatment outcomes. Yet very little research has been done to develop and test treatments to improve outcomes for these patients. Unfortunately, there are currently no known treatment for CUD and comorbid depressive disorders, and it is our hope that this chapter will inspire researchers to develop and test integrated treatments to better help these patients. ICART was developed using evidence-based techniques for CUD and for anxiety disorders specifically to treat patients with comorbid CUD and anxiety disorders and initial results are promising. Further, PFI-NAC is an online intervention that may be useful to intervene with college students with cannabis misuse and elevated anxiety to help these students better manage their cannabis use and anxiety in hopes of helping them meet their academic and other goals.

References

American Psychological Association Task Force on Race and Ethnicity Guidelines in Psychology. (2019). *Race and ethnicity guidelines in psychology: Promoting responsiveness and equity*. http://www.apa.org/about/policy/race-and-ethnicity-in-psychology.pdf

Arias, F., Szerman, N., Vega, P., Mesias, B., Basurte, I., Morant, C., Ochoa, E., Poyo, F., & Babin, F. (2013). Alcohol abuse or dependence and other psychiatric disorders. Madrid study on the prevalence of dual pathology. *Mental Health and Substance Use, 6*(4), 339–350. https://doi.org/10.1080/17523281.2012.748674

Bahorik, A. L., Newhill, C. E., & Eack, S. M. (2013). Characterizing the longitudinal patterns of substance use among individuals diagnosed with serious mental illness after psychiatric hospitalization. *Addiction, 108*(7), 1259–1269. https://doi.org/10.1111/add.12153

Bahorik, A. L., Sterling, S. A., Campbell, C. I., Weisner, C., Ramo, D., & Satre, D. D. (2018). Medical and non-medical marijuana use in depression: Longitudinal associations with suicidal ideation, everyday functioning, and psychiatry service utilization. *Journal of Affective Disorders, 241*, 8–14. https://doi.org/10.1016/j.jad.2018.05.065

Baker, T. B., Piper, M. E., McCarthy, D. E., Majeskie, M. R., & Fiore, M. C. (2004). Addiction motivation reformulated: An affective processing model of negative reinforcement. *Psychological Review, 111*(1), 33–51. https://doi.org/10.1037/0033-295x.111.1.33

Bersani, G., Bersani, F. S., Caroti, E., Russo, P., Albano, G., Valeriani, G., Imperatori, C., Minichino, A., Manuali, G., & Corazza, O. (2016). Negative symptoms as key features of depression among cannabis users: A preliminary report. *European Review for Medical and Pharmacological Sciences, 20*(3), 547–552.

Bonn-Miller, M. O., & Moos, R. H. (2009). Marijuana discontinuation, anxiety symptoms, and relapse to marijuana. *Addictive Behaviors, 34*(9), 782–785. https://doi.org/10.1016/j.addbeh.2009.04.009

Bricker, J. B., Russo, J., Stein, M. B., Sherbourne, C., Craske, M., Schraufnagel, T. J., & Roy-Byrne, P. (2007). Does occasional cannabis use impact anxiety and depression treatment outcomes?: Results from a randomized effectiveness trial. *Depression and Anxiety, 24*(6), 392–398. https://doi.org/10.1002/da.20248

Buckner, J. D., & Carroll, K. M. (2010). Effect of anxiety on treatment presentation and outcome: Results from the Marijuana Treatment Project. *Psychiatry Research, 178*(3), 493–500. https://doi.org/10.1016/j.psychres.2009.10.010

Buckner, J. D., Schmidt, N. B., Lang, A. R., Small, J. W., Schlauch, R. C., & Lewinsohn, P. M. (2008). Specificity of social anxiety disorder as a risk factor for alcohol and cannabis dependence. *Journal of Psychiatric Research, 42*(3), 230–239. https://doi.org/10.1016/j.jpsychires.2007.01.002

Buckner, J. D., Crosby, R. D., Silgado, J., Wonderlich, S. A., & Schmidt, N. B. (2012a). Immediate antecedents of marijuana use: An analysis from ecological momentary assessment. *Journal of Behavior Therapy and Experimental Psychiatry, 43*(1), 297–304. https://doi.org/10.1016/j.jbtep.2011.09.010

Buckner, J. D., Heimberg, R. G., Schneier, F. R., Liu, S., Wang, S., & Blanco, C. (2012b). The relationship between cannabis use disorders and social anxiety disorder in the National Epidemiological Study of Alcohol and Related Conditions (NESARC). *Drug and Alcohol Dependence, 124*, 128–134. https://doi.org/10.1016/j.drugalcdep.2011.12.023

Buckner, J. D., Zvolensky, M. J., Schmidt, N. B., Carroll, K. M., Schatschneider, C., & Crapanzano, K. (2014). Integrated cognitive behavioral therapy for cannabis use and anxiety disorders: Rationale and development. *Addictive Behaviors, 39*(3), 495–496. https://doi.org/10.1016/j.addbeh.2013.10.023

Buckner, J. D., Zvolensky, M. J., Crosby, R. D., Wonderlich, S. A., Ecker, A. H., & Richter, A. A. (2015). Antecedents and consequences of cannabis use among racially diverse cannabis users: An analysis from ecological momentary assessment. *Drug and Alcohol Dependence, 147*, 20–25. https://doi.org/10.1016/j.drugalcdep.2014.12.022

Buckner, J. D., Ecker, A. H., Beighley, J. S., Zvolensky, M. J., Schmidt, N. B., Shah, S. M., & Carroll, K. M. (2016a). Integrated cognitive behavioral therapy for comorbid cannabis use and anxiety disorders. *Clinical Case Studies, 15*(1), 68–83. https://doi.org/10.1177/1534650115590857

Buckner, J. D., Zvolensky, M. J., Ecker, A. H., & Jeffries, E. R. (2016b). Cannabis craving in response to laboratory-induced social stress among racially diverse cannabis users: The impact of social anxiety disorder. *Journal of Psychopharmacology, 30*(4), 363–369. https://doi.org/10.1177/0269881116629115

Buckner, J. D., Walukevich, K. A., Zvolensky, M. J., & Gallagher, M. W. (2017a). Emotion regulation and coping motives serially affect cannabis cessation problems among dually diagnosed outpatients. *Psychology of Addictive Behaviors, 31*(7), 839–845. https://doi.org/10.1037/adb0000310

Buckner, J. D., Zvolensky, M. J., Ecker, A. H., Jeffries, E. R., Lemke, A. W., Dean, K. E., Businelle, M. S., & Gallagher, M. W. (2017b). Anxiety and cannabis-related problem severity among dually diagnosed outpatients: The impact of false safety behaviors. *Addictive Behaviors, 70*, 49–53. https://doi.org/10.1016/j.addbeh.2017.02.014

Buckner, J. D., Zvolensky, M. J., Businelle, M. S., & Gallagher, M. W. (2018). Direct and indirect effects of false safety behaviors on cannabis use and related problems. *The American Journal on Addictions, 27*(1), 29–34. https://doi.org/10.1111/ajad.12659

Buckner, J. D., Zvolensky, M. J., Ecker, A. H., Schmidt, N. B., Lewis, E. M., Paulus, D. J., Lopez-Gamundi, P., Crapanzano, K. A., & Bakhshaie, J. (2019). Integrated cognitive behavioral therapy for comorbid cannabis use and anxiety disorders: A pilot randomized controlled trial. *Behavior Research and Therapy, 115*, 38–45. https://doi.org/10.1016/j.brat.2018.10.014

Buckner, J. D., Zvolensky, M. J., & Lewis, E. M. (2020). On-line personalized feedback intervention for negative affect and cannabis: A pilot randomized controlled trial. *Experimental and Clinical Psychopharmacology, 28*(2), 143–149. https://doi.org/10.1037/pha0000304

Buckner, J. D., Morris, P. E., & Zvolensky, M. J. (2021). Integrated cognitive behavioral therapy for comorbid cannabis use and anxiety disorders: The impact of severity of cannabis use. *Experimental and Clinical Psychopharmacology, 29*, 272–278. https://doi.org/10.1037/pha0000456

Buckner, J. D., Zvolensky, M. J., Ferrie, M. L., & Morris, P. E. (2023). False safety behavior use among Black adults. *Cognitive Behaviour Therapy, 52*(1), 65–74. https://doi.org/10.1080/16506073.2022.2139291

Buckner, J. D., Zvolensky, M. J., & Scherzer, C. R. (in press). Microaggressions and cannabis-related problems among Black adults: The roles of negative affect and cannabis use motives. *Cognitive Therapy and Research*. https://doi.org/10.1007/s10608-023-10375-8

Cornelius, J. R., Bukstein, O. G., Douaihy, A. B., Clark, D. B., Chung, T. A., Daley, D. C., Wood, D. S., & Brown, S. J. (2010). Double-blind fluoxetine trial in comorbid MDD–CUD youth and young adults. *Drug and Alcohol Dependence, 112*(1–2), 39–45. https://doi.org/10.1016/j.drugalcdep.2010.05.010

Courbasson, C. M., & Nishikawa, Y. (2010). Cognitive behavioral group therapy for patients with co-existing social anxiety disorder and substance use disorders: A pilot study. *Cognitive Therapy and Research, 34*(1), 82–91. https://doi.org/10.1007/s10608-008-9216-8

Crane, N. A., Langenecker, S. A., & Mermelstein, R. J. (2015). Gender differences in the associations among marijuana use, cigarette use, and symptoms of depression during adolescence and young adulthood. *Addictive Behaviors, 49*, 33–39. https://doi.org/10.1016/j.addbeh.2015.05.014

Cuttler, C., Spradlin, A., & McLaughlin, R. J. (2018). A naturalistic examination of the perceived effects of cannabis on negative affect. *Journal of Affective Disorders, 235*, 198–205. https://doi.org/10.1016/j.jad.2018.04.054

Danielsson, A.-K., Lundin, A., Agardh, E., Allebeck, P., & Forsell, Y. (2016). Cannabis use, depression and anxiety: A 3-year prospective population-based study. *Journal of Affective Disorders, 193*, 103–108. https://doi.org/10.1016/j.jad.2015.12.045

Dierker, L., Selya, A., Lanza, S., Li, R., & Rose, J. (2018). Depression and marijuana use disorder symptoms among current marijuana users. *Addictive Behaviors, 76*, 161–168. https://doi.org/10.1016/j.addbeh.2017.08.013

Ecker, A. H., Lang, B., Hogan, J., Cucciare, M. A., & Lindsay, J. (2020). Cannabis use disorder among veterans: Comorbidity and mental health treatment utilization. *Journal of Substance Abuse Treatment, 109*, 46–49. https://doi.org/10.1016/j.jsat.2019.11.003

Fairman, B. J., & Anthony, J. C. (2012). Are early-onset cannabis smokers at an increased risk of depression spells? *Journal of Affective Disorders, 138*(1–2), 54–62. https://doi.org/10.1016/j.jad.2011.12.031

Feingold, D., & Weinstein, A. (2021). Cannabis and depression. *Advances in Experimental Medicine and Biology, 1264*, 67–80. https://doi.org/10.1007/978-3-030-57369-0_5

Feingold, D., Weiser, M., Rehm, J., & Lev-Ran, S. (2016). The association between cannabis use and anxiety disorders: Results from a population-based representative sample. *European Neuropsychopharmacology, 26*(3), 493–505. https://doi.org/10.1016/j.euroneuro.2015.12.037

Flórez-Salamanca, L., Secades-Villa, R., Budney, A. J., García-Rodríguez, O., Wang, S., & Blanco, C. (2013). Probability and predictors of cannabis use disorders relapse: Results of the National Epidemiologic Survey on Alcohol and Related Conditions (NESARC). *Drug and Alcohol Dependence, 132*(1–2), 127–133. https://doi.org/10.1016/j.drugalcdep.2013.01.013

Freeman, T. P., Hindocha, C., Baio, G., Shaban, N. D. C., Thomas, E. M., Astbury, D., Freeman, A. M., Lees, R., Craft, S., Morrison, P. D., Bloomfield, M. A. P., O'Ryan, D., Kinghorn, J., Morgan, C. J. A., Mofeez, A., & Curran, H. V. (2020). Cannabidiol for the treatment of cannabis use disorder: A phase 2a, double-blind, placebo-controlled, randomised, adaptive Bayesian trial. *Lancet Psychiatry, 7*(10), 865–874. https://doi.org/10.1016/s2215-0366(20)30290-x

Gage, S. H., Hickman, M., Heron, J., Munafò, M. R., Lewis, G., Macleod, J., & Zammit, S. (2015). Associations of cannabis and cigarette use with depression and anxiety at age 18: Findings from the Avon Longitudinal Study of Parents and Children. *PLoS One, 10*(4), e0122896. https://doi.org/10.1371/journal.pone.0122896

Gobbi, G., Atkin, T., Zytynski, T., Wang, S., Askari, S., Boruff, J., Ware, M., Marmorstein, N., Cipriani, A., Dendukuri, N., & Mayo, N. (2019). Association of cannabis use in adolescence and risk of depression, anxiety, and suicidality in young adulthood: A systematic review and meta-analysis. *JAMA Psychiatry, 76*(4), 426–434. https://doi.org/10.1001/jamapsychiatry.2018.4500

Guillem, E., Arbabzadeh-Bouchez, S., Vorspan, F., & Bellivier, F. (2015). Comorbidity in 207 cannabis users in a specific outpatient setting. *L'Encéphale, 41*(1), S7–S12. https://doi.org/10.1016/j.encep.2014.06.004

Hasin, D. S., Kerridge, B. T., Saha, T. D., Huang, B., Pickering, R., Smith, S. M., Jung, J., Zhang, H., & Grant, B. F. (2016). Prevalence and correlates of DSM-5 Cannabis use disorder, 2012-2013: Findings from the National Epidemiologic Survey on Alcohol and Related Conditions-III. *The American Journal of Psychiatry, 173*(6), 588–599. https://doi.org/10.1176/appi.ajp.2015.15070907

Hides, L., Carroll, S., Catania, L., Cotton, S. M., Baker, A., Scaffidi, A., & Lubman, D. I. (2010). Outcomes of an integrated cognitive behaviour therapy (CBT) treatment program for co-occurring depression and substance misuse in young people. *Journal of Affective Disorders, 121*(1), 169–174. https://doi.org/10.1016/j.jad.2009.06.002

Horwood, L. J., Fergusson, D. M., Coffey, C., Patton, G. C., Tait, R., Smart, D., Letcher, P., Silins, E., & Hutchinson, D. M. (2012). Cannabis and depression: An integrative data analysis of four Australasian cohorts. *Drug and Alcohol Dependence, 126*(3), 369–378. https://doi.org/10.1016/j.drugalcdep.2012.06.002

Hser, Y.-I., Mooney, L. J., Huang, D., Zhu, Y., Tomko, R. L., McClure, E., Chou, C.-P., & Gray, K. M. (2017). Reductions in cannabis use are associated with improvements in anxiety, depression, and sleep quality, but not quality of life. *Journal of Substance Abuse Treatment, 81*, 53–58. https://doi.org/10.1016/j.jsat.2017.07.012

Kay-Lambkin, F. J., Baker, A. L., Lewin, T. J., & Carr, V. J. (2009). Computer-based psychological treatment for comorbid depression and problematic alcohol and/or cannabis use: A randomized controlled trial of clinical efficacy. *Addiction, 104*(3), 378–388. https://doi.org/10.1111/j.1360-0443.2008.02444.x

Kedzior, K. K., & Laeber, L. T. (2014). A positive association between anxiety disorders and cannabis use or cannabis use disorders in the general population--a meta-analysis of 31 studies. *BMC Psychiatry, 14*, 136. https://doi.org/10.1186/1471-244x-14-136

Kerridge, B. T., Pickering, R., Chou, P., Saha, T. D., & Hasin, D. S. (2018). DSM-5 cannabis use disorder in the National Epidemiologic Survey on Alcohol and Related Conditions-III: Gender-specific profiles. *Addictive Behaviors, 76*, 52–60. https://doi.org/10.1016/j.addbeh.2017.07.012

Khantzian, E. J. (1997). The self-medication hypothesis of substance use disorders: A reconsideration and recent applications. *Harvard Review of Psychiatry, 4*(5), 231–244. https://doi.org/10.3109/10673229709030550

Lai, H. M. X., & Sitharthan, T. (2012). Exploration of the comorbidity of cannabis use disorders and mental health disorders among inpatients presenting to all hospitals in New South Wales, Australia. *The American Journal of Drug and Alcohol Abuse, 38*(6), 567–574. https://doi.org/10.3109/00952990.2012.694523

Lees, R., Hines, L. A., D'Souza, D. C., Stothart, G., Di Forti, M., Hoch, E., & Freeman, T. P. (2021). Psychosocial and pharmacological treatments for cannabis use disorder and mental health comorbidities: A narrative review. *Psychological Medicine, 51*(3), 353–364. https://doi.org/10.1017/S0033291720005449

Levin, F. R., Mariani, J., Brooks, D. J., Pavlicova, M., Nunes, E. V., Agosti, V., Bisaga, A., Sullivan, M. A., & Carpenter, K. M. (2013). A randomized double-blind, placebo-controlled trial of venlafaxine-extended release for co-occurring cannabis dependence and depressive disorders. *Addiction, 108*(6), 1084–1094. https://doi.org/10.1111/add.12108

Livingston, N. R., Hetelekides, E., Bravo, A. J., & Looby, A. (2023). Negative affect regulation and marijuana use in college students: Evaluating the mediating roles of coping and sleep motives. *Journal of Psychoactive Drugs, 55*(2), 203–212. https://doi.org/10.1080/02791072.2022.2054747

Marel, C., Sunderland, M., Mills, K. L., Slade, T., Teesson, M., & Chapman, C. (2019). Conditional probabilities of substance use disorders and associated risk factors: Progression from first use to use disorder on alcohol, cannabis, stimulants, sedatives and opioids. *Drug and Alcohol Dependence, 194*, 136–142. https://doi.org/10.1016/j.drugalcdep.2018.10.010

Mason, M. J. (2020). Depressive symptoms moderate cannabis use for young adults in a text-delivered randomized clinical trial for cannabis use disorder. *Addictive Behaviors, 104*, 106259. https://doi.org/10.1016/j.addbeh.2019.106259

Mathews, R. R., Hall, W. D., & Gartner, C. E. (2011). Depression and psychological distress in tobacco smokers and people with cannabis dependence in the National Survey of Mental Health and Wellbeing. *Medical Journal of Australia, 195*, S12–S15. https://doi.org/10.5694/j.1326-5377.2011.tb03259.x

Miller, W. R., & Rollnick, S. (2013). *Motivational interviewing: Helping people change* (3rd ed.). Guilford Press.

Morris, P. E., & Buckner, J. D. (2023). Cannabis-related problems and social anxiety: The roles of sex and cannabis use motives updated. *Addictive Behaviors, 137*. https://doi.org/10.1016/j.addbeh.2022.107528

National Institute on Drug Abuse. (2022). *Marijuana and hallucinogen use among young adults reached all time-high in 2021*. Retrieved October 20, 2022 from https://nida.nih.gov/news-events/news-releases/2022/08/marijuana-and-hallucinogen-use-among-young-adults-reached-all-time-high-in-2021

Onaemo, V. N., Fawehinmi, T. O., & D'Arcy, C. (2021). Comorbid cannabis use disorder with major depression and generalized anxiety disorder: A systematic review with meta-analysis of nationally representative epidemiological surveys. *Journal of Affective Disorders, 281*, 467–475. https://doi.org/10.1016/j.jad.2020.12.043

Ouellette, M. J., Rowa, K., Cameron, D. H., Elcock, A., Soreni, N., Pawluk, E. J., & McCabe, R. E. (2022). Does cannabis use impact cognitive behavioural therapy outcomes for anxiety and related disorders? A preliminary examination. *Journal of Psychiatric Research, 156*, 690–697. https://doi.org/10.1016/j.jpsychires.2022.10.054

Pacek, L. R., Weinberger, A. H., Zhu, J., & Goodwin, R. D. (2020). Rapid increase in the prevalence of cannabis use among people with depression in the United States, 2005-17: The role of differentially changing risk perceptions. *Addiction, 115*(5), 935–943. https://doi.org/10.1111/add.14883

Rasic, D., Weerasinghe, S., Asbridge, M., & Langille, D. B. (2013). Longitudinal associations of cannabis and illicit drug use with depression, suicidal ideation and suicidal attempts among Nova Scotia high school students. *Drug and Alcohol Dependence, 129*(1–2), 49–53. https://doi.org/10.1016/j.drugalcdep.2012.09.009

Riccardi, C. J., Korte, K. J., & Schmidt, N. B. (2017). False safety behavior elimination therapy: A randomized study of a brief individual transdiagnostic treatment for anxiety disorders. *Journal of Anxiety Disorders, 46*, 35–45. https://doi.org/10.1016/j.janxdis.2016.06.003

Salkovskis, P. M., Clark, D. M., & Hackmann, A. (1991). Treatment of panic attacks using cognitive therapy without exposure or breathing retraining. *Behaviour Research and Therapy, 29*(2), 161–166. https://doi.org/10.1016/0005-7967(91)90044-4

Schmidt, N. B., Buckner, J. D., & Keough, M. E. (2007). Anxiety sensitivity as a prospective predictor of alcohol use disorders. *Behavior Modification, 31*(2), 202–219. https://doi.org/10.1177/0145445506297019

Schmidt, N. B., Buckner, J. D., Pusser, A. T., Woolaway-Bickel, K., & Preston, J. L. (2012). Randomized controlled trial of False Safety Behavior Elimination Therapy (F-SET): A unified cognitive behavioral treatment for anxiety psychopathology. *Behavior Therapy, 43*(3), 518–532. https://doi.org/10.1016/j.beth.2012.02.004

Steinberg, K. L., Roffman, R. A., Carroll, K. M., McRee, B., Babor, T. F., Miller, M., Kadden, R., Duresky, D., & Stephens, R. (2005). *Brief counseling for marijuana dependence: A manual for treating adults*. Center for Substance Abuse Treatment, Substance Abuse and Mental Health Services Administration.

Stewart, S. H., & Conrod, P. J. (Eds.). (2008). *Anxiety and substance use disorders: The vicious cycle of comorbidity*. Springer.

Substance Abuse and Mental Health Services Administration. (2021). *Key substance use and mental health indicators in the United States: Results from the 2020 National Survey on Drug Use and Health* (HHS Publication No. PEP21-07-01-003, NSDUH Series H-56). https://www.samhsa.gov/data

Teesson, M., Slade, T., Swift, W., Mills, K., Memedovic, S., Mewton, L., Grove, R., Newton, N., & Hall, W. (2012). Prevalence, correlates and comorbidity of DSM-IV cannabis use and cannabis use disorders in Australia. *Australian & New Zealand Journal of Psychiatry, 46*(12), 1182–1192. https://doi.org/10.1177/0004867412460591

Tomko, R. L., Baker, N. L., Hood, C. O., Gilmore, A. K., McClure, E. A., Squeglia, L. M., McRae-Clark, A. L., Sonne, S. C., & Gray, K. M. (2020). Depressive symptoms and cannabis use in a placebo-controlled trial of N-Acetylcysteine for adult cannabis use disorder. *Psychopharmacology, 237*(2), 479–490. https://doi.org/10.1007/s00213-019-05384-z

Tourjman, S. V., Buck, G., Jutras-Aswad, D., Khullar, A., McInerney, S., Saraf, G., Pinto, J. V., Potvin, S., Poulin, M. J., Frey, B. N., Kennedy, S. H., Lam, R. W., MacQueen, G., Milev, R., Parikh, S. V., Ravindran, A., McIntyre, R. S., Schaffer, A., Taylor, V. H., van Ameringen, M., Yatham, L. N., & Beaulieu, S. (2023). Canadian Network For Mood and Anxiety Treatments (CANMAT) task force report: A systematic review and recommendations of cannabis use in bipolar disorder and major depressive disorder. *The Canadian Journal of Psychiatry, 68*(5), 299–311. https://doi.org/10.1177/07067437221099769

Troup, L. J., Andrzejewski, J. A., Braunwalder, J. T., & Torrence, R. D. (2016). The relationship between cannabis use and measures of anxiety and depression in a sample of college campus cannabis users and non-users post state legalization in Colorado. *PeerJ, 4*, e2782. https://doi.org/10.7717/peerj.2782

Turna, J., Simpson, W., Patterson, B., Lucas, P., & Van Ameringen, M. (2019). Cannabis use behaviors and prevalence of anxiety and depressive symptoms in a cohort of Canadian medicinal cannabis users. *Journal of Psychiatric Research, 111*, 134–139. https://doi.org/10.1016/j.jpsychires.2019.01.024

United Nations Office on Drugs and Crime. (2020). *World Drug Report*. Sales No. E.20.XI.6. https://wdr.unodc.org/wdr2020/index.html

van der Pol, P., Liebregts, N., de Graaf, R., Korf, D. J., van den Brink, W., & van Laar, M. (2013). Facilitators and barriers in treatment seeking for cannabis dependence. *Drug and Alcohol Dependence, 133*(2), 776–780. https://doi.org/10.1016/j.drugalcdep.2013.08.011

Walukevich-Dienst, K., Crapanzano, K. A., Lewis, E. M., & Buckner, J. D. (2019). Cannabis and anxiety: A biopsychosocial model. *Current Addiction Reports, 6*(4), 456–465. https://doi.org/10.1007/s40429-019-00284-w

Walukevich-Dienst, K., Lewis, E. M., & Buckner, J. D. (2020). Cannabis-related impairment and social anxiety: The role of use to manage negative and positive affect in social situations. *Substance Use & Misuse, 55*(2), 271–280. https://doi.org/10.1080/10826084.2019.1664590

Wu, L.-T., Zhu, H., Mannelli, P., & Swartz, M. S. (2017). Prevalence and correlates of treatment utilization among adults with cannabis use disorder in the United States. *Drug and Alcohol Dependence, 177*, 153–162. https://doi.org/10.1016/j.drugalcdep.2017.03.037

Zvolensky, M. J., Rogers, A. H., Manning, K., Hogan, J. B. D., Paulus, D. J., Buckner, J. D., Mayorga, N. A., Hallford, G., & Schmidt, N. B. (2018). Anxiety sensitivity and cannabis use problems, perceived barriers for quitting, and fear of quitting. *Psychiatry Research, 263*, 115–120. https://doi.org/10.1016/j.psychres.2018.03.006

Chapter 4
Treating Comorbid Major Depressive Disorder and Substance Use Disorder

Suzette Glasner and Megan Eastlick

Overview: Co-occurring Substance Use Disorders and Major Depressive Disorder

Substance use disorders (SUDs) and major depressive disorder (MDD) commonly co-occur and, when overlapping, these conditions are associated with greater depressive symptomatology, higher rates of health service utilization, and poorer clinical course and outcomes. While acute and short-term use of substances may result in negative consequences (including cognitive impairment, engagement in risky behaviors, high blood pressure, and respiratory failure), people who use substances chronically are most likely to develop an SUD, as the risk of symptoms including withdrawal, tolerance, social consequences, and health complications increases (Rehm et al., 2013). Major depressive disorder (MDD) is a syndrome comprising persistently depressed mood lasting at least 2 weeks and can include concurrent loss of interest or pleasure derived from activities one used to enjoy (i.e., anhedonia). Symptoms of MDD include sleep disturbance, loss of energy, and recurrent thoughts of death; these symptoms cause significant impairment, and negatively impact one's well-being. Among subgroups of individuals, MDD can be accompanied by anxiety, melancholic features, and may follow seasonal patterns (Otte et al., 2016).

SUDs and MDD are closely linked: depending on the substance, up to 67% of individuals with SUDs meet criteria for MDD (Vujanovic et al., 2017). People with alcohol use disorders (AUDs) are 3.7 times more likely to meet criteria for MDD,

S. Glasner (✉)
UCLA Integrated Substance Abuse Programs, Los Angeles, CA, USA
e-mail: sglasner@ucla.edu

M. Eastlick
Pelago, New York, NY, USA

K. Wolitzky-Taylor (ed.), *Treating Comorbid Substance Use and Emotional Disorders*, CBT: Science Into Practice, https://doi.org/10.1007/978-3-031-62971-6_4

and those with other drug use disorders are 9 times more likely to have co-occurring depression when compared with those who do not have a substance use disorder. Likewise, 40% of those with MDD have also met criteria for AUD, and 17.2% for another substance use disorder (Baskin-Sommers & Foti, 2015).

In light of their association with greater functional impairment, suicidality, and emergency care, innovative and evidence-based treatment strategies are especially critical for addressing co-occurring SUDs and MDD (Baskin-Sommers & Foti, 2015; Vekaria et al., 2021; Watkins et al., 2022). In addition to negatively impacting individuals, SUD and MDD have widespread public health consequences, contributing significantly to disability, loss of productivity, increased demands on healthcare, and increased mortality rates. MDD and SUDs cost the US economy $83.1 billion and $428.1 billion annually, respectively (Baskin-Sommers & Foti, 2015), underscoring the importance of understanding their etiologies and developing scalable approaches to treating both conditions effectively.

Etiology of Co-occurring SUD and MDD

The etiology of concurrent SUD and MDD is complex. Meeting the criteria for one disorder has been found to increase the likelihood of experiencing the other, which has been interpreted as suggesting multiple plausible etiologies (McHugh & Weiss, 2019; Ross et al., 2016; Turner et al., 2018): (1) Depression may lead individuals to self-medicate with alcohol or drugs, leading to the development of an SUD over time. This "self-medication hypothesis" is supported by research demonstrating that among individuals with a diagnosed depressive disorder who report using substances to cope with depression, the risk of SUD 3 years later is 7 times greater relative to those who do not self-medicate with substances (Lazareck et al., 2012). (2) Repeated substance use can lead to depressive symptoms during withdrawal or in between use episodes, and these symptoms can take on a life of their own over time, resulting in the development of a depressive disorder (Ross et al., 2016).

An alternative model suggests that a common third factor may underlie both illnesses (Baskin-Sommers & Foti, 2015; Conner et al., 2009). For example, genetic vulnerability may increase the risk of depression, which in turn, impacts the likelihood of substance use. Likewise, there may be a common neurobiological substrate underlying both SUD and MDD. In particular, both MDD and SUD populations evidence disruptions to their reward system, including key structures underlying reinforcement and pleasure such as the nucleus accumbens (Iqbal et al., 2019). It has been posited that some of the core symptoms of depression (e.g., anhedonia) and SUDs (e.g., compulsive drug-seeking and use despite negative consequences) are the result of pathophysiological changes in the reward system that are associated with both conditions (Baskin-Sommers & Foti, 2015; Brewer et al., 2010). Another common third mechanism comprises the absence of healthy sources of positive reinforcement; among individuals with depression, the lack of motivation and energy coupled with anhedonia and loss of interest in activities can reinforce depression and increase the risk of substance use (Martínez-Vispo et al., 2018). Ongoing research is being conducted to further explore the autonomous vs. compounding influences of SUD and MDD on the brain (Baskin-Sommers & Foti, 2015).

Given that research exploring the causal pathways to SUD—MDD's bidirectional relationship has yielded mixed findings, there are likely subgroups for whom self-medication, the reverse (i.e., SUD trajectories leading to depression), and shared risk factors are explanatory. Nevertheless, understanding the etiologies of co-occurring depressive disorders and SUD, including their temporal sequencing, can support the process of diagnosis and development of treatment recommendations (Baskin-Sommers & Foti, 2015).

Substance-Induced Versus Substance-Dependent MDD

Despite the frequent co-occurrence of SUDs and psychiatric disorders, accurately diagnosing the two conditions can be challenging. Co-occurring symptoms often overlap, reinforce, or disguise one another, resulting in similar behaviors when someone is under the influence of or withdrawing from a substance to those of someone with MDD. For example, it may be unclear during an initial screening whether a person who self-reported substance use has lost interest in pleasurable activities, struggled with sleep disturbances, or endorsed anxiety symptoms as a result of co-occurring substance use and MDD, or whether the depression symptoms are purely driven by substance use, and can be expected to remit with abstinence. In the latter scenario, the symptoms would be considered to be "substance-induced."

Differentiating between substance-induced MDD and MDD independent of substance use can provide additional insight to inform an understanding of the overall diagnostic picture, as well as determining treatment recommendations. The onset of a substance-induced mood disorder typically occurs during intoxication or withdrawal, and the diagnosis is not uncommon among those with SUD. According to Revadigar and Gupta (2020), 40–60% of those with AUD and 55% with opioid use disorder (OUD) meet criteria for substance-induced depression. Diagnosed based on criteria for MDD (Revadigar & Gupta, 2020), patients with substance-induced MDD may experience a reduction in depressive symptoms when they abstain from substances, whereas patients with co-occurring SUD and independent MDD cannot rely on abstaining from substances alone to result in MDD symptom remission (Langås et al., 2013). Whether MDD is substance-induced or present independent of substance use, its frequent co-occurrence with SUDs underscores the transdiagnostic processes that characterize these disorders: those experiencing substance-induced MDD may be more likely to continue using substances, and those with independent MDD may be more likely to resume substance use following a period of abstinence (Magidson et al., 2013).

While a period of continuous abstinence from substances can help improve diagnostic reliability, if untreated, the observed depressive symptoms may themselves trigger continued substance use and treatment disengagement. Therefore, treating the symptoms, whether pharmacologically or using behavioral therapy techniques, may be clinically important to optimize treatment outcomes. To improve diagnostic accuracy, gathering a patient's symptom history retrospectively with reference to prior periods of abstinence from substances (if applicable) and collecting urine toxicology data can provide insights into current symptoms (Iqbal et al., 2019).

Therapeutic Interventions for Co-occurring Disorders

If left untreated, rates of recovery for both SUD and MDD are greatly reduced (Vekaria et al., 2021). Nevertheless, the complex relationship between the two conditions can make effective treatment challenging. Co-occurring MDD symptoms tend to disrupt intervention efforts targeting SUD (Ross et al., 2016), as people with MDD may misuse substances to cope, and those with SUDs may struggle with adhering to treatment recommendations for managing their depressive symptoms, such as taking their antidepressant medication (Vekaria et al., 2021). In addition, the use of other substances while taking mood-stabilizing prescriptions may compromise medication effectiveness, or possibly exacerbate existing depressive symptoms (Han et al., 2017). People actively engaged in SUD treatment with concomitant MDD tend to have poorer treatment outcomes, insufficient care, higher rates of resuming substance use after abstaining for a period of time, and reduced adherence to treatment recommendations than those who meet criteria for one disorder (Martínez-Vispo et al., 2018; Watkins et al., 2022; Yule & Kelly, 2019).

As a result of the intertwined pathologies of these disorders, low likelihood of sustained symptom improvement when addressing just one disorder, and diagnostic challenges, simultaneous management of both SUDs and MDD has emerged as the gold standard (Han et al., 2017; Osilla et al., 2009; Vujanovic et al., 2017; Yule & Kelly, 2019). Integrating SUD and MDD treatment reduces barriers to care, as patients enter only one treatment program to receive support for both disorders, and builds on existing (often finite) resources (Hunter et al., 2012). As stigma cultivates patient reluctance to seek care, incorporating SUD treatment with other mental or physical health services may lessen this concern (Mojtabai et al., 2014). In addition, concurrently addressing SUDs and MDD has been found to reduce symptoms of both disorders, and relapse rates: programs that effectively integrate mental health and substance use treatment have better outcomes than parallel or sequential treatment systems (Vekaria et al., 2021).

Various therapeutic techniques have been found to improve both SUD and MDD symptoms when targeted independently, and the limited research available has suggested promising results for using these approaches to manage co-occurring disorders. This success may be a result of targeting the common psychological, behavioral, and biological processes underlying both disorders simultaneously. For example, increased stress and rumination are strongly associated with both MDD and SUD: people who ruminate tend to have difficulty with cognitive shifting, and are vulnerable to persistent depression and substance use. Likewise, exposure to stress is associated with MDD, substance use, and cravings for substances. Therapeutic approaches that address these vulnerabilities may offer relief from co-occurring symptoms (Brewer et al., 2010). The following sections and integrated case study review methods for treating co-occurring SUDs and MDD concurrently.

Case Study: Max

Max is a 27-year-old single, employed male who works in construction. He started drinking when he was 18, mostly in a binge pattern when he went out and socialized on the weekends. Over the years, he found himself drinking with increasing frequency, leading to daily alcohol use, which he has sustained for the past 3 years. Typically, he drinks between 5 and 10 beers after he comes home from work. Though he has tried to make rules for himself to drink less frequently during the week, he usually ends up breaking them. At most, he has been able to abstain for 1 or 2 days at a time once or twice a month, noting that he experiences withdrawal symptoms including anxiety and insomnia when he tries to cut back or stop drinking.

Although Max has never been in treatment to address his alcohol use, he has received psychotherapy in the past for depression and anxiety. However, his episodes of treatment have been brief, involving a few supportive counseling sessions with different therapists. Max made an evaluation appointment with a therapist, noting that he needed help to stop drinking because it has been causing him to gain weight and having a negative impact on his mood and anxiety. When the therapist asked him what he felt he needed help with the most, he stated, "I've come to recognize that drinking in moderation doesn't work for me. I need to stop but I can't do it on my own."

We'll return to Max's case as we review the different psychosocial evidence-based treatment modalities that benefit individuals with co-occurring substance use disorders and mood or anxiety symptomatology.

Motivational Interviewing

Motivational interviewing (MI) is a person-centered style of counseling that explores patient readiness for change. MI focuses on building the patient-clinician relationship, eliciting change talk, exploring and resolving ambivalence to promote sustainable behavior change. This approach can be delivered as a brief intervention on its own, or used to enrich other skills-based approaches such as cognitive behavioral therapy (Hettema et al., 2005). MI is also the foundation of motivational enhancement therapy (MET); initially designed to promote abstinence from alcohol, MET uses MI techniques to specifically enhance motivation for addressing substance use behaviors. MET is brief in nature, and is typically completed within four to six sessions.

MI is rooted in research demonstrating that the quality of the therapeutic relationship is associated with treatment retention, engagement, and, independent of the actual therapeutic materials covered, outcomes. With this is mind, although MI is typically not used for the purpose of managing psychiatric symptoms, its positive impact on the therapeutic alliance creates a solid foundation on which an individual can develop a treatment plan emphasizing health behavior change. Disorders such as SUD and major depression tend to be chronic, with a variable clinical course; a supportive therapeutic alliance encourages patients to remain in care longer, and to reach out for additional support if needed after the conclusion of treatment. In addition, rapport and trust are fundamental and consistently emphasized throughout the treatment process, making the MI approach ideal to augment content-driven programs. Without a strong therapeutic alliance, patients may miss out on important concepts in content focused interventions due to the premature discontinuation of care (Kelly et al., 2012).

MI promotes autonomy, and encourages patients to set their own intentions; counselors do not use "tricks" to get the patient to do what they think is best, they listen to understand the patient's motivations with the understanding that people generally want to make changes that better themselves (Hettema et al., 2005). In fact, sustain talk (statements endorsing the status quo behaviors) and discord are no longer viewed as resistance; on the contrary, counselors can align these contextual cues with the patient's readiness to change, and adjust their approach to connect with the patient's needs. To elicit change talk, MI promotes the use of:

- Open-ended questions
- Affirming
- Reflective listening
- Summarizing

While meeting with a patient, it is important to listen for change talk, as it can be easy to miss. This dialogue can emerge in various ways, and can provide openings for further exploration. Examples of change talk include:

- *Desire* statements indicating a preference for change: "I would feel so much healthier if I stopped smoking."
- *Ability* statements describing their capability: "I can drink less with some support."
- *Reasons* statements discussing change: "If I didn't smoke, I would be able to exercise for longer."
- *Need* statements explaining the importance of change: "I really should cut back on how much I'm drinking, for my health."

As change talk evolves into planning, the patient will then begin to offer action-based dialogue:

- *Commitment* statements discussing intentions: "I am going to stop using methamphetamine next week."
- *Activation* statements expressing a willingness to change: "I am going to go to a SMART Recovery meeting on Tuesday."
- *Taking steps* statements outlining actions already taken: "This week, I called my counselor."

The Transtheoretical Model

When crafting behavior change plans, understanding a person's readiness to change prompts thoughtful decisions about next steps. The Transtheoretical Model (TTM) parallels motivational interviewing, as it describes a patient's readiness for change and serves as a guide for treatment planning. TTM is not a counseling theory; rather, it breaks behavior change down into psychological stages that shift fluidly in an individual over time. The stages are as follows:

- *Precontemplation* indicates a person has no intention to take action, and/or has no perceived need for change. They may not have adequate information about the negative consequences that can result from their engagement in a behavior, or they may have experienced several "failed" attempts at change and have given up; regardless, it is common for people in this stage to avoid the topic of the problematic behavior.
- *Contemplation* describes those who are considering change, and exploring their ambivalence. They have insight into the pros and cons of the behavior, and have not committed to action or change.
- *Preparation* is characterized by the intent to act; a person has made the decision to change, and is aiming to do so in the near future. They have taken steps to work towards their goal (e.g., researched treatment options, reduced exposure to high-risk situations, talked with their friends, purchased a self-help book, etc.), and are creating a plan for moving forward.
- *Action* consists of overt, observable steps taken to modify behavior. A person in the action stage of change demonstrates effort and commitment over time, and is progressing towards their goal.
- *Maintenance* is the continuation of action steps for more than 6 months. A person in the maintenance stage of change may not need to utilize change processes as often, as they notice their new behaviors becoming automatic, and they feel more confident in their new routine. However, without continued maintenance of protective factors, they will be at risk for resuming previous behavior patterns (*Relapse*).

Although it is typical for a person to sequentially progress through the stages of change, it is also common for people to transfer without order: for example, someone in the maintenance stage may experience an event that leads them back to contemplation. To account for this movement, the TTM stages are often drawn as a spiral relationship (Petrocelli, 2002).

Many SUD treatment programs are designed to be action-oriented; this is an excellent fit for people in the preparation and action stages of change, and may not be adequate support for others who have not committed to change. Some people who are engaging in care for their substance use or other psychiatric condition have external motivation for doing so (e.g., family, friends, courts) and present to treatment in the precontemplation and contemplation stages of change. Because these individuals may not be ready for action, they are often labeled as "unmotivated" or "resistant." TTM challenges that conception, and instead puts the burden on the treatment providers to better meet the person where they are in their readiness to change.

Using MI to Engage Max

In Max's case, the therapist uses core MI techniques to engage him in treatment for his co-occurring alcohol use and depressive and anxiety disorder symptoms, and to reinforce the connection he has already observed between them.

Therapist I'm hearing you say that your ideal scenario is being able to drink alcohol in moderation, but you're learning through experience that it's really hard to make that work.

Max Yeah, as time goes by, I feel less and less in control, and that's not a good feeling.

Therapist You're less in control over how much you drink.

Max True, but it's not just that. It's also how drinking affects me.

Therapist Can you say more about that?

Max Well, I feel sad for no reason for at least the first half or even three quarters of the day after I drink a lot, and I'm all jittery when I wake up. That didn't used to happen to me.

In the above dialogue, the therapist used reflective listening and open-ended questions to facilitate Max's openness about his goal to control his alcohol use. In doing so, she establishes the psychological safety that Max needs to open up about his experience of loss of control over drinking, as well as his insights about the negative consequences of his use. In this next section, the therapist helps him to explore his ambivalence about change and figure out some reasonable next steps he can take to approach the change process in a way that feels comfortable to him.

Therapist It sounds like you're struggling with wanting to control your drinking and feeling like at times you're not able to. From what you've described, you're also noticing that as this happens more, you're feeling less and less like yourself psychologically.

Max Yes, exactly.

Therapist I want you to know that this is not at all uncommon. When drinking increases, your body and mind's response to alcohol entering and leaving your system can intensify. It sounds like when alcohol is wearing off, it affects your mood and anxiety, which is normal. But now that you're drinking more than before, those changes in your mood are more pronounced and uncomfortable.

Max Yeah, it's pretty bad. Does this mean I can't drink anymore?

Therapist Well, that's one approach, but it's not your only option. Let's think about that. How do you think it would change things for you if you were to stop drinking?

Max Well, at this point, I feel like quitting might be my only option, because nothing changes when I try to cut back; I can't seem to do it. If I were to quit, I'm hoping that I would feel less sad and anxious and more like myself again.

Therapist You're starting to generate a list of reasons why quitting could be the best goal for you right now, and eliminating sadness and anxiety are at the top. Let's explore what else would be on this list.

In the second part of the dialogue, the therapist continued to use motivational techniques to explore Max's ambivalence about the issue of controlling versus quitting drinking. Leaving the options up to Max, he started to make what are referred to as *self-motivational statements* about changing his drinking and why quitting might be a better suited goal to help him overcome his psychological problems. These types of statements, also known as "change talk," are associated with positive behavior change and treatment outcomes (Magill et al., 2018). As Max begins to discuss how quitting drinking might improve his mental health, the therapist uses the opportunity to engage him in a "Reasons for Quitting" exercise, in which he will build motivation by exploring additional anticipated benefits of changing his alcohol use.

Cognitive Behavioral Therapy

Cognitive behavioral therapy (CBT) is a structured intervention approach that focuses on the present, and the interacting dynamics of a person's thoughts, feelings, and behaviors. According to the cognitive behavioral model, dysfunctional thoughts arise as a result of an individual's core beliefs about themselves, their world, and their future (Fenn & Byrne, 2013). From the perspective that dysfunctional thought patterns cultivate psychological disorders, coupled with the tendency to interpret situations based on how one *perceives* events (which can at times be illogical), CBT encourages patients to identify unhelpful thoughts or emotional responses to various cues, and replace them with healthy coping techniques (Fenn & Byrne, 2013). In the context of substance use and depression, patients use CBT-based skills to reframe core dysfunctional thoughts and beliefs that drive behavior, such as exploring negative thoughts stimulated by specific cues that exacerbate depression symptoms, or interrupting thoughts about using a substance that may lead a person to engage in unhealthy behaviors, such as drinking or using drugs (Osilla et al., 2009; Vujanovic et al., 2017).

Apart from recognizing and challenging one's unhealthy thoughts, another goal of CBT is to provide patients with problem-solving skills. In problem-solving, patients learn to identify the issue, utilize appropriate coping skills, reflect on what worked and what didn't to solve the problem, and adjust accordingly for the next challenge that arises. To achieve this, counselors use a "guided discovery" approach that prompts self-awareness without clinical instructions (Fenn & Byrne, 2013). Elements of CBT used in SUD treatment include case conceptualization, functional analysis, cognitive and motivational strategies, and skills training (McHugh et al., 2010). Similar approaches are used in CBT for depression such as increasing participation in daily activities (e.g., tracking daily activities, using positive reinforcers, setting SMART goals, and journaling), social competency skills (e.g., improving self-confidence, solving problems, engaging in helping behavior), and cognitive techniques (e.g., recognizing that thoughts are not facts, understanding the connection between thoughts, emotions, and behaviors, approaching problems objectively, and identifying automatic thoughts) (Lehner-Adam & Dudas, 2013). Similar to MI, CBT relies on therapeutic alliance, grounded in the clinician's expression of genuineness and empathy (Fenn & Byrne, 2013). Psychoeducation is another critical component of CBT, as patients are provided information on their diagnoses, the therapeutic process, and stress management and relaxation techniques (Khoury & Ammar, 2014).

Useful CBT exercises include:

- Recognizing cognitive distortions
- ABC functional analysis
- Journaling
- Practicing healthy coping techniques
- Recording and challenging dysfunctional thoughts
- Pleasant activity scheduling
- Mindfulness-based techniques

Using CBT to Help Max Build Relapse Prevention Skills

Max decided that he's ready to start working towards the goal of abstaining from alcohol. His therapist provides some education around relapse triggers, which can be external (i.e., tied to cues in the environment that can lead to temptation to drink, such as people he usually drinks with), or internal (i.e., emotions or other internal states that lead to the desire to drink).

Therapist You mentioned that sometimes your mood can trigger drinking. Can you say a little more about how that unfolds?

Max Well, sometimes when I feel sad, I just get this overwhelming feeling that it won't go away, and the only thing I feel I can do in those moments is drink.

Therapist That's a really good insight to help us understand how sadness and drinking are connected for you. I'd like to "unpack" that a little more if you're willing.

Max Sure, we can try.

Therapist There's a way that we understand how triggers lead to certain behaviors that people want to change, like drinking. Usually there's a trigger first (like that sad and overwhelmed feeling), and that trigger leads to a thought. The thought is often the key to understanding how and why you make the decision to drink, even if you're not fully aware of that connection at the time when the decision is made. It sounded to me like the thought might be about the overwhelming feeling, and whether there's any way to make it stop. Is that right?

Max Yes, that sounds right. The thought is "This is never going to go away."

Therapist And what feeling is connected to that?

Max I think it's a hopeless feeling. Does that make sense?

Therapist That makes a lot of sense—if you think you're stuck with a really uncomfortable feeling indefinitely, that would naturally lead to feeling hopeless. So it sounds like feeling overwhelmed leads you to have thoughts that there's really no solution to it, and that brings on a hopeless feeling.

Max Yeah, and it's that hopeless feeling that makes me want to drink.

In the above dialogue, the therapist helped Max understand the sequence of Trigger → Thought → Emotion → Behavior (Drinking). Now that he has broken that process down, the therapist can work with him to generate some alternative thoughts about the overwhelmed feeling (e.g., "I have tools that can help me resolve this," or "I have come out of this feeling before, even though it isn't easy") and teach him some coping skills that he can practice when he is feeling this way, including thought challenging, seeking social support, mindfulness meditation, and other activities that may be helpful in those moments to replace drinking behavior.

Substantial research on the long-term outcomes of CBT indicates this approach leads to durable and sustainable behavior change (Fenn & Byrne, 2013). This approach has been validated by an extensive history of strong empirical evidence, and demonstrates efficacy at reducing depression (including minor symptoms), substance use, and consequences due to substance use (HIDES et al., 2010; Osilla et al., 2009). Given its individual positive impact on SUDs and MDD, as well as its overlapping procedures/approaches for both disorders, utilizing CBT for co-occurring SUD and MDD is a logical step. Ongoing research will continue to build on the known effectiveness of CBT, as well as its compared efficacy to other psychotherapies.

Behavioral Activation

Behavioral Activation (BA) aims to increase engagement in healthy coping skills, and simultaneously decrease maladaptive behaviors (Martínez-Vispo et al., 2018). Developed initially as an evidence-based approach to alleviating depressive symptoms, BA targets positive reinforcement from pleasant activities, which individuals with depression often feel unmotivated to initiate, fueling the cycle of inactivity, few rewards or reinforcers to lift one's mood, and sustained depression. BA has been modified to also treat SUDs, as many people with these co-occurring disorders have inadequate environmental positive reinforcements (Vujanovic et al., 2017). Studies have found that people with SUDs have limited exposure to activities that do not focus on substance use, and encouraging engagement in such activities (such as exercise, journaling, painting, and other pleasurable hobbies) produces reductions in substance use (Martínez-Vispo et al., 2018).

Targeting the similar biological mechanisms of both MDD and SUDs on positive reinforcement, this approach seeks to reduce behavioral responses to depression (such as avoidance and inactivity), overcome positive and negative reinforcements of substance use, and promote pleasure in experiences outside of substance use (Pott et al., 2022). BA demonstrates its CBT origins by incorporating a variety of behavioral therapy approaches, including scheduling daily pleasant activities decreasing avoidance, and promoting relaxation, use of problem-solving skills, and use of self-monitoring strategies (Pott et al., 2022; Vujanovic et al., 2017). In addition to addressing maladaptive behaviors, newer approaches to BA explore factors that contribute to behavior change, such as individual relationships, strengths, and values. Different variations of BA highlight different treatment needs; for example, Brief Behavioral Activation Treatment for Depression (BATD) focuses on treating depression symptoms, while Behavioral Activation Treatment for Smoking (BATS) emphasizes abstinence from tobacco. Both of these programs have reported promising health outcomes; in addition, preliminary results from other BA programs demonstrate reduced severity of depression and improved residential SUD treatment retention (Vujanovic et al., 2017).

Patient exercises that support a BA approach include:

- Monitoring daily activities
- Identifying patient values and goals, building an action plan that aligns with these strengths
- Scheduling activities that bring joy and pleasure
- Proactively identifying and solving barriers that may prevent healthy activity engagement

Using Behavioral Activation to Help Max Engage in Pleasurable Activities

Max has been working with his therapist to better understand the connection between his internal mood states and his alcohol cravings and use patterns. To more fully address his complaints about depressed mood, the therapist explores how behavioral activation techniques might play a role in his treatment.

Therapist I'd like to spend some time talking about the sources of pleasure in your life, and the types of activities that you do or used to do that you find enjoyable.

Max Well, I used to do a lot more things for fun and to feel good than I am doing right now.

Therapist	Do you know why you are doing less of those things right now?
Max	I think that when I'm down, it's just hard to find the energy and motivation to do more than the bare minimum.
Therapist	That is understandable. You have to push yourself and sometimes it feels too hard to do that.
Max	Yeah. I'm not very good at pushing myself.
Therapist	Well, if you were to push yourself, what sorts of things would you be trying to do more of?
Max	I really enjoy mountain biking; I used to go every weekend and sometimes even after work during the week, but I haven't been out riding for over 4 months.
Therapist	That's a great example of a pleasurable activity, because not only is it something you enjoy, but studies show that exercise can have a very positive effect on mood. Can you describe what goes through your mind when the idea of biking comes up for you?
Max	At first, I tell myself, "I should go biking," but then I start thinking of all the steps and the effort it will take, and I just lose my enthusiasm.
Therapist	You feel like it's just too much trouble.
Max	I guess I know it's good for me, but it doesn't feel worth the effort, and I wonder if when I'm biking, I'm going to feel so out of shape that my stamina will be low, and then that will make me feel even worse about myself.
Therapist	It sounds like you are making a lot of assumptions about how it will go and what you will feel like if you do it. This is a really common cycle when a person is feeling depressed and unmotivated; it's natural to make predictions about what things will be like when you do them, but when you're feeling down, you're much more likely to imagine things going badly than well.
Max	That's probably true.
Therapist	One of the treatment approaches we can explore is called "behavioral activation." It's based on the idea that when people are down, they feel less motivated to do things, but by eliminating pleasurable activities, they lose access to many of the things that used to lift their mood. This can become a vicious cycle and worsen depression.

Max's therapist helped him recognize how his mood has been impacting his engagement in pleasant activities, and she provided some education about the Behavioral Activation therapy model. Towards the end of the dialogue, she provided the rationale for Pleasure Predicting, an exercise in which individuals rate the amount of pleasure they expect to experience from an activity, and they rate the actual pleasure during and immediately after the activity. This enables the individual to: (1) objectively evaluate how their mood affects their expectations about an activity, and (2) gather data to inform which activities they actually enjoy and should continue pursuing versus those that do not bring them as much pleasure. Cognitions at each stage can also be recorded as part of this exercise, to examine how common thinking errors affect the ability to feel pleasure, and where indicated, work on challenging irrational thoughts (for example "I'm not good at this, I might as well give up.").

Although the research on BA for co-occurring SUD and MDD is somewhat limited, the current evidence suggests that it is a promising approach with positive preliminary outcomes (Pott et al., 2022).

Mindfulness-Based Relapse Prevention

Mindfulness-based relapse prevention (MBRP) is a blend of mindfulness techniques with CBT-based relapse prevention skills training designed to promote awareness of the moment-to-moment experiences that lead to relapse vulnerability. This enables the individual to "respond mindfully" rather than react in a habitual or automatized way that leads to recurrent substance use. Building on the mindfulness-based cognitive therapy intervention for depression, MBRP fosters the understanding of high-risk situations, and the use of tools such as the practice of self-compassion and acceptance while managing stress, to reduce the likelihood of resuming substance use (Penberthy et al., 2015; Zemestani & Ottaviani, 2016).

The use of mindfulness can be traced back to traditional practices in a variety of cultures and religions, such as Buddhism (Penberthy et al., 2015). According to Jon Kabat-Zinn, "Mindfulness is the awareness that arises from paying attention, on purpose, in the present moment, non-judgmentally." Essentially, mindfulness is a universal construct that promotes awareness of the present moment. This state of mind fosters curiosity without judgment; it awakens those on autopilot, and drives intentional actions (Brewer et al., 2010). Clinically, mindfulness-based interventions have demonstrated therapeutic benefits for those with SUDs, borderline personality disorder (BPD), depression, anxiety, and stress. For individuals with SUDs, mindfulness exercises have been particularly helpful to mitigate the abstinence violation effect, a common error in thinking during the process of addiction recovery, in which an individual who experiences any return to substance involvement interprets the event as a failure in their recovery, and decides to continue using substances as a result. The core nonjudgmental approach that characterizes mindfulness challenges thoughts of "failure," and encourages people to learn from each experience rather than succumb to perceptions of inability to avoid use of a substance (Penberthy et al., 2015).

MBRP fosters self-awareness in understanding both acute (high-risk situations, abstinence violation effect, lack of coping skills) and nonacute (lack of support, environmental challenges, urges, or cravings) risk factors for returning to substance involvement. The relapse prevention (RP) component of MBRP connects insights gained through mindfulness, with practical skills to minimize relapse risk, such as planning ahead for relapse triggers and healthy coping strategies. As a structured therapy, MBRP typically consists of eight 2-h sessions that explore skill-building, meditation, and reflections. The development of self-efficacy through these exercises provides additional protection against relapse (Penberthy et al., 2015).

MBRP has been shown in studies to effectively address both SUD and MDD symptoms in patients with co-occurring symptoms (Glasner-Edwards et al., 2017). This is likely in part accounted for by its focus on affect regulation. MBRP provides tools for managing urges and cravings, allowing patients to acknowledge the craving is happening without reacting to it. Over time, this new response to cravings may lead to reduced intensity in thoughts to use substances (Zemestani & Ottaviani, 2016).

MBRP consists of three primary components (Ramadas et al., 2021):

- Formal mindfulness practice
  - Body scans
  - Sitting meditation (focusing on breath, body, emotions, and thoughts)
  - Loving-kindness meditation
- Informal practice
  - Urge surfing
  - SOBER breathing exercises
  - Mindfulness movement, of daily activities
- Coping strategies
  - Adapting and utilizing informal practice techniques outside of therapeutic settings
  - Establishing coping skills that enhance a patient's capability and confidence to manage challenges

Using MBRP to Help Max Cope with Cravings

To help expand Max's skill set for coping with psychological discomfort without drinking, his therapist introduces the concept of mindfulness meditation in the dialogue below.

Therapist One theme that has come up many times since we started working together is that mood and anxiety symptoms can be triggering for you.

Max Yeah, that's true.

Therapist Sometimes behaviors that aren't really helpful or healthy can become like habits, so much so that you may find yourself doing them without even knowing how you got there. Does this sound like something you've experienced with drinking?

Max At times, yes. I don't really think about it every time I do it, I just sometimes do it. Is that what you mean?

Therapist Yes. And I'll take it one more step. It's not just that you find yourself doing it, but from what you've described, you probably find yourself

	drinking when you're anxious or sad. It's like you're on "auto pilot" sometimes without realizing it.
Max	That's probably right. How do I break that habit?
Therapist	It starts with what we call *mindful awareness*. It takes practice to make this second nature, but you can start by intentionally paying attention to what you're thinking and feeling when you have an urge to drink. Right now, you're probably avoiding those uncomfortable experiences by giving into the urge and reaching for a drink.
Max	So, when I feel the urge to drink, I should pay attention to my thoughts?
Therapist	Yes. But that's hard to do. First, we can work together to train your mind to pay attention to how you're feeling, and the way to "build that muscle" in your brain is to do meditation exercises.
Max	I'm not sure if that will help, but I'm willing to try it.
Therapist	Your willingness to try is the most important part. Let's start with a meditation called the "Body Scan." This will help you learn to pay attention, nonjudgmentally, to different sensations in your body.
Max	Okay!

Max's therapist will start introducing the Body Scan meditation in session, and will conduct what is known as "Inquiry" after completion of meditation exercises. The Inquiry process will help Max describe what he noticed during the meditation (i.e., what were some of the challenging aspects of paying attention in this particular way? What did he observe in his body? Was this familiar?). Over time, Max will be introduced to other meditations (e.g., meditations focusing on the breath, as well as on thoughts, and compassion or loving-kindness), including the SOBER breathing exercise (Bowen et al., 2021; Glasner-Edwards, 2015). The SOBER breathing exercise can be used in a tempting moment to help Max observe what he is experiencing that leads to his craving, and to anchor himself to his breath for a few moments before choosing a course of action. The goal of this exercise is to move away from "reacting" to temptation and instead, engaging in a "mindful response," after he has observed and gained a better understanding of what was driving the craving.

Other Evidence-Based Approaches

Pharmacotherapy is another evidence-based approach to treatment of co-occurring MDD and SUD. Both addiction pharmacotherapy and medications targeting depression can be very helpful for individuals who are experiencing the conditions concurrently. According to a recent study, after 1 year, people prescribed medications for alcohol use disorder were less likely to utilize emergency care services (for a psychiatric or other condition), and evidenced higher psychiatric medication adherence (Yule & Kelly, 2019). Antidepressant medications appear to be most appropriate for those with depression experiencing moderate to severe symptoms, including selective serotonin reuptake inhibitors (SSRIs) and other medications (such as tricyclic antidepressants). For some, outcomes may be optimized from a combination of medication and psychotherapy (Iqbal et al., 2019), and possibly more than one medication—such as an antidepressant along with addiction pharmacotherapy (e.g., naltrexone) (Han et al., 2017).

Peer and community support organizations may offer an additional protective factor for those with co-occurring disorders. Although less common, a variety of peer groups exist to specifically support those with both SUD and MDD, including Dual Recovery Anonymous, Double Trouble in Recovery, and Dual Diagnosis Anonymous; SUD-specific groups, such as Alcoholics Anonymous, have also demonstrated some benefits for those with both AUD and MDD. Recently, there has also been an expansion in digital platforms offering peer support, including chat rooms and online groups that break down geographic barriers. Although more research is needed to assess the effectiveness of these peer support options, patients should be encouraged to explore their best fit options (Yule & Kelly, 2019).

Strategies for Strengthening Integrated Care

Despite robust evidence supporting the concurrent treatment of SUD and MDD, merely 11% of adults received integrated care for their mental health and substance use disorder (Vekaria et al., 2021), owing largely to a variety of challenges that limit the availability of integrated care options. For example, treatment programs have traditionally operated in silos with a focus on determining the "primary" disorder and referring patients to another treatment setting for the "secondary" disorder. In addition, clinician training for integrating treatments targeting SUD and mood disorders is limited (Yule & Kelly, 2019). While it can be challenging to determine the temporal sequencing and relative severity of primary and secondary disorder onset, ultimately a primary versus secondary determination of SUD and MDD may be irrelevant once symptoms have set in (Ross et al., 2016).

Further complicating implementation of integrated treatments, extant research on evidence-based approaches to addressing co-occurring SUD and MDD have various methodological limitations, including potential confounding factors such as results that may be impacted by clinician licensure, individual versus group therapy modalities, and level of community collaboration (Osilla et al., 2009). Moreover, systematic reviews have found both a limited number of quality studies evaluating interventions for co-occurring disorders, and a wide range of variables (e.g., patient, clinician, and treatment-related factors) that vary from study to study and limit robust conclusions (HIDES et al., 2010). In the sections that follow, we consider approaches that may help to overcome these barriers.

Screening and Brief Intervention for Substance Use Disorders

Screenings for various health conditions (e.g., hypertension, diabetes, cancer) are a routine part of primary care. However, screenings for SUDs have been minimal, particularly for certain vulnerable subgroups including adolescents and racial and ethnic minorities (Yule & Kelly, 2019).

Validated screening tools for identifying substance use issues in primary care settings include:

- Alcohol Use Disorders Identification Test (AUDIT)
- Tobacco, Alcohol, Prescription Medication, and Other Substance Use (TAPS)
- National Institute on Drug Abuse (NIDA) Quick Screen
- Brief Screener for Tobacco, Alcohol, and Other Drugs (BSTAD) for adolescents

Screening, Brief Intervention, and Referral to Treatment (SBIRT), a motivational intervention designed to reduce risky substance use, mitigate progression to substance use disorder, and link people who currently have an SUD to specialty treatment, has demonstrated efficacy for reducing unhealthy alcohol use in emergency department and primary care settings, particularly among those with low or moderate levels of use (Barata et al., 2017). In addition, in the first large multi-site randomized clinical trial evaluating the SBIRT approach in mental health treatment settings, SBIRT effectively reduced the frequency of heavy alcohol use and stimulant use, relative to an attention control condition among individuals receiving mental health treatment (Karno et al., 2021). Implementing brief screening protocols such as SBIRT in routine care settings can facilitate higher rates of SUD-MDD detection and treatment.

Incorporate Psychiatric Symptom Screening in SUD Assessments

Co-occurring MDD is common among those with SUDs, and the severity of depression symptoms is associated with poorer treatment adherence and heightened substance relapse risk. Because psychiatric symptoms can worsen SUD clinical course and outcomes, identifying those in SUD treatment settings who need additional support to address mental health difficulties may break down barriers to care and improve outcomes. As such, SUD care entry presents a critical opportunity for MDD screenings (Yule & Kelly, 2019). Clinicians should explore patient history of psychiatric conditions, family history, and refer for evaluation of other health conditions such as hypothyroidism as appropriate; in cases where patient self-reports are inconsistent, gathering collateral information from family and friends may be appropriate to fill in historic gaps (DeVido & Weiss, 2012).

Given that co-occurring SUDs and MDD can be independent of each other (i.e., depressive symptoms persist even after substance use or withdrawal symptoms have ceased) or dependent (i.e., depression symptoms are the result of substance intoxication or withdrawal, and may abate with sustained abstinence from substances), obtaining a timeline to understand temporal sequencing and persistence of symptoms during any periods of abstinence or sobriety can be helpful diagnostically. Ongoing reassessments can be completed over a period of time to gain a deeper understanding of the time course of an individual's symptoms (Yule & Kelly, 2019). Well validated depression screening instruments include the Patient Health Questionnaire-9 item scale (PHQ-9), Hamilton Depression Rating Scale, and Center for Epidemiological Studies-Depression Scale (CES-D).

Blend Evidence-Based Treatment Methods

Many of the therapies discussed have common threads that connect and can be readily integrated or combined. Rather than creating new manuals for each disorder (CBT for depression, CBT for anxiety), these transdiagnostic approaches target maladaptive mechanisms in co-occurring disorders to address shared processes seen in both SUD and MDD, including negative affect, anhedonia, rumination, experiential avoidance, emotion regulation, and distress tolerance (Vujanovic et al., 2017).

Therapies may also improve outcomes when used in conjunction with another; for example, CBT and MI are often integrated to offer comprehensive support for co-occurring disorders (Wüsthoff et al., 2014). These approaches complement each other well: utilizing MI throughout care mobilizes and sustains motivation over time, and CBT offers action steps that strengthen behavior changes. Likewise, research has found a combination of MI and CBT may be more effective in reducing alcohol use, managing depression, and increasing medication adherence than usual care (Naar & Safren, 2017).

Although it can be a standalone intervention, blending psychoeducation is another technique for enhancing other therapeutic approaches. Psychoeducation provides patients and their families with information about their diagnosis, and has been used in treatments for depression and SUDs to increase patient knowledge about symptom management and treatment benefits (Ekhtiari et al., 2017). Psychoeducation can increase patient insight into their disorder, which in turn, supports behavior change. This may be delivered in various modalities, including individual, group, or community-based programs, either through bibliotherapy or therapist-facilitated efforts. Individual and family psychoeducation is often provided after the determination of a depression diagnosis to encourage medication adherence and engagement in healthy activities, while group psychoeducation is a commonly used modality in SUD treatment (Sarkhel et al., 2020).

Integrate Technology

The use of technology in healthcare has historically been adapted to support the management of various illnesses (including diabetes), medication management, and smoking cessation. Recent research has found similar advantages to using technology in behavioral health treatment. Digital interventions that target behavioral health have been found to effectively elicit change, while offering many benefits, including reduced cost, remote monitoring, minimized patient concerns about stigma, and increased patient autonomy in deciding how they prefer to engage in treatment. Moreover, given the shortage of clinicians trained to work with concurrently diagnosed patients, technology-based treatments break down barriers to accessing evidence-based care for high need populations such as those with co-occurring disorders. Digital platforms can offer on-demand access to support, skills-based learning, and coping skills training; their programs can also be tailored, so people can find what they need in that moment (for example, access to guided meditations when a patient is experiencing cravings to drink). New research and reviews are actively determining best practices for digital interventions, which appear to be a feasible and efficacious option for people with co-occurring SUDs and MDD (Bonfiglio et al., 2022; Glasner et al., 2018; Kay-Lambkin et al., 2011). Therapeutic components include some level of clinician-facilitated support to augment digitally delivered therapeutic content, tailoring, contingency management, and gamification (Tofighi et al., 2018).

Reviewing Max's Case

The challenges Max faced when managing his substance misuse and depression symptoms are relatable to many with co-occurring disorders. During his initial assessment, Max acknowledged his past engagement in therapy did not adequately address his concerns, as his depression was not considered within the context of his alcohol use. Through the use of motivational interviewing, Max's therapist used reflective listening and open-ended questions to encourage self-motivational statements until Max felt ready to set goals around reducing symptoms of his co-occurring disorders. He then explored how he would go about abstaining from alcohol, as his therapist utilized Cognitive Behavioral Therapy to help him uncover clues about his triggers to drink (such as his depressed mood), the thoughts associated with that cue, and the resulting behavior (drinking alcohol).

With this insight, Max began to establish healthy alternative coping strategies that met the need (managing depression symptoms) he was attempting to address, albeit unsuccessfully, with alcohol use. Max's therapist incorporated Behavioral Activation to promote Max's engagement in enjoyable activities, such as biking, which in turn, could improve his mood. To further expand his toolbox for working through psychological discomfort, Max learned mindfulness-based relapse prevention techniques (such as meditation) to (a) recognize urges and cravings to drink, and (b) promote mindful responses rather than autopilot reactions. These therapeutic approaches may be integrated throughout sessions and enhanced with the use of psychoeducation and a motivational interviewing style. Max may also discuss with his therapist options for pharmacotherapy and/or peer support, depending on his preferences.

Conclusion

Given the high prevalence of overlapping SUDs and mood disorders, leveraging evidence-based strategies for managing major depression concurrently with alcohol and other substance use disorders is important to optimize treatment engagement and outcomes. Some of the most well-studied approaches to treatment of these co-occurring disorders include motivational interviewing combined with various empirically based interventions such as cognitive behavioral therapy, mindfulness-based relapse prevention, and behavioral activation treatment. In this chapter, we reviewed each of these treatments, examined a clinical case in which they were implemented, and considered the overarching integrated treatment model in which therapies addressing psychiatric symptoms and substance use are delivered concurrently. Pharmacotherapy addressing both SUD and depressive symptoms can be an efficacious component of treatment for this high need population, and should be considered along with patient needs, acuity, and preferences. Finally, there is promising evidence suggesting that many of the intervention approaches that are effective in ameliorating depressive symptoms and substance use can be delivered digitally, expanding patient options for care delivery access and modalities.

References

Barata, I. A., Shandro, J. R., Montgomery, M., Polansky, R., Sachs, C. J., Duber, H. C., Weaver, L. M., Heins, A., Owen, H. S., & Josephson, E. B. (2017). Effectiveness of SBIRT for alcohol use disorders in the emergency department: A systematic review. *Western Journal of Emergency Medicine, 18*(6), 1143.

Baskin-Sommers, A. R., & Foti, D. (2015). Abnormal reward functioning across substance use disorders and major depressive disorder: Considering reward as a transdiagnostic mechanism. *International Journal of Psychophysiology, 98*(2), 227–239.

Bonfiglio, N. S., Mascia, M. L., & Penna, M. P. (2022). Digital treatment paths for substance use disorders (SUDs). *International Journal of Environmental Research and Public Health, 19*(12), 7322.

Bowen, S., Chawla, N., Grow, J., & Marlatt, G. A. (2021). *Mindfulness-based relapse prevention for addictive behaviors*. Guilford Publications.

Brewer, J. A., Bowen, S., Smith, J. T., Marlatt, G. A., & Potenza, M. N. (2010). Mindfulness-based treatments for co-occurring depression and substance use disorders: What can we learn from the brain? *Addiction, 105*(10), 1698–1706. https://doi.org/10.1111/j.1360-0443.2009.02890.x

Conner, K. R., Pinquart, M., & Gamble, S. A. (2009). Meta-analysis of depression and substance use among individuals with alcohol use disorders. *Journal of Substance Abuse Treatment, 37*(2), 127–137.

DeVido, J. J., & Weiss, R. D. (2012). Treatment of the depressed alcoholic patient. *Current Psychiatry Reports, 14*, 610–618.

Ekhtiari, H., Rezapour, T., Aupperle, R. L., & Paulus, M. P. (2017). Neuroscience-informed psychoeducation for addiction medicine: A neurocognitive perspective. *Progress in Brain Research, 235*, 239–264.

Fenn, K., & Byrne, M. (2013). The key principles of cognitive behavioural therapy. *InnovAiT, 6*(9), 579–585. https://doi.org/10.1177/1755738012471029

Glasner, S., Kay-Lambkin, F., Budney, A. J., Gitlin, M., Kagan, B., Chokron-Garneau, H., Ang, A., & Venegas, A. (2018). Preliminary outcomes of a computerized CBT/MET intervention for depressed cannabis users in psychiatry care. *Cannabis (Research Society on Marijuana), 1*(2), 36.

Glasner-Edwards, S. (2015). *The addiction recovery skills workbook: Changing addictive behaviors using CBT, mindfulness, and motivational interviewing techniques*. New Harbinger Publications.

Glasner-Edwards, S., Mooney, L. J., Ang, A., Garneau, H. C., Hartwell, E., Brecht, M. L., & Rawson, R. A. (2017). No title. Mindfulness based relapse prevention for stimulant dependent adults: A pilot randomized clinical trial. *Mindfulness, 8*(1), 126–135.

Han, B., Olfson, M., & Mojtabai, R. (2017). Depression care among adults with co-occurring major depressive episodes and substance use disorders in the United States. *Journal of Psychiatric Research, 91*, 47–56.

Hettema, J., Steele, J., & Miller, W. R. (2005). Motivational interviewing. *Annual Review of Clinical Psychology, 1*, 91–111.

Hides, L., Samet, S., & Lubman, D. I. (2010). Cognitive behaviour therapy (CBT) for the treatment of co-occurring depression and substance use: Current evidence and directions for future research. *Drug and Alcohol Review, 29*(5), 508–517. https://doi.org/10.1111/j.1465-3362.2010.00207.x

Hunter, S. B., Watkins, K. E., Hepner, K. A., Paddock, S. M., Ewing, B. A., Osilla, K. C., & Perry, S. (2012). Treating depression and substance use: A randomized controlled trial. *Journal of Substance Abuse Treatment, 43*(2), 137–151.

Iqbal, M. N., Levin, C. J., & Levin, F. R. (2019). Treatment for substance use disorder with co-occurring mental illness. *FOCUS, 17*(2), 88–97. https://doi.org/10.1176/appi.focus.20180042

Karno, M. P., Rawson, R., Rogers, B., Spear, S., Grella, C., Mooney, L. J., Saitz, R., Kagan, B., & Glasner, S. (2021). Effect of screening, brief intervention and referral to treatment for unhealthy alcohol and other drug use in mental health treatment settings: A randomized controlled trial. *Addiction, 116*(1), 159–169.

Kay-Lambkin, F., Baker, A., Lewin, T., & Carr, V. (2011). Acceptability of a clinician-assisted computerized psychological intervention for comorbid mental health and substance use problems: Treatment adherence data from a randomized controlled trial. *Journal of Medical Internet Research, 13*(1), e1522.

Kelly, T. M., Daley, D. C., & Douaihy, A. B. (2012). Treatment of substance abusing patients with comorbid psychiatric disorders. *Addictive Behaviors, 37*(1), 11–24.

Khoury, B., & Ammar, J. (2014). Cognitive behavioral therapy for treatment of primary care patients presenting with psychological disorders. *Libyan Journal of Medicine, 9*(1), 24186. https://doi.org/10.3402/ljm.v9.24186

Langås, A., Malt, U. F., & Opjordsmoen, S. (2013). Independent versus substance-induced major depressive disorders in first-admission patients with substance use disorders: An exploratory study. *Journal of Affective Disorders, 144*(3), 279–283. https://doi.org/10.1016/j.jad.2012.10.008

Lazareck, S., Robinson, J. A., Crum, R. M., Mojtabai, R., Sareen, J., & Bolton, J. M. (2012). A longitudinal investigation of the role of self-medication in the development of comorbid mood and drug use disorders: Findings from the national epidemiologic survey on alcohol and related conditions (NESARC). *The Journal of Clinical Psychiatry, 73*(5), 10579.

Lehner-Adam, I., & Dudas, B. (2013). Cognitive behavioral therapy (CBT) of depressive disorders. *Mood Disorders, 61*.

Magidson, J. F., Wang, S., Lejuez, C. W., Iza, M., & Blanco, C. (2013). Prospective study of substance-induced and independent major depressive disorder among individuals with substance use disorders in a nationally representative sample. *Depression and Anxiety, 30*(6), 538–545. https://doi.org/10.1002/da.22122

Magill, M., Apodaca, T. R., Borsari, B., Gaume, J., Hoadley, A., Gordon, R. E., Tonigan, J. S., & Moyers, T. (2018). A meta-analysis of motivational interviewing process: Technical, relational, and conditional process models of change. *Journal of Consulting and Clinical Psychology, 86*(2), 140.

Martínez-Vispo, C., Martínez, Ú., López-Durán, A., Fernandez del Rio, E., & Becoña, E. (2018). Effects of behavioural activation on substance use and depression: A systematic review. *Substance Abuse Treatment, Prevention, and Policy, 13*(1), 1–13.

McHugh, R. K., & Weiss, R. D. (2019). Alcohol use disorder and depressive disorders. *Alcohol Research: Current Reviews, 40*(1).

McHugh, R. K., Hearon, B. A., & Otto, M. W. (2010). Cognitive behavioral therapy for substance use disorders. *Psychiatric Clinics, 33*(3), 511–525.

Mojtabai, R., Chen, L., Kaufmann, C. N., & Crum, R. M. (2014). Comparing barriers to mental health treatment and substance use disorder treatment among individuals with comorbid major depression and substance use disorders. *Journal of Substance Abuse Treatment, 46*(2), 268–273.

Naar, S., & Safren, S. A. (2017). *Motivational interviewing and CBT: Combining strategies for maximum effectiveness*. Guilford Publications.

Osilla, K. C., Hepner, K. A., Muñoz, R. F., Woo, S., & Watkins, K. (2009). Developing an integrated treatment for substance use and depression using cognitive–behavioral therapy. *Journal of Substance Abuse Treatment, 37*(4), 412–420.

Otte, C., Gold, S. M., Penninx, B. W., Pariante, C. M., Etkin, A., Fava, M., Mohr, D. C., & Schatzberg, A. F. (2016). Major depressive disorder. *Nature Reviews Disease Primers, 2*(1), 1–20.

Penberthy, J. K., Konig, A., Gioia, C. J., Rodríguez, V. M., Starr, J. A., Meese, W., Worthington-Stoneman, D., Kersting, K., & Natanya, E. (2015). Mindfulness-based relapse prevention: History, mechanisms of action, and effects. *Mindfulness, 6*, 151–158.

Petrocelli, J. V. (2002). Processes and stages of change: Counseling with the transtheoretical model of change. *Journal of Counseling & Development, 80*(1), 22–30.

Pott, S. L., Delgadillo, J., & Kellett, S. (2022). Is behavioral activation an effective and acceptable treatment for co-occurring depression and substance use disorders? A meta-analysis of randomized controlled trials. *Journal of Substance Abuse Treatment, 132*, 108478.

Ramadas, E., de Lima, M. P., Caetano, T., Lopes, J., & dos Dixe, M. A. (2021). Effectiveness of mindfulness-based relapse prevention in individuals with substance use disorders: A systematic review. *Behavioral Sciences, 11*(10), 133.

Rehm, J., Marmet, S., Anderson, P., Gual, A., Kraus, L., Nutt, D. J., Room, R., Samokhvalov, A. V., Scafato, E., & Trapencieris, M. (2013). Defining substance use disorders: Do we really need more than heavy use? *Alcohol and Alcoholism, 48*(6), 633–640.

Revadigar, N., & Gupta, V. (2020). *Substance induced mood disorders*. StatPearls Publishing.

Ross, J., Teesson, M., Lejuez, C., Mills, K., Kaye, S., Brady, K., Dore, G., Prior, K., Larkin, X., & Cassar, J. (2016). The efficacy of behavioural activation treatment for co-occurring depression and substance use disorder (the activate study): A randomized controlled trial. *BMC Psychiatry, 16*, 1–14.

Sarkhel, S., Singh, O. P., & Arora, M. (2020). Clinical practice guidelines for psychoeducation in psychiatric disorders general principles of psychoeducation. *Indian Journal of Psychiatry, 62*(Suppl 2), S319.

Tofighi, B., Abrantes, A., & Stein, M. D. (2018). The role of technology-based interventions for substance use disorders in primary care: A review of the literature. *Medical Clinics, 102*(4), 715–731.

Turner, S., Mota, N., Bolton, J., & Sareen, J. (2018). Self-medication with alcohol or drugs for mood and anxiety disorders: A narrative review of the epidemiological literature. *Depression and Anxiety, 35*(9), 851–860.

Vekaria, V., Bose, B., Murphy, S. M., Avery, J., Alexopoulos, G., & Pathak, J. (2021). Association of co-occurring opioid or other substance use disorders with increased healthcare utilization in patients with depression. *Translational Psychiatry, 11*(1), 265.

Vujanovic, A. A., Meyer, T. D., Heads, A. M., Stotts, A. L., Villarreal, Y. R., & Schmitz, J. M. (2017). Cognitive-behavioral therapies for depression and substance use disorders: An overview of traditional, third-wave, and transdiagnostic approaches. *The American Journal of Drug and Alcohol Abuse, 43*(4), 402–415. https://doi.org/10.1080/00952990.2016.1199697

Watkins, L. E., Patton, S. C., Drexler, K., Rauch, S. A. M., & Rothbaum, B. O. (2022). Clinical effectiveness of an intensive outpatient program for integrated treatment of comorbid substance abuse and mental health disorders. *Cognitive and Behavioral Practice*. https://doi.org/10.1016/j.cbpra.2022.05.005

Wüsthoff, L. E., Waal, H., & Gråwe, R. W. (2014). The effectiveness of integrated treatment in patients with substance use disorders co-occurring with anxiety and/or depression-a group randomized trial. *BMC Psychiatry, 14*(1), 1–12.

Yule, A. M., & Kelly, J. F. (2019). Integrating treatment for co-occurring mental health conditions. *Alcohol Research: Current Reviews, 40*(1).

Zemestani, M., & Ottaviani, C. (2016). Effectiveness of mindfulness-based relapse prevention for co-occurring substance use and depression disorders. *Mindfulness, 7*(6), 1347–1355.

Chapter 5
Treating Comorbid Posttraumatic Stress Disorder and Substance Use Disorder

Chantel T. Ebrahimi, Jordan A. Gette, Tanya C. Saraiya, and Denise A. Hien

Prevalence of Posttraumatic Stress Disorder and Substance Use Disorders

Posttraumatic stress disorder (PTSD) may develop following exposure to a Criterion "A" traumatic event (i.e., either directly experienced, witnessed, or learned about affecting a close family or friend) and results in experiencing four distinct symptom clusters: intrusive thoughts, avoidance, negative cognitions and mood, and hyperarousal (American Psychiatric Association, 2013). In the *Diagnostic and Statistical Manual of Mental Disorders*—Fifth edition (*DSM-5*; American Psychiatric Association, 2013), a substance use disorder (SUD) diagnosis is defined as 11 symptoms falling in four broad domains of impaired control of use, impairment in quality of life due to substance use, increased tolerance or physical dependence on substances, and risky use that cover 11 different criteria or symptoms associated with the substance use. PTSD and SUDs are often comorbid disorders. In other words, these two separate disorders frequently occur simultaneously. The prevalence of these comorbid disorders has been rising over the last two decades. In the early 2000s, the prevalence rate of a current PTSD diagnosis among SUD patients was around 30–40% (Bonin et al., 2000; Kessler et al., 2005). Inversely, 50–75% of

C. T. Ebrahimi
Department of Psychology, The New School for Social Research, New York, NY, USA

J. A. Gette · T. C. Saraiya
Center of Alcohol and Substance Use Studies, Rutgers University, New Brunswick, NJ, USA
e-mail: denise.hien@rutgers.edu

D. A. Hien (✉)
Department of Psychiatry and Behavioral Sciences, Medical University of South Carolina, Charleston, USA

K. Wolitzky-Taylor (ed.), *Treating Comorbid Substance Use and Emotional Disorders*, CBT: Science Into Practice, https://doi.org/10.1007/978-3-031-62971-6_5

veterans with PTSD also had a SUD diagnosis (Kulka et al., 1990). In 2012, the prevalence rate of PTSD in SUD patients was on average around 40% and ranged from 10% to 86% in non-SUD patients (Gielen et al., 2012). In 2016, from the National Epidemiologic Survey on Alcohol and Related Conditions–III, individuals with SUD were 1.6 times more likely to have a PTSD diagnosis than those without a SUD (Grant et al., 2016). In veterans, the likelihood for comorbidity with AUD and PTSD was 2.1 times greater and for other SUD and PTSD was 3.1 times greater (Goldstein et al., 2016; Grant et al., 2016).

Comorbid PTSD-SUD is associated with a more severe profile versus either disorder alone. For example, PTSD can interfere with nighttime sleep and thereby contribute to a feeling of "numbness" or irritability during the day. As a result, an individual with comorbid PTSD-SUD may understandably turn to substances to cope with their difficulties sleeping. Unfortunately, this habitual trend can ironically only worsen the severity of their PTSD symptoms. Compared to either disorder presenting alone, comorbid PTSD-SUD is associated with a wider range of difficulties, including a poorer treatment prognosis (Najt et al., 2011), greater likelihood for readmission to treatment (Ouimette et al., 1997), lower treatment compliance (Bradizza et al., 2006), and higher rates of suicide (McCauley et al., 2012). In addition, healthcare costs associated with treating PTSD-SUD are rising above $2 billion annually (Davis et al., 2022). Use of empirically supported treatments for PTSD-SUD could mitigate the public health burden associated with these disorders and substantially improve the quality of life for individuals with these disorders.

Brief Treatment History

With these high rates of comorbid PTSD-SUD, treatment studies across the globe have been implemented to help reduce PTSD and SUD symptoms individually, with a recent focus on concurrent treatment which we will elaborate on in this chapter. PTSD treatment, historically, has primarily only focused on trauma processing (i.e., "trauma-focused therapy"; Hien et al., 2022, 2023) such as Prolonged Exposure (PE; Foa et al., 2019) or Cognitive Processing Therapy (CPT; Resick et al., 2016). Seeking Safety (Najavits, 2002) emerged as a non-trauma-focused PTSD-SUD treatment that engages skill building to help live a better, sustainable life, as opposed to engaging in trauma processing or "re-living the trauma." Substance use treatments can be categorized in two domains: (1) abstinence models and (2) harm reductionist models. Historically, treatment for SUD was rooted in the medical model and designed as an abstinence-based programs (e.g., Alcoholics Anonymous or other 12-step treatment programs). Harm reduction models emerged in the early 2000s and shifted the focus from zero-use to identifying self-compassionate, pragmatic approaches to reducing harm associated with use and improving quality of life (Tatarsky, 2002).

Several decades of research show that treating these disorders independently leads to poorer treatment outcomes than treating them together (Hien et al., 2015;

Norman et al., 2019; Ruglass et al., 2017). There are three predominant models that theorize the connection between PTSD and SUD. The "self-medication hypothesis" (Khantzian, 1997) suggests that individuals with trauma exposure or PTSD symptoms may use substances to alleviate trauma-related distress. Put another way, dysregulated affect and distress in the wake of trauma drive substance misuse. The second explanatory model is the "high-risk hypothesis," which states that substance use may increase risk for exposure to traumatic events as it may place individuals in higher risk situations (Windle, 1994; Haller & Chassin, 2014). Proponents of the "high-risk hypothesis" may also suggest that individuals who use substances are further at risk for harm due to their impaired awareness and may not easily detect danger in their environment (Davis et al., 2009). Lastly, the "susceptibility hypothesis" suggests that individuals who use substances may increase their risk for developing PTSD following a traumatic event as their substance use problems may impair their emotion regulation skills or managing other PTSD symptoms (Chilcoat & Breslau, 1998). This may increase their anxiety (Stewart et al., 1998) or increase their avoidance of their trauma memories impairing their ability to process the trauma material (Kaysen et al., 2011). In particular, the self-medication hypothesis is largely supported by patient feedback, ecological momentary assessment studies, and the order of onset where the traumatic event precedes the onset of substance use (Back et al., 2014; Hawn et al., 2020).

The Sequential Model of Co-occurring PTSD & SUD Treatment

The sequential model of PTSD-SUD treatment focuses on treatment of the SUD(s) followed by treatment of PTSD after a period of sustained abstinence from substance use (McCauley et al., 2012). The underlying rationale for the sequential model is that continued substance use during PTSD treatment could interfere with PTSD treatment progress or that engagement in PTSD treatment could result in substance use relapse (Nace, 1998; Pitman et al., 1991). It is thought that if individuals engage in PTSD treatment prior to developing effective coping and relapse prevention skills, the increases in negative affect and hyperarousal associated with PTSD treatment could result in SUD relapse (Souza & Spates, 2008). Below, we review cognitive-behavioral approaches and treatment protocols for PTSD and SUD.

Cognitive Behavioral Therapy (CBT) Approaches to SUD

CBT for the treatment of SUDs span a wide range of approaches. Common elements underlying these treatments stem from the conceptualization that substance use reinforces or rewards behavior through positive (e.g., enhancing experiences) and negative (e.g., decreasing negative affect) reinforcement (McHugh et al., 2010). CBTs for SUD aim to weaken the reinforcing effects by cognitively restructuring thoughts that maintain use, enhancing behavioral skills, and introducing alternative reinforcers. Many approaches to SUD incorporate functional analysis (or behavioral chains) that help individuals identify the antecedents and consequences associated with substance use, or colloquially referred to as the ABCs (antecedents, behaviors, consequences). These functional chains serve as the basis for developing an individualized treatment plan to address substance use cognitively and behaviorally. Below, we provide an overview of two approaches to the treatment of SUDs: Relapse Prevention and Contingency Management.

Relapse Prevention

Relapse prevention (RP) is an individual or group CBT approach that targets substance use by altering responses to substance use cues (Kadden et al., 1992). Though RP can vary in session number, treatment length, and format, RP has two primary components: (1) identifying high-risk situations and triggers; and (2) skills development (Douaihy et al., 2007). Using functional analysis, individuals identify situations in which they are at higher risk of engaging in substance use (e.g., spending time with substance using peers). The patient and therapist work to identify internal and external cues associated with use and develop plans to either prevent or manage these situations. For example, in seemingly irrelevant decisions, the clinician and patient discuss a narrative that may increase risk of use. An example narrative is that a patient may drive by a bar in which they often drink with friends on their route home for work. Passing the bar on their commute could trigger an urge to drink or meet up with a peer who drinks. As such, creating a new commute home could serve as a tool for reducing the number of drinking cues the patient is exposed to. Cognitively, patients challenge thoughts related to substance use such as perceived benefits (e.g., "a drink will make this event more fun") and rationalization (e.g., "I can use just this once and be fine"). Behaviorally, patients may be encouraged to engage in experiments such as abstaining from use during a social gathering to aid in the cognitive restructuring. Patients also engage in behavioral components such as drug refusal, coping, and problem-solving skills. Across randomized controlled trials, RP has demonstrated small treatment effect sizes (Magill & Ray, 2009).

Recent modifications to traditional RP also incorporate mindfulness-based strategies to assist individuals with managing thoughts and physiological responses to substance use cues. Additional skills learned in mindfulness-based RP include nonjudgmental awareness and "urge surfing" which encourages patients to "ride the wave" of craving and observe it without engaging in use and without judging themselves (Witkiewitz et al., 2014). Mindfulness-based RP has gained strong empirical support for SUDs treatment (Grant et al., 2017). In particular, this approach may be particularly helpful in addressing withdrawal/craving symptoms and decreasing consequences associated with use. See Table 5.1 for main concepts and therapeutic skills learned in RP.

Contingency Management

Contingency management (CM) is a behavioral intervention that draws from operant conditioning to encourage changes in substance use in exchange for a reward (e.g., gift card). Generally, CM protocols seek negative urine drug screens in exchange for a monetary incentive. However, the targeted behavior can vary (e.g., attending session, bringing receipts from alcohol purchases, keeping a substance use log) depending on patient need and goals. Reinforcement can remain consistent or escalate over time with consecutive behavioral goals being met. For example, a patient may receive $5 for 1–3 consecutive negative screens, $10 for 4–6 consecutive screens, and $15 for 7+ consecutive screens. CM has resulted in moderate effect sizes with substance use treatment outcomes and may be particularly effective for opioids and cocaine (Prendergast et al., 2006). CM is a behavioral intervention and does not inherently include cognitive skills or broader skills development, however these skills can be incorporated into CM. CM can be presented as a stand-alone treatment or may be combined with other approaches such as RP.

Table 5.1 Concepts, treatment targets, and skills in relapse prevention

Concept	Treatment target	Therapy skills and tools
Relapse is a process	Identify warning signs and triggers including environmental, cognitive, and affecti7ve cues	Functional analysis Daily activity, thoughts, and mood logs
Understanding high-risk situations	Develop coping skills to mitigate risk	Refusal self-efficacy Interpersonal effectiveness Cognitive restructuring Mindfulness Positive activity planning
The role of social relationships in recovery	Develop supportive social relationships	Problem-solving Interpersonal effectiveness Behavioral experiments
Affect and relapse	Identify links between emotional states, substance urges, and behavior	Psychoeducation, identifying emotions Cognitive restructuring Mindfulness
Environment and relapse	Identify "people, places, and things" associated with substance use urges	Functional analysis Daily activity logs Problem-solving

CBT Approaches to PTSD

Exposure-Based Therapies

Exposure-based approaches to the treatment of PTSD developed from theories of fear responding and principles of operant conditioning (Mowrer, 1960). In this framework, contextual stimuli associated with the traumatic event are conditioned to generate a fear response. As such, exposure to the event or stimuli can evoke feelings of fear, anxiety, and panic, even if nonthreatening in the moment. To cope with these feelings, an individual with PTSD naturally avoids these cues. However, avoidance of these cues creates a negative reinforcement feedback loop by which escaping from or eliminating exposure to trauma cues reinforces the fear response and increases its intensity over time. This model was expanded upon to include cognitions that develop in response to trauma. Emotional processing theory (Foa & Kozak, 1986; Foa & McNally, 1986; Foa et al., 2006) posits that individuals exposed to traumatic events may develop broadened associations between trauma-related stimuli that are presently nonthreatening (e.g., memories, places, situations). Additionally, they may ascribe meanings to the trauma or parts of the trauma that hinder their current functioning (e.g., "the world is dangerous" or "I cannot trust anyone"). Behavioral approaches to PTSD aim to modify the fear structure by activating the fear response and presenting contradictory information (Foa & Kozak, 1986). The goal is for individuals to incorporate the new information to alter trauma-related beliefs and attain habituation in which exposures to the feared stimuli result in diminished physiological and emotional responses. Examples of exposure-based therapies for PTSD include Prolonged Exposure Therapy, Trauma-Focused Cognitive Behavioral Therapy, and Written Exposure Therapy. Here, we provide additional details on Prolonged Exposure.

Prolonged Exposure Therapy Prolonged exposure therapy (PE; Foa et al., 2019) is an 8–15 session treatment that where sessions are typically 90 minutes long and occur either weekly or twice per week. PE is structured to consist of: (1) psychoeducation about PTSD and the rationale for PE; (2) breathing retraining; (3) in vivo exposures; and (4) imaginal exposures. Psychoeducation is used to educate the patient about the underpinnings of PTSD from an emotional processing therapy framework, describe the process of exposures for habituation, and outline expectations for PE. Breathing retraining is used to give patients skills for managing hyperarousal. However, it is important to note that this skill is not recommended to be used during exposures as it may interfere with the requisite elevations in arousal needed to stimulate the fear response.

Most PE sessions focus on the in vivo and imaginal exposures, as these are considered the active ingredients for these treatment protocol. For imaginal exposures, the patient closes their eyes and recites the index trauma memory aloud in detail including sensory details, thoughts, and physiological responses to their clinician. The patient reports their subjective units of distress (SUDS) every 5 minutes to the clinician. Imaginal exposures are repeatedly continued in each session from session 3 and onwards to experience a reduction in arousal. Starting in session 2, for in vivo exposures, the provider and patient work together to develop an exposure hierarchy in which situations eliciting a fear response are ranked in order of intensity and are completed in ascending order until each exposure can be completed with minimal arousal and distress. The exposures on the hierarchy should have varying degrees of associated distress and should be able to elicit the fear response without compromising the patient's safety. Hierarchies should not involve physically dangerous situations. For example, an individual with a history of physical assault may avoid crowds or public spaces may have items on their hierarchy that include walking through a quiet park (lower distress) or going to a grocery store on a Saturday afternoon (moderate-to-high distress) followed by crowds (high distress). Patients engage in exposures as homework between sessions. Overall, homework in PE includes listening to audio recordings of the most recent session, listening to imaginal exposure recordings once a day, practicing breathing retraining, and completing in vivo exposures. PE has consistently showed strong evidence for treating PTSD across meta-analytic studies examining PE and PE + pharmacotherapy (Levinson et al., 2022; Powers et al., 2010; Zhou et al., 2020). See Table 5.2 for details on the session content.

Table 5.2 Prolonged exposure session content

Session number	Primary focus	Session elements and homework
1–2	Psychoeducation, breathing retraining, develop in vivo hierarchy, begin in vivo exposures	PTSD and treatment rationale Breathing retraining Learn in vivo exposures Practice first in vivo exposure Listen to session recordings
3	Psychoeducation, in vivo and first imaginal exposures	Rationale for imaginal exposures Review of in vivo homework and continued exposures Listen to session recordings Listen to imaginal exposure every day
4–9	In vivo exposures, imaginal exposures	Listen to imaginal exposure recording daily Continue in vivo exposures Practice breathing retraining Listen to session recordings
Final session (10 or 12)	PTSD relapse prevention, termination	Imaginal exposure Review skills Termination and review progress/growth PTSD relapse prevention Concluding treatment

Cognition-Based Therapies

There are several underlying theories of cognition posited in the context of PTSD including the social cognitive theory of PTSD. Similar to behavioral theories, the social cognitive theory of PTSD suggests that avoidance of trauma-related stimuli and maladaptive appraisals of the event result in nonrecovery of PTSD. This nonrecovery occurs through the process of assimilation in which individuals try to incorporate the traumatic event into existing cognitive schema, particularly their beliefs about the self, others, and the world. The assimilation process is thought to be an attempt to view traumatic events as predictable or within our personal control to make sense of the event. Several maladaptive cognitions can emerge during the assimilation process such as "just-world" cognitions (e.g., "bad things do not happen to good people and therefore, I must be bad"), hindsight bias, and the belief that the event would not have occurred had a different action been taken (Fischhoff, 1975; Payne et al., 2007). Maladaptive cognitions may also occur through the process of overaccommodation, the process of changing beliefs to fit the traumatic event (McCann & Pearlman, 1990; Payne et al., 2007). Overaccommodation, may lead individuals to generalize their experience beyond the context of the traumatic event (e.g., "no one is to be trusted"), impacting current functioning. The goal of cognitive approaches to PTSD is to address maladaptive beliefs developed through assimilation and overaccommodation by directly modifying the beliefs, rather than through the processes of habituation (Resick et al., 2016).

Cognitive Processing Therapy Cognitive processing therapy (CPT; Resick et al., 2016) is a 12-session individual or group trauma protocol that utilizes cognitive restructuring strategies to address maladaptive beliefs ("stuck points") associated with traumatic experiences. CPT is divided into three phases: education, trauma processing, and challenging cognitions. Cognitive restructuring in CPT is achieved by challenging maladaptive thoughts until the thought is eliminated or replaced by a more balanced belief. To achieve this, clients engage in Socratic dialogue in which the provider helps guide the client through use of open-ended questions. Types of questions include clarification, challenging assumptions, evaluating the objective evidence, and challenging core beliefs. Open-ended questions are used to address cognitive distortions and to aid clients in distinguishing between thoughts, emotions, and behaviors. Though cognitive restructuring is used in the treatment of many disorders, CPT focuses on thoughts about the trauma such as approaching trauma-related stimuli, one's ability to cope with the trauma and future events, beliefs about the trauma itself, and current thoughts that developed from the trauma. CPT includes the option of completing a written trauma narrative to be read daily, similar to exposure-based treatments; however, the narrative is not considered a requirement of CPT and outcome studies have found CPT to be equally as efficacious without the inclusion of a narrative (Walter et al., 2014). Like PE, CPT has garnered strong empirical support for the treatment of PTSD across samples and formats (Asmundson et al., 2019; Tran et al., 2016). See Table 5.3 for details on the session content for a 12-week CPT treatment.

Integrated or Concurrent Model

In contrast to the sequential model of treatment, the integrated or concurrent model of treatment for co-occurring SUD and PTSD aims to target both conditions simultaneously given their mutual reinforcement of one another. Importantly, there is little support to suggest that individuals are at higher risk of relapse if PTSD and SUD are addressed concurrently and few patients report a preference for a sequential model of PTSD-SUD treatment (Back et al., 2006). Accordingly, most integrated or concurrent approaches are designed based in principles of the self-medication hypothesis (Khantzian, 1997) in which substance use is seen as a maladaptive form of coping with PTSD symptoms. Formalized research on integrated treatment models arose in the 1990s and extant literature shows four major treatment approaches to date: (1) Seeking Safety (Najavits, 2021), (2) Concurrent Treatment of PTSD and SUD Using Prolonged Exposure (COPE; Back et al., 2014); (3) Integrated Cognitive Behavioral Therapies, including Cognitive Processing Therapy (Resick et al., 2016); and (4) the combination of medications for SUD with behavioral treatments for PTSD. It should be noted that there are other treatment approaches that have focused on individuals with co-occurring SUD and PTSD, but

Table 5.3 Cognitive processing therapy session content

Session number	Primary focus	Session elements and homework
1	Psychoeducation, introduction to stuck points	PTSD and treatment rationale Stuck points Writing an impact statement
2–3	Self-monitoring of thoughts, emotions, and behaviors; introduction to Socratic questioning	Daily monitoring of events, thoughts, emotions, and behaviors Trauma narrative and daily reading of narrative (optional)
4–11	Challenging questions and patterns of problematic thinking including beliefs about safety, trust, power, and control	Daily monitoring of events, thoughts, emotions, and behaviors Challenging beliefs worksheets Challenging questions worksheets Behavioral homework (e.g., self-care tasks) Post-treatment impact statement
12 (Final session)	Assignment review, future plans	Review skills Review progress/growth PTSD relapse prevention Concluding treatment and plans for future therapy

here, we mention the major treatments. For a full review of these treatments and their comparative efficacy to one another, please see Hien et al. (2022, 2023) and Kline et al. (2022).

Seeking Safety Seeking Safety (Najavits, 2021) was one of the first manualized integrated treatments that simultaneously attended to both SUD and co-occurring PTSD. Developed by Dr. Lisa Najavits, Seeking Safety is a 25-session cognitive behavioral group therapy that was originally designed for women with PTSD and SUD. Since its inception, it has expanded to be flexibly adapted to any individual with co-occurring PTSD and SUD as well as in an individual therapy format. At present, the manual provides 25 different topics that can be selected in the clinician and patient's desired order, where treatment can consist of 25 or fewer sessions. The treatment and associated topics focus on developing coping skills, safety, and awareness for SUD and PTSD. For instance, one topic is titled "taking back power from PTSD" and another is titled "setting boundaries in relationships" (Najavits, 2021). Each group session is further organized to consist of a check in and review of coping skills from the last session, an inspirational quote to start the group's session, the discussion of new content with group members utilizing handouts and practicing skills, and a check out that includes each group member's commitment to practice a skill prior to the next session.

A recent meta-analysis compared the outcomes of 12 randomized clinical trials of Seeking Safety versus wait-list controls or alternative treatments (e.g., psychoeducational groups or Relapse Prevention therapy). Results showed that across studies, there was a medium effect size of reduction in PTSD symptoms across both treatment control conditions and a small effect size of reduction in substance use across treatment control conditions (Lenz et al., 2016). Findings suggest that Seeking Safety can be helpful in the reduction of PTSD symptoms among those with PTSD and SUD and importantly is a flexible treatment that can be implemented in diverse treatment settings.

Concurrent Treatment of PTSD and SUD Using Prolonged Exposure (COPE) A notable difference between Seeking Safety and the next treatment that focuses on co-occurring SUD and PTSD is the degree of focus on the traumatic experience that led to PTSD symptoms. As Hien et al. (2022, 2023) stated, Seeking Safety is a "non-trauma-focused" therapy where sessions do not require the patient to discuss the traumatic experience(s) that led to the development of PTSD symptoms. In contrast, "trauma-focused" therapies focus on the patient sharing the traumatic experience(s) they experienced with their provider in a systematic manner to alleviate distress. One trauma-focused integrated treatment is Concurrent Treatment of PTSD and SUD Using Prolonged Exposure or COPE (Back et al., 2014). COPE is an integrated, trauma-focused, cognitive behavioral treatment that combines two evidence-based treatments: Prolonged Exposure therapy (Foa et al., 2019) with Relapse Prevention therapy (Kadden et al., 1992).

COPE consists of 12, 90-minute sessions of individual therapy where each session has content focused on PTSD and substance use. Importantly, COPE does not require abstinence, but instead adopts a harm reduction approach. A typical session in COPE focuses on 45–60 minutes of Prolonged Exposure therapy followed by 30–45 minutes on a Relapse Prevention skill. Over four randomized clinical trials have shown that COPE is significantly superior at reducing PTSD symptoms and moderately better at reducing substance use relative to active control conditions, such as Relapse Prevention therapy and Seeking Safety (Back et al., 2019; Ruglass et al., 2017; Mills et al., 2016; Norman et al., 2019). Importantly, none of these studies have shown an increase in substance use and these results have led COPE to be certified by the *Treatments That Work* Series by Oxford University Press. Emerging work on COPE has begun to examine whether the combination of COPE with medications, such as Oxytocin, may additionally improve outcomes (Back et al., 2023) as well as how COPE may be adapted to adolescents with co-occurring SUD and PTSD (Mills et al., 2020).

Integrated Cognitive Behavioral Therapy An additional group of treatments that have concurrently targeted PTSD and SUD are integrated cognitive behavioral treatments. One of these treatments is Integrated Cognitive Behavioral Therapy, an 8-session manualized intervention that focuses on cognitive behavioral approaches to cope with PTSD symptoms and reduce substance use. Two randomized clinical trials have shown mixed findings on outcomes. One study showed significant reductions in PTSD symptoms for the Integrated Cognitive Behavioral Therapy treatment group relative to standard care in substance use treatment (McGovern et al., 2011) and the other found no group differences in PTSD symptoms across treatment groups, but solely reductions in substance use for the Integrated Cognitive Behavioral Therapy treatment group relative to the control condition receiving standard care in substance use treatment programs (McGovern et al., 2015).

Due to these mixed findings, there has been limited additional work on Integrated Cognitive Behavioral Therapy. However, akin to the combination of Prolonged Exposure therapy with Relapse Prevention in COPE, novel work has begun to examine the combination of Cognitive Processing Therapy with Relapse Prevention therapy as an additional integrated treatment. This integrated treatment, titled the Treatment of Integrated Posttraumatic Stress and Substance Use (TIPSS) consists of 12, 60-minute individual therapy sessions with content combining Cognitive Processing Therapy and Relapse Prevention. The first pilot trial on this intervention and an associated case study (Vujanovic et al., 2018; Vujanovic et al., 2019) are ongoing, and thus, results are forthcoming. If evidence shows significant reductions in PTSD symptoms and SUD, TIPPS may provide further support to the advantage of trauma-focused integrated treatments rather than non-trauma-focused integrated treatments.

Combination Therapies The last major group of integrated treatment approaches to PTSD and co-occurring SUD consists of the combination of psychotherapy interventions with pharmacotherapies to boost intervention effects. For instance, Hien et al. (2015) combined Seeking Safety with sertraline and compared it to Seeking Safety with placebo. The authors found that the experimental group of Seeking

Safety with sertraline showed significantly greater reductions in PTSD symptoms than the placebo control group; the groups did not differ in alcohol use disorder outcomes. In addition, Foa et al. (2013) compared Prolonged Exposure, naltrexone, the combination of Prolonged Exposure and naltrexone, and supportive counseling to one another. The authors found that the combination of Prolonged Exposure therapy with naltrexone showed the greatest long-term, sustained, reductions in PTSD and co-occurring alcohol use disorder.

Emerging research has also begun to examine how the combination of N-acetylcysteine with Relapse Prevention therapy may reduce PTSD and co-occurring alcohol use disorder (Back et al., 2020). These results are promising given that other research has shown that the combination of medication with trauma-focused treatment seems to be the most promising treatment approach for co-occurring PTSD and SUD. Hien et al. (2022, 2023) harmonized 36 randomized clinical trials of treatments for PTSD and co-occurring SUD and found the largest effect sizes for trauma-focused treatments combined with medications. While the authors found medium to large effect sizes for other treatment approaches as well, such as integrated cognitive behavioral treatments, this finding suggests future work may benefit from examining how to best combine medications with trauma-focused treatments to advance care in PTSD and SUD.

Clinical Guidelines

As we have described above, there are numerous modalities and treatment types to draw upon for individuals struggling with co-occurring PTSD + SUD and the emotion dysregulation problems which accompany these conditions. We recommend that the clinician engage in treatment planning as a collaborative process following a strong assessment and deliberative consultation with the patient. Many of the above-mentioned treatments are a manualized 12-session treatment that can appear as a one-size-fits-all. Although rigorously tested, there may be patients who cannot engage in the treatment in the set 12-session structure and need modifications. For example, a patient engaged in COPE may not be ready to engage in in vivo trauma exposure in the third session and perhaps needs to review the contents of sessions 1 and 2 before the in vivo exposure occurs or perhaps the patient slipped, and the focus of the session is on relapse prevention as opposed to imaginal exposures. Clinical judgement, flexibility, and consultation are imperative when working PTSD-SUD patients. We provide an example at the end of this chapter. Adopting an integrative treatment framework (Hien et al., 2019) recognizes the importance of linking traumatic stress and substance use disorders and provides an overarching model for clinical care which focuses on the individual needs and wishes of the client, while also centering the therapeutic relationship between the patient and clinician in collaborating on the plan for care.

Historically, prior to the past two decades, prevailing guidance suggested that the patient should first achieve abstinence to proceed with treatment for their mental health conditions (Nass et al., 2019). However, since then, empirical evidence testing the benefits of sequential versus integrated models have shown the converse, that sequential models were not necessary to prevent substance use relapse. Recommendations for those with trauma, emotional dysregulation, and related mental health conditions such as depression or anxiety disorders were clear that there was no need to wait to receive care for their mental health conditions, including PTSD symptoms, separate from their substance use issues (Hien et al., 2015; Norman et al., 2019; Ruglass et al., 2017). The bulk of empirical evidence supports conceptualizing and treating traumatic stress and substance use issues contemporaneously (e.g., Hien et al., 2023; Roberts et al., 2022; Simpson et al., 2021).

However, even within the integrative treatment framework, decisions regarding how to implement care for both sets of conditions can involve decisions and choices that the patient and clinician should make together. Also, it should be noted that adopting a sequential approach where one disorder would be treated first, prior to the start of treatment the other condition, technically could be viewed as a single-disorder treatment. For example, in a case where a patient is in early- or middle-stage recovery and either has had significant help with their substance use or is concurrently receiving separate care at a substance use clinic but has not previously been diagnosed with PTSD, or ever talked about their trauma, a clinician may recommend an initial focus on their trauma. In this case of sequential care, the patient and clinician, together, would select the best type of treatment (i.e., cognitive processing therapy, PE, etc.) that fits the patient's treatment goals at the time. Or, for a client who is using alcohol throughout the day to a level where there is concern that stopping use or even reducing use could result in significant withdrawal symptoms, selecting to treat the alcohol use disorder with an inpatient detoxification treatment before embarking on trauma work would still be a clinically sound treatment recommendation. In many cases, especially when there is not a clear need for stabilization; however, selecting an integrated treatment which helps the clinician and client keep both conditions in mind during each session would be the best choice. As evidenced, there is no one way to treat a PTSD-SUD patient and treatment plan largely depend on the patient's clinical presentation and severity of diagnoses.

An integrated approach could involve implementing an evidence-based model such as those discussed above (i.e., COPE, TIPSS, or Seeking Safety) which all seek to address the trauma and substance use material in each session as the client unfolds through the treatment process. But even within an integrated model, decisions can be made about which material to organize the sessions around. For example, one might decide that since the patient has active and heavy use of alcohol or stimulants, the sessions on managing craving, urge surfing and dealing with high-risk situations common to all integrated models, could also be conducted earlier in the treatment process and might be most beneficial to the patient.

Thus, the options and choice of a sequential model versus an integrated one may revolve around (but are not limited to) consideration of the following:

- Client readiness and motivation to address either their substance use or trauma material
- The client's previous treatment history and how much or how comfortable they are with techniques such as relapse prevention, or conversely, whether they have previously worked with their trauma using a psychoeducational or trauma-processing model
- Level of acute symptoms and need for stabilization in one domain or the other
- Supports available (i.e., are they connected to self-help groups, do they have a sponsor or anyone in their life who they can rely upon)
- Availability of expertise/costs of care in cases where the therapist may need to refer for collateral treatments
- Client choice of how they would like to work on their issues as they conceptualize them
- Clinician recommendations for the client based on their assessment of client readiness, or level of avoidance

Complex Trauma

The aforementioned PTSD treatments only focus on, and have been empirically validated for, traumatic events that meet Criterion A in the *DSM-5* (APA, 2013), as discussed earlier in the chapter. In recent years, there is a growing body of evidence that acknowledges that some traumatic events are not only one-time, isolated events, but can also be chronic and repeated, often occurring throughout the lifespan. This experience of trauma is referred to as complex trauma (Briere & Scott, 2015). Experiencing racism-related events, or racial trauma, is a form of complex trauma (Cénat, 2022) as well as discrimination due to gender, sexuality, religion, etc. Exposure to racial trauma can be a one-time event or long-lasting where its impact builds up over time and is associated with increased alcohol use (Desalu et al., 2019), suicidal behaviors (Polanco-Roman et al., 2022), development of PTSD symptoms (Kirkinis et al., 2021), and other adverse mental health outcomes (Pieterse & Powell, 2016). There is increasing evidence showing the positive associations between media-exposure of racial trauma and subsequent depressive and PTSD symptoms (Tynes et al., 2019). The race-based traumatic stress model (Carter, 2007) has helped to explain the observed health disparities in Black, Indigenous, and People of Color (BIPOC) where both poor mental and physical health are observed (Phelan & Link, 2015, Paradies et al., 2015). Carter's model parallels the PTSD model suggesting that exposure to racist-related events throughout one's life may result in increased distress, hypervigilance, avoidance of people or places, etc. In alignment with the "self-medication hypothesis" it is also thought that individuals exposed to racist-related events may use substances to cope with the pain and negative emotions associated with the event(s) suggesting the need for treatment.

Despite the empirical evidence that suggests the overlap of complex trauma to *DSM-5* PTSD trauma, much of the racial trauma treatment remain theoretical in nature making it difficult for clinicians to translate into practice. The difficulty with racial trauma treatment is that patients may be experiencing stress but are unaware of their experiences with racism or their racial identity is less well-developed. Given the need for care, the National Center for PTSD complied a set of over-arching treatment guidelines for clinicians working with individuals dealing with racial trauma: seek opportunities that are empowering, find alignment with their values, engage in self-care and lifestyle changes, seek support, and limit their media exposure (Galvoski et al., 2022). Unfortunately, these guidelines may still leave clinicians ill-equipped to navigate healing from racial trauma symptoms in therapy. There are two treatment models that have recently emerged to help clinicians gain the necessary skills to work with this form of complex trauma. Williams and Wetterneck (2022) released the "Racial Trauma Treatment: A 12-Session CBT Protocol" for individuals dealing with racial trauma. This treatment begins with the use of validated scales to assess racial stress and trauma and moves towards providing psychoeducation on racism, building coping strategies and a support network, understanding the patient's internalized racism, building skills to combat racism, and engaging in social activism and activism.

The KNIFFLEY Racial Trauma Therapy Model (KRTTM) has emerged as another racial trauma treatment protocol to increase the number of community-based clinicians fit to treat racial trauma (Kniffley et al., 2023). This training consists of three modules that starts at gaining an overview of the frequency of racist-related events for BIPOC individuals and the mental health challenges providing language for clinicians to use, the second module teaches clinician's how to navigate around trauma memories and trauma symptomatology, and the last module provides a comprehensive training in the 12-session Kniffley Racial Trauma Therapy manual, which is currently being evaluated for its efficacy. This is a burgeoning treatment area and further research is required especially for comorbid trauma and substance use patients.

Concrete Guidelines and Best Practices

Beyond selection of a sequential or integrated model, below are some of our suggestions for working with dual-diagnosed PTSD-SUD patients that apply to all the reviewed treatment approaches:

Capture a Thorough Background

During the first session, it is important to understand the patient's background including the history of the trauma and substance use as well as their current living conditions and context. Clinicians should inquire *gently* about the trauma incident(s) and go beyond a traditional Criterion A traumatic event including multiple traumatic events (i.e., emotional abuse, neglect) and other forms of complex trauma. It is not advisable to engage the patient in the reenactment of their trauma, but rather observe their physical and emotional reactions. Something to consider during the initial session or intake is determining the patient's "window of tolerance" (Ogden & Minton, 2000). The "window of tolerance" is an emotional range in which the patient is not too hyperaroused or hypoaroused and their cognitive capacities remain intact and ready to process their trauma. See Fig. 5.1 for a depiction of this "window of tolerance." The description of the "window of tolerance" might serve as a helpful psychoeducational tool early on and throughout treatment to refer to as patients engage in their trauma narrative or their in vivo exposures.

It is also important to capture a thorough substance use history inquiring about their individual use (type, duration, pattern, etc.), substance use history in the family, and if relevant, their social groups that may use substances. It is important to understand the patient's relationship to their substance use and learn how long the substance use has served a purpose in their life. It is important to also gauge severity of use—i.e., type of substance, route of administration, frequency of use, where it is purchased, length of use per session, duration of use in lifetime. Engaging in motivational interviewing skills (Miller & Rollnick, 2013) in the intake session and the following sessions is helpful to build rapport and reduce any judgement-prone language regarding their level of use.

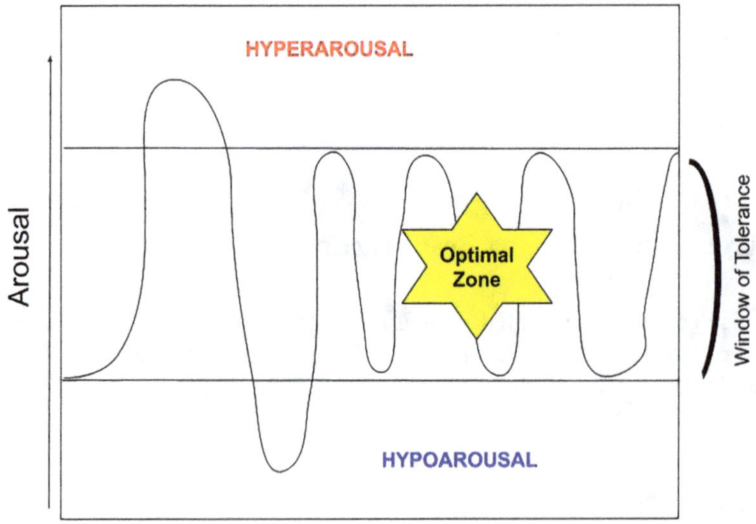

Fig. 5.1 Window of tolerance

Assess Safety

Next, it is imperative to determine the patient's risk level for violence and harm to self and others before and during treatment. Clinicians should complete a thorough suicide risk assessment inquiring about any present and past thoughts of suicide ideation, plan, and/or attempt(s) as well as non-suicidal self-injurious behaviors and any intent or plan to harm others. Shea's (1999) "*The Practical Art of Suicide Assessment: A Guide for Mental Health Professionals and Substance Abuse Counselors*" is helpful book to guide clinicians in ascertaining level of risk. If the level of risk is considered high and the patient's ideation is active, the clinician must complete a collaborative safety plan with the patient and document it. Some resources are: Collaborative Assessment & Management of Suicidality (CAMS) or Stanley-Brown Safety Plan. If the patient is at risk to harm themselves or others, it is imperative that you stay with the patient until safety is achieved in the therapy room and/or if hospitalization is required.

A form of safety that is often forgotten about is assessment of intimate partner violence (IPV), including domestic, sexual, physical violence, and/or stalking by an intimate partner. Women (41%) are more likely to be victims of IPV compared to men (26%; Leemis et al., 2022). It is important to ascertain where and when the violence occurs to reduce injury, negative consequences, and even death (Stockman et al., 2015). If working with a patient with IPV, it is important to provide the requisite psychoeducation and safety skills in efforts to create protective environments (i.e., victim-centered services, housing programs, change of physical and social settings) early in treatment to decrease the risk of re-experiencing IPV and potential relapse (Niolon et al., 2017).

Determine Assessments

The use of assessments is helpful to track the severity of PTSD and SUD symptoms as patients engage in the treatment. The frequency of assessments is also something to consider as some clinicians may prefer to administer the same assessments each week, where others may prefer to space out the assessments at weeks 1, 6, and 12 of treatments. This is up to the clinician's discretion. Below are some commonly used assessments:

A. *Urine Drug Screen*: This is very easy to complete every week and can corroborate self-report data on patient's use. This is particularly helpful in abstinence-based treatment models as it is an easy way to track goals of no use, but it may negatively impact the treatment alliance especially if the patient continues using while engaging in an abstinence-based treatment model. If taking a harm reduction approach, urine drug screens may be less helpful unless abstinence is a patient's identified goal. One harm reduction way in which urine drug screens can be helpful is to reduce harm associated with supply. Some clinicians have used toxicology reports to help track and identify "healthy" suppliers versus "unhealthy" suppliers if the patient is purchasing unregulated substances. For example, Mr. F presented to substance use treatment to reduce his opioid use. Mr. F had a significant trauma history, but it was determined by the treatment team that a sequential model may be more helpful to establish safety as he had three prior opioid-related overdoses. Mr. F began individual therapy for relapse prevention and methadone, a medication used to treat opioid use disorder (MOUD). In the early sessions, it was apparent that Mr. F could not trust his opioid supplier and questioned whether fentanyl was being laced in with the heroin he was purchasing. Together, the patient and clinician determined to implement urine drug screens weekly to narrow down the supplier who he can trust to reduce his chance of consuming fentanyl and overall reduce harms around his use. After establishing safety and a less harmful approach to his opioid use, Mr. F was better prepared to engage in reducing his PTSD symptoms.

B. *Addiction Severity Index (ASI)*: The ASI (McLellan et al., 1980) is a structured-interview that aims to understand the level substance use in seven problem areas (e.g., medical, employment, drug use, alcohol use, legal status, family/social status, psychiatric status) that takes around 1-hour to complete. At the end of the interview, the clinician should have a better sense of the severity of the substance use and a comprehensive overview of the areas in which their substance use interferes with their life. The scores in each problem area can be used to develop a treatment plan that best assesses the patient's needs; often scores of 4 or greater can indicate an area of treatment or specific treatment goal. Although the ASI provides a comprehensive overview of the substance use issues, it is time-consuming in nature and long which may have drawbacks depending on the patient. Because of the length of the interview, it is not advisable to complete at every session, but rather at key points during the treatment protocol (i.e., session 1 and session 12).

C. *PTSD Checklist for DSM-5 (PCL-5)*: The PCL-5 is a 20-item self-report measure the assesses for 20 *DSM-5* symptoms of PTSD (Weathers et al., 2013b). This scale serves multiple purposes—it can help monitor symptom change throughout treatment as well as screen and provide a provisional diagnosis for PTSD. This checklist takes about 5–10 minutes to complete and is an easy metric to provide patients weekly to determine level of PTSD symptom severity. It is important that patients anchor their responses to a Criterion A event when completing this assessment; the Life Events Checklist for *DSM-5* (LEC-5; Weathers et al., 2013c) is a good tool to determine the Criterion A event. For instance, Mr. J was in a cognitive-based trauma only treatment where the PCL was used at the start of every session to determine the level of PTSD symptom severity he was experiencing in the past week. This was a helpful tool for both the clinician and Mr. J as they collaboratively set an agenda for the session that reflected and centered on the current impact of his PTSD symptoms. Mr. J reported finding it helpful to put a number on how he was feeling.

D. *Clinician-Administered PTSD Scale for DSM-5 (CAPS-5)*: The CAPS-5, a 30-item structured interview, is the "gold standard" to assess PTSD (Weathers et al., 2013a). Usually the LEC-5 is used before the CAPS-5 to determine the Criterion A event(s). The full interview can take between 45 and 60 minutes to administer where it can make a current (past month) or lifetime diagnosis of PTSD as well as assess PTSD symptoms in the last week. Unlike the PCL-5, the CAPS-5 can assess the onset and duration of symptoms, subjective distress, and the impact of the symptoms on daily functioning. The advantage of the CAPS-5 is that it provides a severity score for each symptom cluster, which helps clinician's tailor their treatment plans. Due to the length of the interview, this assessment tool may be most beneficial at the start and end of treatments.

E. *Other Options*: The Timeline Follow-Back (TLFB) Tool (Robinson et al., 2012) is another assessment that can either be completed through an interview, self-administered, or administered by the computer. It asks patients to retrospectively recall their drug use in the past week up to 2 years before the session date. Tracking their use can serve as a motivational feedback tool for patients as they learn more about their substance use and identify their antecedents of use. In addition to the TLFB, there are several other substance use measures that can be used. Some examples are the AUDIT, DUDIT, SIPS, ASSIST, DAST and several specific drug craving questionnaires. This is up to the clinician's discretion to determine which measure best serves the needs of the patient.

Timing of Trauma Work Relative to SUD Reductions

Sometimes a sequential approach may be advantageous depending on the patient's clinical profile. Mrs. C presented to therapy for support around her PTSD symptoms and was increasingly experiencing recurrent nightmares of the traumatic event and avoiding certain places. Her alcohol use increased after the traumatic event and at the start of treatment, Mrs. C was drinking 6–8 alcohol drinks per day. In the case of Mrs. C, addressing her PTSD at the start of treatment, while also working on reducing her alcohol use may increase the risk of relapse or continued increased use (Nass et al., 2019). In addition, Mrs. C was ambivalent about reducing her alcohol use. Through consultation with others, the clinician decided to work on reducing Mrs. C's alcohol use through motivational interviewing and relapse prevention skills to establish stability and preparedness for trauma work. Mrs. C was able to reduce her alcohol use to a controlled level and reported feeling "ready" to process her trauma. Clinicians may also consider the use of pharmacotherapy for either PTSD or the substance of focus at the start of treatment to stabilize the patient as they embark on engaging with trauma.

Establishing Safety

Establishing safety is crucial not only with every patient, but especially important in PTSD-SUD patients. Many patients may feel reticent to share their trauma story as it may be associated with feelings of shame, guilt, fear, and anger. Paired with the telling of their trauma is the acceptance of the damage it has caused not only to their psychological and physical health, but also the distances it has created in their social circles. Clinicians should be acutely aware of the multifaceted impact trauma had on the patient's life and should not ask the patient to tell their whole trauma story in the first session. Using the "window of tolerance" framework, it is important for the clinician to determine a comfortable pace for the patient to engage in their trauma. Additionally, the clinician should constantly be validating the patient's experience of the traumatic event while providing psychoeducation to normalize their experiences.

Relatedly, many patients in the first session may not want to change their substance use and show resistance or hesitation towards change. Clinicians must remember that regardless of how harmful the patient's level of use may be, that substance use can be syntonic to an individual and typically serves a purpose—whether it be numbing, masking feelings, escaping, etc. To build safety and alliance, clinicians must accept the patient's current substance use and any resistance towards change in a nonjudgmental manner. In these scenarios, engaging in motivational interviewing can be helpful to build more curiosity about the patient's current level of use and the impact on their daily functioning. Building acceptance towards the patient's trauma and substance use can help pair these two experiences together and increase intrinsic motivation for change. Again, this is more easily done when the clinician is nonjudgmental, normalizing, and accepting.

Lastly, the quality of the therapeutic alliance is the strongest predictor for treatment success (Safran & Muran, 2000; Bauer et al., 2022). In other words, the therapeutic relationship can be healing for many patients. It is important to remember that the therapeutic relationship may be the only, or some of the few, compassionate, accepting, validating, and empowering relationships the patient has. The first couple of sessions should be focused on accepting and validating the patient's trauma and substance use to build rapport and strengthen the alliance for the work to come. The therapeutic alliance can also be helpful in the development of treatment goals where it can be conducted in a collaborative manner with the patient. If there is not enough safety established in the therapy room, there may be obstacles preventing the patient from fully engaging in the therapy, development of treatment goals, and/or with the clinician.

Clinical Vignette

Here we present a treatment case of a patient with co-occurring PTSD-SUD:

Ms. B presented for treatment in her early 40 s, a Latina woman, divorced, unemployed, with a significant history of depression. She was a mother of several school age children and currently living with her boyfriend in a turbulent, and sometimes physically violent relationship.

Her chief complaint was: "I need help. I can't think. I don't know what to do."

Ms. B's trauma history included being beaten by her mother and her violent mentally ill father. Subsequently she became involved with a verbally and physically abusive man, with whom she had her children beginning at age 19. She reported being molested by a relative at age 7.

The patient reported a range of primarily depressive, anxious symptoms, and emotional dysregulation. She complained of feeling sad and depressed, crying all the time, feeling overwhelmed by problems, exhausted, not motivated, confused, unable to focus, and she reported passive suicidal ideation, with no previous attempts. She experienced low self-esteem, excessive shame, and guilt, and had difficulty trusting her own judgement. She met criteria for PTSD, but her treatment was focused on the instability surrounding her substance use. She did report hypervigilance and struggling with memories of her childhood abuse that would come to mind at random times and interfere with her ability to sleep.

Ms. B reported episodic, binge drinking; she also reported binge eating to self soothe. She used cannabis every night to help her sleep and keep away her bad memories. She denied any other self-injurious behavior.

Ms. B participated in individual psychotherapy, pharmacotherapy, and group therapy designed to help her understand the impact of her traumatic past on her current life. Pharmacotherapy helped regulate her mood and ensured stability prior to engaging in her trauma processing. A concurrent treatment model was used in the case of Ms. B as her substance use wasn't impairing with her daily functioning, but rather was more episodic in nature. In her Seeking Safety group, she developed several skills including mindfulness to build awareness of her emotions, distracting and self-soothing techniques when faced with traumatic memories of her childhood, countering negative self-statements and learning to be more compassionate with herself, learning to be a more consistent parent, and involving herself in more activities outside of the home. In addition, Ms. B learned relapse prevention strategies that helped to reduce her binge drinking and cannabis use.

In conjunction with her Seeking Safety group, Ms. B saw an individual therapist and expressed intrusive thoughts of her childhood that she "wanted to have more control over". At this point, the clinician provided a few trauma-focused interventions options and together Ms. B and clinician discussed the various options and decided on Prolonged Exposure. Ms. B stated, "I'm ready to remember what happened to me. I want to talk about it."

The clinician deviated from the 12-week Prolonged Exposure protocol as Ms. B was a parent to small children and treatment involved constant crisis management regarding the care of her children when she would either relapse, decompensate, or was at risk for either. This patient had a supportive family; however, the patient was in a constant cycle of feeling relief that they could provide help and desperation to be more independent from them. In these instances, the manualized treatment went on pause and the focus of the treatment turned to reducing shame around her relapse, creating a list of trusted family members and friends she can call on for support, and reflecting on her role as a mother. These were moments when the clinician had to practice flexibility and attunement towards the patient's needs and the focus was not on the in vivo *or imaginal exposures.*

Several weeks of crisis management had to occur before the exposures began again. Treatment was aimed at helping her achieve greater stability but was often challenging and her clinicians felt alternatively hopeful and helpless. She would do well for significant periods of time, be hopeful and motivated, moving toward employment and housing and being able to care for her children and herself, but could still become easily triggered by her traumatic past. She was easily dysregulated and demonstrated impulsive decision-making and poor judgement.

At this point, the clinician had to put aside the Prolonged Exposure protocol to work on skill building and incorporated many of the Seeking Safety core concepts with Ms. B. Learning to assert herself, to set appropriate boundaries and to communicate more effectively became central to much of her therapeutic work, especially as Ms. B became aware of how her rage often followed periods of allowing others in her life to take advantage of her. For example, Ms. B's partner was frequently erratic and manipulative, on and off drugs, and even stealing from her to support his habit. Other "friends" relied on her "availability" recognizing that she would never say no when asked to watch their kids or help out somehow, even when they had demonstrated that they were grossly taking advantage of her. As a parent it was also very difficult to set limits for her children. See dialogue below of clinician teaching Ms. B the skill of setting boundaries:

Ms. B	I don't know why I can't say no. I always feel like I have to help everyone, and no one is here to help me. Ugh, this makes me so mad!
Therapist	Can you tell me more about the need to always help everyone?
Ms. B	I feel pulled to take care of others, like it's my job. But my job is to take care of my kids and myself. I'm working really hard to be a good mother.
Therapist	Yes, I can see how hard you're working. Let's practice writing down some phrases to help you say "no" when you feel pulled to take care of others.
Ms. B	Yes. I remember we discussed this in my Seeking Safety skills group, but I think it's time to revisit this. I guess I could say, 'I really wish I could help you, but I cannot at this time.'
Therapist	That's a great start! What are you telling yourself when you set that boundary.
Ms. B	I guess I'm saying, 'I can't focus on myself if I'm being pulled in multiple directions.' Or 'setting this boundary is for the both of us.'
Therapist	Yes, I like these phrases. I can see how much you value boundary setting. Let's do some role play so that you can practice some of these phrases?

In a particularly difficult reversal, Ms. B found herself becoming the primary caretaker to her now aging mother. Although still furious over her mother's abusive and neglectful behavior toward her, she was unable to set boundaries in this relationship, or to enlist more equal responsibility for her mother's care with her siblings. With this boundary setting, she felt ready to re-engage in the trauma processing work. This was when the clinician restarted Prolonged Exposure. At this point, Ms. B was stable enough to engage in the exposures and began to see reduced emotional distress around her childhood trauma as well as reduced sleep disturbances.

Overall, Ms. B made gradual strides toward setting boundaries that were better for her, enabling her to become more independent, and to feel better about herself as a person. This, along with some more directed anger management skills, helped Ms. B to feel that her anger and frustration could be managed and expressed more appropriately with fewer outbursts.

Noteworthy is the way in which Ms. B presented her chief complaint: "I need help. I can't think. I don't know what to do." Some clients predominant experience is numbness, preventing them from identifying how they might be feeling. Moreover, the overarching experience of being overwhelmed is often the fog that clinicians go through with their patients for some time early in treatment, as they and their clinicians sort out the emotional and cognitive components to their distress, trauma, and substance use. Patients with complex trauma histories rarely present a linear path between their traumatic past (and sometimes traumatic present) and what they are experiencing today.

At the end of treatment, Ms. B was able to identify and maintain her boundaries, she no longer felt disturbed by her traumatic memories, felt a sense of accomplishment as a mother, and engaged in less episodic binge drinking.

References

American Psychiatric Association (Ed.). (2013). *Diagnostic and Statistical Manual of Mental Disorders* (5th ed.). American Psychiatric Association.

Asmundson, G. J., Thorisdottir, A. S., Roden-Foreman, J. W., Baird, S. O., Witcraft, S. M., Stein, A. T., et al. (2019). A meta-analytic review of cognitive processing therapy for adults with posttraumatic stress disorder. *Cognitive Behaviour Therapy, 48*(1), 1–14.

Back, S. E., Brady, K. T., Jaanimägi, U., & Jackson, J. L. (2006). Cocaine dependence and PTSD: A pilot study of symptom interplay and treatment preferences. *Addictive Behaviors, 31*(2), 351–354.

Back, S. E., Flanagan, J. C., Killeen, T., Saraiya, T. C., Brown, D. G., Jarnecke, A. M., Foa, E. B., Yusko, D. A., McLean, C. P., Suvak, M. K., Bux, D. A., Jr., Oslin, D., O'Brien, C. P., Imms, P., Riggs, D. S., & Volpicelli, J. (2013). Concurrent naltrexone and prolonged exposure therapy for patients with comorbid alcohol dependence and PTSD: a randomized clinical trial. *JAMA, 310*(5), 488–495. https://doi.org/10.1001/jama.2013.8268

Back, S. E., Foa, E. B., Killeen, T., Mills, K., Teesson, M., Dansky Cotton, B., Carroll, K. M., & Brady, K. T. (2014). *Concurrent treatment of PTSD and substance use disorders using prolonged exposure (COPE): Therapist manual*. Oxford University Press. https://doi.org/10.1093/med:psych/9780199334513.001.0001

Back, S. E., Killeen, T., Badour, C. L., Flanagan, J. C., Allan, N. P., Ana, E. S., Lozano, B., Korte, K. J., Foa, E. B., & Brady, K. T. (2019, Mar). Concurrent treatment of substance use disorders and PTSD using prolonged exposure: A randomized clinical trial in military veterans. *Addictive Behaviors, 90*, 369–377. https://doi.org/10.1016/j.addbeh.2018.11.032

Back, S. E., Gray, K., Santa Ana, E., Jones, J. L., Jarnecke, A. M., Joseph, J. E., Prisciandaro, J., Killeen, T., Brown, D. G., Taimina, L., Compean, E., Malcolm, R., Flanagan, J. C., & Kalivas, P. W. (2020). N-acetylcysteine for the treatment of comorbid alcohol use disorder and posttraumatic stress disorder: Design and methodology of a randomized clinical trial. *Contemporary Clinical Trials, 91*, 105961. https://doi.org/10.1016/j.cct.2020.105961

Back, S. E., Flanagan, J. C., Killeen, T., Saraiya, T. C., Brown, D. G., Jarnecke, A. M., Rothbaum, A. O., Joseph, J., Santa Ana, E., & de Arellano, A. (2023). COPE and oxytocin for the treatment of co-occurring PTSD and alcohol use disorder: Design and methodology of a randomized controlled trial in US military veterans. *Contemporary Clinical Trials, 126*, 107084.

Bauer, A. G., Ruglass, L. M., Shevorykin, A., Saraiya, T. C., Robinson, G., Cadet, K., Julien, L., Chao, T., & Hien, D. (2022). Predictors of therapeutic alliance, treatment feedback, and clinical outcomes among African American women in treatment for co-occurring PTSD and SUD. *Journal of Substance Abuse Treatment, 139*, 108766. https://doi.org/10.1016/j.jsat.2022.108766

Bonin, M. F., Norton, G. R., Asmundson, G. J. G., Dicurzio, S., & Pidlubney, S. (2000). Drinking away the hurt: The nature and prevalence of PTSD in substance abuse patients attending a community-based treatment program. *Journal of Behavior Therapy and Experimental Psychiatry, 31*(1), 55–66. https://doi.org/10.1016/S0005-7916(00)00008-2

Bradizza, C. M., Stasiewicz, P. R., & Paas, N. D. (2006). Relapse to alcohol and drug use among individuals diagnosed with co-occurring mental health and substance use disorders: A review. *Clinical Psychology Review, 26*(2), 162–178. https://doi.org/10.1016/j.cpr.2005.11.005

Briere, J., & Scott, C. (2015). Complex trauma in adolescents and adults. *Psychiatric Clinics of North America, 38*(3), 515–527. https://doi.org/10.1016/j.psc.2015.05.004

Carter, R. T. (2007). Racism and psychological and emotional injury: Recognizing and assessing race-based traumatic stress. *The Counseling Psychologist, 35*(1), 13–105. https://doi.org/10.1177/0011000006292033

Cénat, J. M. (2022). Complex racial trauma: Evidence, theory, assessment, and treatment. *Perspectives on Psychological Science: A Journal of the Association for Psychological Science, 18*(3), 17456916221120428. https://doi.org/10.1177/17456916221120428

Chilcoat, H. D., & Breslau, N. (1998). Investigations of causal pathways between PTSD and drug use disorders. *Addictive Behaviors, 23*(6), 827–840. https://doi.org/10.1016/s0306-4603(98)00069-0

Davis, K. C., Stoner, S. A., Norris, J., George, W. H., & Masters, N. T. (2009). Women's awareness of and discomfort with sexual assault cues: Effects of alcohol consumption and relationship type. *Violence Against Women, 15*, 1106–1125. https://doi.org/10.1177/1077801209340759

Davis, L. L., Schein, J., Cloutier, M., Gagnon-Sanschagrin, P., Maitland, J., Urganus, A., Guerin, A., Lefebvre, P., & Houle, C. R. (2022). The economic burden of posttraumatic stress disorder in the United States from a societal perspective. *The Journal of Clinical Psychiatry, 83*(3), 21m14116. https://doi.org/10.4088/JCP.21m14116

Desalu, J. M., Goodhines, P. A., & Park, A. (2019). Racial discrimination and alcohol use and negative drinking consequences among Black Americans: A meta-analytical review. *Addiction (Abingdon, England), 114*(6), 957–967. https://doi.org/10.1111/add.14578

Douaihy, A., Stowell, K. R., Park, T. W., & Daley, D. C. (2007). Relapse prevention: Clinical strategies for substance use disorders. In *Therapist's guide to evidence-based relapse prevention* (pp. 37–71). Academic Press.

Fischhoff, B. (1975). Hindsight is not equal to foresight: The effect of outcome knowledge on judgment under uncertainty. *Journal of Experimental Psychology: Human Perception and Performance, 1*(3), 288.

Foa, E. B., & Kozak, M. J. (1986). Emotional processing of fear: exposure to corrective information. *Psychological Bulletin, 99*(1), 20.

Foa, E. B., & McNally, R. J. (1986). Sensitivity to feared stimuli in obsessive-compulsives: A dichotic listening analysis. *Cognitive Therapy and Research, 10*(4), 477–485.

Foa, E. B., Huppert, J. D., & Cahill, S. P. (2006). Emotional processing theory: An update. In B. O. Rothbaum (Ed.), *Pathological anxiety: Emotional processing in etiology and treatment* (pp. 3–24). The Guilford Press.

Foa, E. B., Chrestman, K. R., & Gilboa-Schechtman, E. (2008). *Prolonged exposure therapy for adolescents with PTSD emotional processing of traumatic experiences, therapist guide*. Oxford University Press.

Foa, E. B., Yusko, D. A., McLean, C. P., Suvak, M. K., Bux, D. A., Jr, Oslin, D., O'Brien, C. P., Imms, P., Riggs, D. S., & Volpicelli, J. (2013). Concurrent naltrexone and prolonged exposure therapy for patients with comorbid alcohol dependence and PTSD: a randomized clinical trial. JAMA, 310(5), 488–495. https://doi.org/10.1001/jama.2013.8268

Foa, E. B., Hembree, E. A., Rothbaum, B. O., & Rauch, S. A. M. (2019). *Prolonged exposure therapy for PTSD: Emotional processing of traumatic experiences – Therapist guide* (2nd ed.). Oxford University. https://www.oxfordclinicalpsych.com/view/10.1093/med-psych/9780190926939.001.0001/med-9780190926939

Galvoski, T., Kaysen, D., McClendon, J., & Garcia, N. (2022). *Provider guide to addressing patient reactions to race-based violence during PTSD treatment*. Veteran Affairs. https://www.ptsd.va.gov/professional/treat/specific/patient_reactions_race_violence.asp

Gielen, N., Havermans, R. C., Tekelenburg, M., & Jansen, A. (2012). Prevalence of post-traumatic stress disorder among patients with substance use disorder: It is higher than clinicians think it is. *European Journal of Psychotraumatology, 3*. https://doi.org/10.3402/ejpt.v3i0.17734

Goldstein, R. B., Smith, S. M., Chou, S. P., Saha, T. D., Jung, J., Zhang, H., Pickering, R. P., Ruan, W. J., Huang, B., & Grant, B. F. (2016). The epidemiology of DSM-5 posttraumatic stress disorder in the United States: Results from the National Epidemiologic Survey on Alcohol and Related Conditions-III. *Social Psychiatry and Psychiatric Epidemiology, 51*(8), 1137–1148. https://doi.org/10.1007/s00127-016-1208-5

Grant, B. F., Saha, T. D., Ruan, W. J., Goldstein, R. B., Chou, S. P., Jung, J., Zhang, H., Smith, S. M., Pickering, R. P., Huang, B., & Hasin, D. S. (2016). Epidemiology of DSM-5 drug use disorder: Results from the National Epidemiologic Survey on Alcohol and Related Conditions-III. *JAMA Psychiatry, 73*(1), 39–47. https://doi.org/10.1001/jamapsychiatry.2015.2132

Grant, S., Colaiaco, B., Motala, A., Shanman, R., Booth, M., Sorbero, M., & Hempel, S. (2017). Mindfulness-based relapse prevention for substance use disorders: A systematic review and meta-analysis. *Journal of Addiction Medicine, 11*(5), 386.

Haller, M., & Chassin, L. (2014). Risk pathways among traumatic stress, posttraumatic stress disorder symptoms, and alcohol and drug problems: A test of four hypotheses. *Psychology of Addictive Behaviors: Journal of the Society of Psychologists in Addictive Behaviors, 28*(3), 841–851. https://doi.org/10.1037/a0035878

Hawn, S. E., Cusack, S. E., & Amstadter, A. B. (2020). A systematic review of the self-medication hypothesis in the context of posttraumatic stress disorder and comorbid problematic alcohol use. *Journal of Traumatic Stress, 33*(5), 699–708. https://doi.org/10.1002/jts.22521

Hien, D. A., Levin, F. R., Ruglass, L. M., López-Castro, T., Papini, S., Hu, M. C., Cohen, L. R., & Herron, A. (2015, Apr). Combining seeking safety with sertraline for PTSD and alcohol use disorders: A randomized controlled trial. *Journal of Consulting and Clinical Psychology, 83*(2), 359–369. https://doi.org/10.1037/a0038719

Hien, D. A., Litt, L., Lopez-Castro, T., & Ruglass, L. (2019). Treatment of addictions (25 pages). In C. Courtois & J. Ford (Eds.), *Treatment of complex trauma: A sequenced relationship based approach* (2nd ed.). Guilford Press.

Hien, D. A., Fitzpatrick, S., Saavedra, L. M., Ebrahimi, C. T., Norman, S. B., Tripp, J., Ruglass, L. M., Lopez-Castro, T., Killeen, T. K., Back, S. E., & Morgan-López, A. A. (2022). What's in a name? A data-driven method to identify optimal psychotherapy classifications to advance treatment research on co-occurring PTSD and substance use disorders. *European Journal of Psychotraumatology, 13*(1), 2001191. https://doi.org/10.1080/20008198.2021.2001191

Hien, D. A., Morgan-López, A. A., Saavedra, L. M., Ruglass, L. M., Ye, A., López-Castro, T., Fitzpatrick, S., Killeen, T. K., Norman, S. B., Ebrahimi, C. T., & Back, S. E. (2023). Project harmony: A meta-analysis with individual patient data on behavioral and pharmacologic trials for comorbid posttraumatic stress and alcohol or other drug use disorders. *American Journal of Psychiatry, 180*(2). https://doi.org/10.1176/appi.ajp.22010071

Kadden, R., Carroll, K., Donovan, D., Cooney, N., Monti, P., Abrams, D., Litt, M., & Hester, R. (1992). *Cognitive-behavioral coping skills therapy manual: A clinical research guide for therapists treating individuals with alcohol abuse and dependence*. National Institute on Alcohol Abuse and Alcoholism.

Kaysen, D., Atkins, D. C., Moore, S. A., Lindgren, K. P., Dillworth, T., & Simpson, T. (2011). Alcohol use, problems, and the course of posttraumatic stress disorder: A prospective study of female crime victims. *Journal of Dual Diagnosis, 7*(4), 262–279. https://doi.org/10.1080/15504263.2011.620449

Kessler, R. C., Berglund, P., Demler, O., Jin, R., Merikangas, K. R., & Walters, E. E. (2005). Lifetime prevalence and age-of-onset distributions of DSM-IV disorders in the National Comorbidity Survey Replication. *Archives of General Psychiatry, 62*(6), 593–602. https://doi.org/10.1001/archpsyc.62.6.593

Khantzian, E. J. (1997). The self-medication hypothesis of substance use disorders: A reconsideration and recent applications. *Harvard Review of Psychiatry, 4*(5), 231–244. https://doi.org/10.3109/10673229709030550

Kirkinis, K., Pieterse, A. L., Martin, C., Agiliga, A., & Brownell, A. (2021). Racism, racial discrimination, and trauma: A systematic review of the social science literature. *Ethnicity & Health, 26*(3), 392–412. https://doi.org/10.1080/13557858.2018.1514453

Kline, A. C., Panza, K. E., Lyons, R., Kehle-Forbes, S. M., Hien, D. A., & Norman, S. B. (2022). Trauma-focused treatment for comorbid post-traumatic stress and substance use disorder. *Nature Reviews Psychology, 2*(1), 24–39. https://doi.org/10.1038/s44159-022-00129-w

Kniffley, S., Crosby, S. D., Jones, K. V., Middleton, J., & Caine, A. (2023). Bridging the gap: Evaluating the efficacy of racial trauma therapy training for community mental health clinicians. *Psychological Trauma: Theory, Research, Practice, and Policy*. No Pagination Specified. https://doi.org/10.1037/tra0001467

Kulka, R. A., Schlenger, W. E., Fairbank, J. A., Hough, R. L., Jordan, B. K., Marmar, C. R., & Weiss, D. S. (1990). *Trauma and the Vietnam war generation: Report of findings from the National Vietnam Veterans Readjustment Study* (p. xxix, 322). Brunner/Mazel.

Leemis, R. W., Friar, N., Khatiwada, S., Chen, M. S., Kresnow, M., Smith, S. G., Caslin, S., & Basile, K. C. (2022). *The national intimate partner and sexual violence survey: 2016/2017 report on intimate partner violence*. National Center for Injury Prevention and Control, Centers for Disease Control and Prevention.

Lenz, A. S., Henesy, R., & Callender, K. (2016). Effectiveness of seeking safety for co-occurring posttraumatic stress disorder and substance use. *Journal of Counseling & Development, 94*, 51–61. https://doi.org/10.1002/jcad.12061

Levinson, D. B., Halverson, T. F., Wilson, S. M., & Fu, R. (2022). Less dropout from prolonged exposure sessions prescribed at least twice weekly: A meta-analysis and systematic review of randomized controlled trials. *Journal of Traumatic Stress, 35*(4), 1047–1059.

Magill, M., & Ray, L. A. (2009). Cognitive-behavioral treatment with adult alcohol and illicit drug users: A meta-analysis of randomized controlled trials. *Journal of Studies on Alcohol and Drugs, 70*(4), 516–527.

McCann, I. L., & Pearlman, L. A. (1990). Vicarious traumatization: A framework for understanding the psychological effects of working with victims. *Journal of Traumatic Stress, 3*, 131–149.

McCauley, J. L., Killeen, T., Gros, D. F., Brady, K. T., & Back, S. E. (2012). Posttraumatic stress disorder and co-occurring substance use disorders: Advances in assessment and treatment. *Clinical Psychology: Science and Practice, 19*(3), 283.

McGovern, M. P., Lambert-Harris, C., Alterman, A. I., Xie, H., & Meier, A. (2011). A randomized controlled trial comparing integrated cognitive behavioral therapy versus individual addiction counseling for co-occurring substance use and posttraumatic stress disorders. *Journal of Dual Diagnosis, 7*(4), 207–227. https://doi.org/10.1080/15504263.2011.620425

McGovern, M. P., Lambert-Harris, C., Xie, H., Meier, A., McLeman, B., & Saunders, E. (2015). A randomized controlled trial of treatments for co-occurring substance use disorders and post-traumatic stress disorder. *Addiction (Abingdon, England), 110*(7), 1194–1204. https://doi.org/10.1111/add.12943

McHugh, R. K., Hearon, B. A., & Otto, M. W. (2010). Cognitive behavioral therapy for substance use disorders. *Psychiatric Clinics, 33*(3), 511–525.

McLellan, A. T., Luborsky, L., O'Brien, C. P., & Woody, G. E. (1980). An improved diagnostic instrument for substance abuse patients: The addiction severity index. *Journal of Nervous & Mental Diseases, 168*, 26–33.

Miller, W. R., & Rollnick, S. (2013). *Motivational interviewing: Helping people change* (3rd ed.). Guilford Press.

Mills, K. L., Barrett, E. L., Merz, S., Rosenfeld, J., Ewer, P. L., Sannibale, C., Baker, A. L., Hopwood, S., Back, S. E., Brady, K. T., & Teesson, M. (2016, Nov 15). Integrated exposure-based therapy for co-occurring post traumatic stress disorder (PTSD) and substance dependence: Predictors of change in PTSD symptom severity. *Journal of Clinical Medicine, 5*(11). https://doi.org/10.3390/jcm5110101

Mills, K. L., Barrett, E., Back, S. E., Cobham, V. E., Bendall, S., Perrin, S., Brady, K. T., Ross, J., Peach, N., Kihas, I., Cassar, J., Schollar-Root, O., & Teesson, M. (2020, Nov 30). Randomised controlled trial of integrated trauma-focused psychotherapy for traumatic stress and substance use among adolescents: trial protocol. *BMJ Open, 10*(11), e043742. https://doi.org/10.1136/bmjopen-2020-043742

Mowrer, O. H. (1960). Two-factor learning theory: Versions one and two. In O. H. Mowrer (Ed.), *Learning theory and behavior* (pp. 63–91). Wiley. https://doi.org/10.1037/10802-003

Nace, E. P. (1998). Posttraumatic stress disorder and substance abuse. Clinical issues. *Recent Developments in Alcoholism, 6*(9), 9–26. https://doi.org/10.1007/978-1-4615-7718-8_1

Najavits, L. M. (2002). *Seeking safety: A treatment manual for PTSD and substance abuse* (p. xiv, 401). Guilford Press.

Najavits, L. M. (2021). *Seeking safety: A treatment manual for PTSD and substance abuse*. Guilford Publications.
Najt, P., Fusar-Poli, P., & Brambilla, P. (2011). Co-occurring mental and substance abuse disorders: A review on the potential predictors and clinical outcomes. *Psychiatry Research, 186*(2–3), 159–164. https://doi.org/10.1016/j.psychres.2010.07.042
Nass, G. C. M., van Rens, L. W., & Dijkstra, B. A. G. (2019). Clinicians' perceptions for indicating and contra-indicating integrated treatment for SUD and comorbid PTSD, a vignette study. *Substance Abuse Treatment, Prevention, and Policy, 14*(1), 7. https://doi.org/10.1186/s13011-019-0194-5
Niolon, P. H., Kearns, M., Dills, J., Rambo, K., Irving, S., Armstead, T., & Gilbert, L. (2017). *Preventing intimate partner violence across the lifespan: A technical package of programs, policies and practices*. National Center for Injury Prevention and Control, Centers for Disease Control and Prevention.
Norman, S. B., Trim, R., Haller, M., Davis, B. C., Myers, U. S., Colvonen, P. J., Blanes, E., Lyons, R., Siegel, E. Y., Angkaw, A. C., Norman, G. J., & Mayes, T. (2019, Apr 24). Efficacy of integrated exposure therapy vs integrated coping skills therapy for comorbid posttraumatic stress disorder and alcohol use disorder: A randomized clinical trial. *JAMA Psychiatry, 76*(8), 791–799. https://doi.org/10.1001/jamapsychiatry.2019.0638
Ogden, P., & Minton, K. (2000). Sensorimotor psychotherapy: One method for processing traumatic memory. *Traumatology, 6*(3), 149–173. https://doi.org/10.1177/153476560000600302
Ouimette, P. C., Ahrens, C., Moos, R. H., & Finney, J. W. (1997). Posttraumatic stress disorder in substance abuse patients: Relationship to 1-year posttreatment outcomes. *Psychology of Addictive Behaviors, 11*(1), 34–47. https://doi.org/10.1037/0893-164X.11.1.34
Paradies, Y., Ben, J., Denson, N., Elias, A., Priest, N., Pieterse, A., Gupta, A., Kelaher, M., & Gee, G. (2015). Racism as a Determinant of Health: A Systematic Review and Meta-Analysis. *PLOS ONE, 10*(9), e0138511. https://doi.org/10.1371/journal.pone.0138511
Payne, A. J., Joseph, S., & Tudway, J. (2007). Assimilation and accommodation processes following traumatic experiences. *Journal of Loss and Trauma, 12*(1), 75–91.
Phelan, J. C., & Link, B. G. (2015). Is Racism a Fundamental Cause of Inequalities in Health. *Annual Review of Sociology, 41*(1), 311–330. https://doi.org/10.1146/annurev-soc-073014-112305
Pieterse, A., & Powell, S. (2016). A theoretical overview of the impact of racism on people of color. In *The cost of racism for people of color: Contextualizing experiences of discrimination* (pp. 11–30). American Psychological Association. https://doi.org/10.1037/14852-002
Pitman, R. K., Altman, B., Greenwald, E., Longpre, R. E., Macklin, M. L., & Steketee, G. S. (1991). Psychiatric complications during flooding therapy for posttraumatic stress disorder. *Journal of Clinical Psychiatry., 52*(1), 17–20.
Polanco-Roman, L., DeLapp, R. C., Dackis, M. N., Ebrahimi, C. T., Mafnas, K. S., Gabbay, V., & Pimentel, S. S. (2022). Racial/ethnic discrimination and suicide-related risk in a treatment-seeking group of ethnoracially minoritized adolescents. *Clinical Child Psychology and Psychiatry, 28*(4), 13591045221132682. https://doi.org/10.1177/13591045221132682
Powers, M. B., Halpern, J. M., Ferenschak, M. P., Gillihan, S. J., & Foa, E. B. (2010). A meta-analytic review of prolonged exposure for posttraumatic stress disorder. *Clinical Psychology Review, 30*(6), 635–641.
Prendergast, M., Podus, D., Finney, J., Greenwell, L., & Roll, J. (2006). Contingency management for treatment of substance use disorders: A meta-analysis. *Addiction, 101*(11), 1546–1560.
Resick, P. A., Monson, C. M., & Chard, K. M. (2016). Cognitive processing therapy for PTSD: A comprehensive manual. .
Roberts, N. P., Lotzin, A., & Schäfer, I. (2022). A systematic review and meta-analysis of psychological interventions for comorbid post-traumatic stress disorder and substance use disorder. *European Journal of Psychotraumatology, 13*(1), 2041831. https://doi.org/10.1080/20008198.2022.2041831

Robinson, S. M., Sobell, L. C., Sobell, M. B., & Leo, G. I. (2012, Dec 31). Reliability of the timeline followback for cocaine, cannabis, and cigarette use. *Psychology of Addictive Behaviors*. Advance online publication. https://doi.org/10.1037/a0030992

Rothbaum, A. O., Joseph, J., Ana, E. S., de Arellano, A., Shoemaker, H. L., Dixon, R. A., Nietert, P. J., & Brady, K. T. (2023). COPE and oxytocin for the treatment of co-occurring PTSD and alcohol use disorder: Design and methodology of a randomized controlled trial in U.S. military veterans. *Contemporary Clinical Trials, 126*, 107084. https://doi.org/10.1016/j.cct.2023.107084

Ruglass, L. M., Lopez-Castro, T., Papini, S., Killeen, T., Back, S. E., & Hien, D. A. (2017). Concurrent treatment with prolonged exposure for co-occurring full or subthreshold posttraumatic stress disorder and substance use disorders: A randomized clinical trial. *Psychotherapy and Psychosomatics, 86*(3), 150–161. https://doi.org/10.1159/000462977

Safran, J. D., & Muran, J. C. (2000). *Negotiating the therapeutic alliance: A relational treatment guide*. Guilford Press.

Shea, S. C. (1999). *The practical art of suicide assessment: A guide for mental health professionals and substance abuse counselors*. Wiley.

Simpson, T. L., Goldberg, S. B., Louden, D. K. N., Blakey, S. M., Hawn, S. E., Lott, A., Browne, K. C., Lehavot, K., & Kaysen, D. (2021). Efficacy and acceptability of interventions for co-occurring PTSD and SUD: A meta-analysis. *Journal of Anxiety Disorders, 84*, 102490. https://doi.org/10.1016/j.janxdis.2021.102490

Souza, T., & Spates, C. R. (2008). Treatment of PTSD and substance abuse comorbidity. *The Behavior Analyst Today, 9*(1), 11–26. https://doi.org/10.1037/h0100643

Stewart, S. H., Pihl, R. O., Conrod, P. J., & Dongier, M. (1998). Functional associations among trauma, PTSD, and substance-related disorders. *Addictive Behaviors, 23*(6), 797–812. https://doi.org/10.1016/s0306-4603(98)00070-7

Stockman, J. K., Hayashi, H., & Campbell, J. C. (2015). Intimate Partner Violence and its Health Impact on Ethnic Minority Women [corrected] [published correction appears in J Womens Health (Larchmt). 2015 Mar;24(3):256]. *Journal of Womens Health (Larchmt), 24*(1), 62–79. https://doi.org/10.1089/jwh.2014.4879

Tatarsky, A. (Ed.). (2002). *Harm reduction psychotherapy: A new treatment for drug and alcohol problems*. Jason Aronson.

Tran, K., Moulton, K., Santesso, N., & Rabb, D. (2016). *Cognitive processing therapy for post-traumatic stress disorder: A systematic review and meta-analysis*. Canadian Agency for Drugs and Technologies in Health.

Tynes, B. M., Willis, H. A., Stewart, A. M., & Hamilton, M. W. (2019). Race-related traumatic events online and mental health among adolescents of color. *Journal of Adolescent Health, 65*(3), 371–377. https://doi.org/10.1016/j.jadohealth.2019.03.006

Vujanovic, A. A., Smith, L. J., Green, C. E., Lane, S. D., & Schmitz, J. M. (2018). Development of a novel, integrated cognitive-behavioral therapy for co-occurring posttraumatic stress and substance use disorders: A pilot randomized clinical trial. *Contemporary Clinical Trials, 65*, 123–129. https://doi.org/10.1016/j.cct.2017.12.013

Vujanovic, A. A., Smith, L. J., Tipton, K. P., & Schmitz, J. M. (2019). A novel, integrated cognitive-behavioral therapy for co-occurring posttraumatic stress and substance use disorders: A case study. *Cognitive and Behavioral Practice, 26*(2), 307–322. https://doi.org/10.1016/j.cbpra.2018.03.003

Walter, K. H., Dickstein, B. D., Barnes, S. M., & Chard, K. M. (2014). Comparing effectiveness of CPT to CPT-C among US veterans in an interdisciplinary residential PTSD/TBI treatment program. *Journal of Traumatic Stress, 27*(4), 438–445.

Weathers, F. W., Blake, D. D., Schnurr, P. P., Kaloupek, D. G., Marx, B. P., & Keane, T. M. (2013a). *The clinician-administered PTSD scale for DSM-5 (CAPS-5).* [Assessment] Available from www.ptsd.va.gov

Weathers, F. W., Litz, B. T., Keane, T. M., Palmieri, P. A., Marx, B. P., & Schnurr, P. P. (2013b). *The PTSD checklist for DSM-5 (PCL-5)*. Scale available from the National Center for PTSD at www.ptsd.va.gov

Weathers, F. W., Blake, D. D., Schnurr, P. P., Kaloupek, D. G., Marx, B. P., & Keane, T. M. (2013c). *The life events checklist for DSM-5 (LEC-5)*. Instrument available from the National Center for PTSD at www.ptsd.va.gov

Williams, M. T., & Wetterneck, C. (2022). *Racial trauma treatment: A 12-session CBT protocol*. PESI.

Windle, M. (1994). Substance use, risky behaviors, and victimization among a US national adolescent sample. *Addiction, 89*(2), 175–182. https://doi.org/10.1111/j.1360-0443.1994.tb00876.x

Witkiewitz, K., Warner, K., Sully, B., Barricks, A., Stauffer, C., Thompson, B. L., & Luoma, J. B. (2014). Randomized trial comparing mindfulness-based relapse prevention with relapse prevention for women offenders at a residential addiction treatment center. *Substance Use & Misuse, 49*(5), 536–546.

Zhou, Y., Sun, L., Wang, Y., Wu, L., Sun, Z., Zhang, F., & Liu, W. (2020). Developments of prolonged exposure in treatment effect of post-traumatic stress disorder and controlling dropout rate: A meta-analytic review. *Clinical Psychology & Psychotherapy, 27*(4), 449–462.

Chapter 6
Affect Management Training for Substance Use Disorders: A Transdiagnostic Approach to Treating Co-occurring Emotional Disorder Symptoms and Substance Use

Alexandra Tanner, Isabelle Lanser, and Kate Wolitzky-Taylor

Introduction

Over the last several years the field has shifted from a categorical model of diagnosis to a dimensional model (Cuthbert, 2014). A dimensional model of emotional disorders emphasizes the mechanism that contribute to the development and maintenance of the disorders, rather than discrete symptoms. Focusing on mechanisms allows for treatments developed from this approach to be transdiagnostic as many disorders share overlapping mechanisms, thereby leading to more parsimonious, streamlined, and integrated interventions that cut across multiple psychopathologies that often co-occur (see Sauer-Zavala et al., 2017, for a review). Emotional disorders (ED), such as anxiety disorders and depressive disorders, share many of the same mechanisms. For example, both anxiety and depressive disorders are the result of, and are maintained by, maladaptive reactivity to negative affect. Negative affect is defined as the broad spectrum of negative emotions (i.e., sadness, worry, disgust, anger, fear). Maladaptive reactivity to that negative affect refers to responding to these emotions in a way that is unhelpful and ultimately serves to maintain the emotional difficulties/emotional disorder symptoms.

Avoidance behaviors are a common maladaptive response to negative affect in both anxiety and depressive disorders. In anxiety disorders, the experience of fear motivates avoidance of the feared stimulus, preventing inhibitory learning from occurring and increasing the fear response in future encounters with this stimulus. In depressive disorders, avoidance often manifests as behavioral inactivation due to

A. Tanner · I. Lanser · K. Wolitzky-Taylor (✉)
Department of Psychiatry and Biobehavioral Sciences and Semel Institute for Neuroscience and Human Behavior, Integrated Substance Abuse Programs, Los Angeles, CA, USA
e-mail: tannera@ucla.edu; ilanser@g.ucla.edu; kbtaylor@mednet.ucla.edu

K. Wolitzky-Taylor (ed.), *Treating Comorbid Substance Use and Emotional Disorders*, CBT: Science Into Practice, https://doi.org/10.1007/978-3-031-62971-6_6

anhedonia or beliefs that the activity will not yield positive affect or will increase negative affect. Thus, targeting avoidance by teaching approach responses via exposure for anxiety disorders and behavioral activation for depression addresses the same maladaptive response to negative affect, resulting in improvements in functioning and reductions in symptoms.

Substance use disorders (SUD) and ED have a high comorbidity and typically demonstrate poorer treatment outcomes than SUD alone (Burns et al., 2005; Kushner et al., 2005; Magidson et al., 2012). Individuals with ED experience greater negative affect and perceive negative emotions as more distressing than individuals without ED (Brown & Barlow, 2009; Roemer et al., 2005). As a result, they tend to rely on strategies to eliminate or suppress negative emotions to cope with these experiences, which in turn maintains and exacerbates their distress (Barlow et al., 2014; Aldao & Nolen-Hoeksema, 2010; Baker et al., 2004; Sauer-Zavala et al., 2012). Substance use represents one maladaptive strategy for eliminating or suppressing negative affect. Further, a number of constructs representing maladaptive responses to negative affect have been identified as transdiagnostic processes implicated in the onset and maintenance of both ED and SUD, with some found to mediate the association between ED and SUD (Buckner et al., 2007; Howell et al., 2010; Wolitzky-Taylor et al., 2015; Wolitzky-Taylor et al., 2016). These transdiagnostic processes include anxiety sensitivity (the perception of anxiety symptoms as dangerous or harmful); distress intolerance (the perceived inability to tolerate or cope with distress); and several facets of emotion dysregulation (i.e., cognitive misappraisal, negative urgency and avoidance). Taken together, emerging research reveals that these transdiagnostic constructs that represent various maladaptive cognitive, behavioral, and emotional reactions to negative affect may account for, or statistically explain, the high comorbidity between ED and SUD.

Treatments that target the shared mechanisms thought to underlie both ED and SUD are likely to improve treatment outcomes for both SUD and comorbid SUD and ED. Further, intervening during critical stages of development, such as adolescence and early adulthood (i.e., emerging adulthood), may help to prevent the onset of SUD and improve long-term outcomes. Adolescence through early adulthood represent times of rapid neurological and emotion regulation development, as well as increased experimentation and risk-taking behaviors, including illicit drug use (SAMHSA, 2014). Among adolescents, cannabis is the most frequently used illicit drug and CUD is the most prevalent SUD (Johnston et al., 2000; Wittchen et al., 2007). Moreover, CUD in adolescence is associated with ED (Wittchen et al., 2007; McGee et al., 2000), and ED during adolescence predict the onset of SUD in emerging adulthood (Wolitzky-Taylor et al., 2012). Thus, targeting both CUD and ED among adolescents and early adults may improve outcomes for SUD more broadly.

This chapter reviews and describes a novel treatment called Affect Management Training (AMT), originally developed for emerging adults targeting the mechanisms hypothesized to underlie both ED and CUD with the goal of reducing cannabis use (Fig. 6.1). This intervention demonstrated efficacy in a clinical trial of 18- to 25-year olds with CUD and elevations in negative affect and constructs representing maladaptive reactivity to negative affect (Wolitzky-Taylor et al., 2022). Given that CUD is the most prevalent SUD among emerging adults, AMT was initially evaluated in a CUD population. However, there is empirical support for the

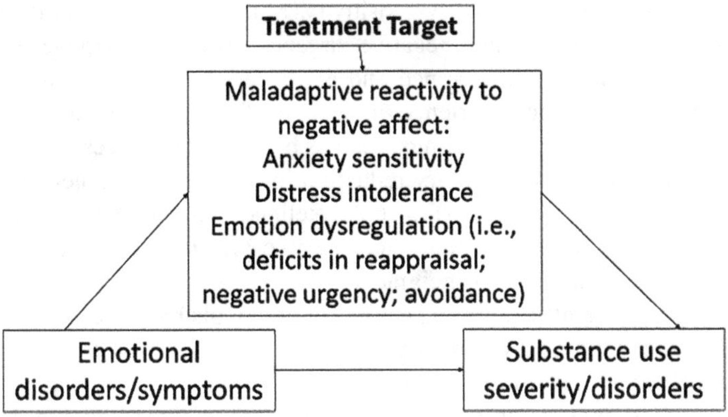

Fig. 6.1 Theoretical model of affect management training targeting the constructs of maladaptive reactivity to negative affect hypothesized to underlie and mediate the relation between emotional disorders and substance use disorders

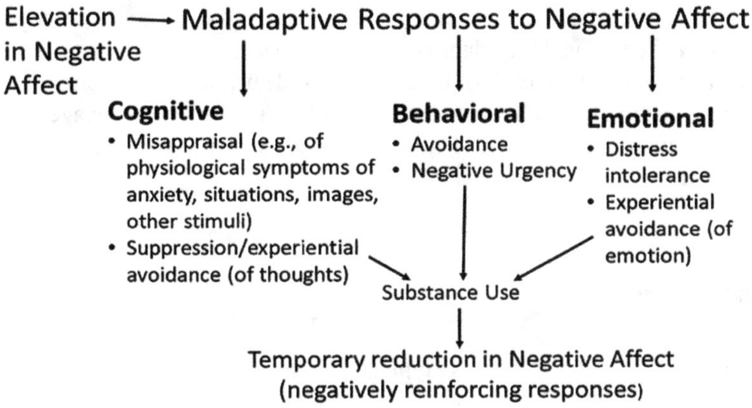

Fig. 6.2 Theoretical model demonstrating the reinforcing cycle of how maladaptive responses to negative affect lead to substance use and temporary reductions in negative affect

model underlying the premise of AMT for a variety of other substances of dependence (see Fig. 6.2), suggesting that AMT is likely effective for the treatment of other SUD manifestations. Thus, CUD was considered the test case for demonstrating the effectiveness of AMT for comorbid ED and SUD.

Affect Management Training (AMT) Model

The specific constructs of maladaptive reactivity to negative affect can be divided into three categories: maladaptive cognitive, behavioral, and emotional responding to negative affect. Maladaptive cognitive responding to negative affect includes cognitive misappraisals and anxiety sensitivity. Maladaptive behavioral responses include avoidance coping and negative urgency. And maladaptive emotional responses include distress intolerance and experiential avoidance. Each of these constructs contribute to the experience of negative affect and motivate behaviors to eliminate or suppress negative feelings, such as by using substances. Substance use in this context results in a temporary reduction in negative affect, negatively reinforcing substance use behaviors (Fig. 6.2). Reliance on avoidance strategies for coping, such as substance use, maintain negative affect by reinforcing the very mechanisms contributing to the heightened distress and substance use: negative beliefs about negative affect (i.e., misappraisals), low distress tolerance, increased fear of anxiety symptoms (i.e., anxiety sensitivity), negative urgency, and ongoing avoidance behaviors. Additionally, with continued substance use over time, individuals with SUD may begin to experience cravings and urges to use, both as a result of increased substance dependence and tolerance, as well as a conditioned response to the experience of negative affect itself, exacerbating ED and creating a vicious cycle between the experience of negative affect and substance use.

Understanding maladaptive reactivity to negative affect as a driver of substance use highlights several avenues for change. AMT is designed to target the cognitive, behavioral, and emotional maladaptive responses to negative affect by teaching clients adaptive responses in each of these domains. Thus, utilizing a combination of cognitive, behavioral, mindfulness and acceptance strategies to manage negative affect and cannabis cravings, AMT aims to reduce substance use and symptoms of both ED and SUD simultaneously.

Distinctions with CBT

Traditional models of CBT for SUD typically focus on strategies more directly tied to use behaviors, such as identifying high-risk situations and triggers, positive coping skills, coping in high-stress situations, identifying distorted thinking related to urge to use, drug refusal skills, social support, and communication skills. These treatment models fail to address the overlapping symptomology in clients with comorbid emotional disorders, and the transdiagnostic constructs that functionally link negative affect to substance use. These omissions likely lead to poorer outcomes for these clients relative to clients with SUD alone. In contrast, the transdiagnostic framework of AMT allows it to be effective for a wide spectrum of emotional and substance use disorders where negative affect reactivity is a primary etiological and maintenance mechanism. Additionally, this treatment approach helps clients understand their substance use in the broader context of their emotional difficulties rather than as a stand-alone issue.

Intervention and Case Example

AMT is a 12-session individual therapy for emerging adults (aged 18–25) who meet the diagnostic criteria for cannabis use disorder, endorse elevated negative affect and demonstrate maladaptive responding to negative affect. AMT is designed to target the core mechanisms hypothesized to link SUD (including CUD) with ED (i.e., anxiety and depression). This manualized intervention focuses on helping clients build skills to target maladaptive responding to negative affect (i.e., anxiety sensitivity, distress intolerance, and emotion dysregulation) in the context of reducing cannabis use.

All intervention components/strategies included in AMT are based on cognitive and behavioral principles, thus all therapists are expected to have background and training in cognitive behavior therapies, specifically for anxiety disorders, and familiarity with mindfulness and acceptance strategies is preferred. Additionally, prior to delivery, all therapists should be trained in AMT and demonstrate competency to deliver each treatment component.

The AMT manual includes a summary for each session highlighting the session goals, materials needed for the session, a brief agenda and a detailed session outline. While manualized, the treatment sessions are not scripted; rather, therapists use the manual handouts combined with Socratic questioning and guided discovery to help clients understand the connections between their negative affect, maladaptive reactivity to negative affect and cannabis use, as well as learn new skills to manage negative affect and reduce cannabis use. All session materials, including handouts for in-session exercises and between-session practices, can be found in the manual appendix.

AMT includes six primary treatment components: education, mindfulness/acceptance, cognitive reappraisal skills, problem solving/coping skills, preparing for exposures and affect management in the context of exposures. Each component is designed to specifically address at least one of the transdiagnostic targets linking SUD to ED (see Fig. 6.3 from AMT manual). Additionally, each skill is introduced as a strategy to replace cannabis use in the context of experiencing negative emotions and cannabis cravings.

The following case example will demonstrate the components of AMT and its application for managing emotional distress and reducing cannabis use.

> Sylvia is a 22-year-old, cisgender, bisexual, Latina female in her 3rd year at a large, public university. She began using cannabis in high school, and since then uses a cannabis vape frequently throughout the day, every day. Sylvia has previously received treatment for social anxiety disorder and major depressive disorder but says that pharmacotherapy didn't work for her in the past and prefers using cannabis to manage her symptoms. Recently, she has noticed that she is running through her vape cartridges much faster than in the past, has been struggling to fall asleep, and is experiencing loss of appetite and restlessness. Sylvia presented to treatment because her parents and friends have started to comment on her cannabis use and are concerned that she is going to her on-campus job and her classes while high.

Component	Description	Transdiagnostic Target
Education	Components of negative affect, adaptive v. maladaptive ways to respond to negative affect, how maladaptive responding to negative affect and cannabis use mutually maintain each other, how cannabis use is tied to these components, self-monitoring, general education about cannabis use and substance use disorders	Avoidance and misappraisal
Mindfulness/ acceptance	Understanding concept of mindful and nonjudgmental awareness of emotional experience, practicing mindfulness techniques, how to use mindfulness in the context of reducing cannabis use	Experiential avoidance, suppression, distress intolerance
Cognitive reappraisal skills	Identifying automatic thoughts, downward arrow, challenging odds, decatastropizing, using cognitive reappraisal in the context of negative affect-inducing situations that result in cannabis craving	Misappraisal
Problem solving/ coping skills	Coping in the context of decatastrophizing, problem solving/decision making, distress tolerance skills (attentional refocusing, self-care), applying problem solving and coping skills in high risk situations for cannabis use	Avoidance and negative urgency
Preparing for exposure	Rationale, interoceptive assessment, identifying distressing stimuli, constructing hierarchy of distressing/avoided stimuli, preparing for and planning exposure	Avoidance (behavioral and experiential)
Affect management in the context of experiencing distressing stimuli	In-session skill and exposure practice, continued assigning and reviewing of homework assignments to work through hierarchy and refine skills; relapse prevention in the context of managing negative affect as a trigger for cannabis use	Avoidance, negative urgency, distress intolerance, misappraisal (including anxiety sensitivity)

Fig. 6.3 Description of each treatment component of AMT and the corresponding transdiagnostic mechanisms targeted

Treatment Components and Case Dialogue

Session 1

The education component of treatment occurs across the first two sessions of AMT and includes motivational enhancement, psychoeducation, and an introduction to self-monitoring to target avoidance and misappraisal. In addition to orienting clients to the treatment, the primary aim of the first session is to use motivational interviewing techniques to increase motivation for reducing cannabis use and identify treatment goals. Clients explore their cannabis use and expectations using the "Does cannabis use meet my expectations?" form. Next, the "Problem Brainstorming" worksheet is used to explore any ways cannabis is causing problems for clients or interfering in their life. Lastly, the "Pros and Cons Balance Sheet" asks clients to consider the pros and cons of their current use vs. reducing their use. Lastly, clients are asked to identify a concrete goal for changing their cannabis use for homework.

Therapist You mentioned that you've been using cannabis to "self-medicate," can you tell me what that means to you?

Sylvia Sure, when I first started vaping, I noticed that I immediately felt more calm and less anxious. I felt like I could study without getting worried about failing or whether I was smart enough to pass my classes. I also was less worried about the future in general. I felt light, happy, and everything was more enjoyable. When I tried antidepressants, I didn't

	feel any of those effects and I still needed to vape in order to feel better, so I decided to stop the medication since it wasn't helping anyway.
Therapist	So, when you were prescribed medication in the past, you didn't feel much of a difference in your overall mood and anxiety unless you used cannabis?
Sylvia	Exactly. Weed is the only thing that makes me feel like myself.
Therapist	I'm curious how cannabis fits in to your day now. What do you do in a typical day and how does using cannabis change what you do?
Sylvia	I usually wake up around 9am, scroll on my phone in bed and use my weed pen to help me start off my day in a relaxed way. Then, I get up brush my teeth and get ready. I usually skip breakfast because I'm not really hungry in the morning and head to class. I like to listen to music as I walk to campus and I usually use my vape on my walk over to keep myself from getting too in my head. I usually have 2 hours of class time and then get some lunch before my next class. On my way home from campus I listen to music, vape, and think about what I want to do when I get home. Once I'm home, I usually talk to my roommates before I get ready for work.
Therapist	You're using cannabis pretty consistently throughout the day. How does it help you get through your day?
Sylvia	It helps me not be bothered by everything so much. Like I said, it helps me get out of my head.
Therapist	You mentioned that you've been using cannabis for quite a long time now, and you have some expectations of how you want it to help you get through the day. How much does cannabis actually help you in the way you expect it to?
Sylvia	I definitely feel more relaxed after taking a hit, I don't even get high anymore. Sometimes though I still feel anxious and sad, especially by the end of the day. It's like I have to keep using it to keep my mood up, otherwise the worries start flooding back.
Therapist	Cannabis keeps the worries at bay, but doesn't get rid of them completely, is that right?
Sylvia	For sure, I know that if I stopped vaping or if I used less I would be a nervous wreck all the time.
Therapist	You've told me how cannabis helps you get through the day, I'm wondering if there's anything that cannabis gets in the way of or ways that it might actually cause problems for you?
Sylvia	I mean it's definitely expensive and has only gotten more expensive now that I'm using more cartridges every week.
Therapist	Okay, so it's causing some financial difficulties. Anything else?
Sylvia	Yeah, I guess my friends have said they feel like I'm not paying attention to them or they don't feel as supported by me because I'm so relaxed all the time. They've also said that they're concerned that I use before going to class and work and my parents have said the same thing.
Therapist	What are your friends and parents concerned about?

Sylvia	They worry that other people can tell that I'm high even though I told them I don't even get high anymore. They also said that they worry about me using before driving.
Therapist	They're worried you might get into an accident.
Sylvia	Exactly, and that I'm not making a good impression on my boss or my professors and that's going to make it difficult for me to get recommendation letters when I graduate. But I told them they're the only ones who seem to comment on it or notice even.
Therapist	It seems like your cannabis use is also causing some conflicts with your friends and family because you disagree over how it's affecting you.
Sylvia	Definitely.
Therapist	Are there any physical or medical consequences that you've noticed?
Sylvia	I guess I'm more winded than I used to be when I walk to campus or go up stairs. I also have noticed that I tend to cough more and have phlegm in my throat more often than not. I think it helps me with my sleep but sometimes I'm not sure.
Therapist	Can you say more about that?
Sylvia	Yeah, I usually like to take a hit of my weed pen before I go to sleep because it helps me relax. But, sometimes I notice that I have really bad dreams or I wake up more frequently if I've used a lot before bed.
Therapist	I see, so in addition to noticing some breathing difficulty and coughing, sometimes using actually makes it harder for you to stay asleep even though you're using before bed to help you sleep.
Sylvia	Yeah, there's definitely a sweet spot that I need to be in, otherwise I have terrible sleep.
Therapist	Okay, thank you for sharing these problems with me. I'd like to now explore the pros and cons of continuing to use and changing your use. What do you see as the benefits of continuing to use the way you are right now?
Sylvia	Well, I won't be anxious. I also will be in a good mood—
Therapist	What does a "good mood" mean to you?
Sylvia	Relaxed, not stressed, calm, chill
Therapist	Okay, any other benefits?
Sylvia	I'm just more fun to be around, I laugh more, I'm not so serious all the time.
Therapist	And what about the cons?
Sylvia	It's expensive. My friends and family are worried about me. I guess the sleep thing, too.
Therapist	Okay, so on the one hand if you continue to use the way you are now, you'll get to feel less stressed and you're more fun to be around. But on the other hand, it's expensive, your friends and family are concerned, and sometimes it makes it difficult for you to sleep. Let's think about the cons of changing your use.
Sylvia	That's easy, I'll be super stressed all the time. I'll be in a bad mood and I won't enjoy anything anymore.

Therapist What will you be stressed about?

Sylvia Everything. School, my family, my dog, my future, whether I'll ever be in a relationship…everything.

Therapist I see. And are there any pros to changing your use?

Sylvia I'll probably save money. It also might be nice to not feel anxious when I can't vape. I might feel more energetic. Being relaxed is nice but I definitely take longer to do things.

Therapist Alright, it seems like the main con of changing your use is mood related, you're worried you'll feel more anxious and not be able to enjoy things. On the other hand, you think you'll save money, have more energy, and not experience anxiety when you're not able to vape. When you look at all the pros and cons, what do you take from this exercise?

Sylvia I guess the main thing is I can see why it's been so hard for me to want to stop or change my cannabis use. I'm really scared of feeling how I felt before I found cannabis. That was a really dark time for me and cannabis really helped me get through it. I can also see that there are ways it's not helping me right now that I tend to ignore.

Therapist Sometimes what worked for us at one point in our lives stops working or doesn't work as well as it used to. It sounds like that's where you're at right now with your cannabis use.

Sylvia Yeah, I think so.

Session 2

The second treatment session focuses on providing psychoeducation on the AMT treatment model, specifically how maladaptive responding to negative affect through cannabis use maintains negative affect. Clients are given education on the short-term and long-term effects of cannabis on mood, cognitive functioning and physiology. The "It's Just Marijuana" checklist is used to dispel common myths regarding the benefits of cannabis. Clients learn about the three components (thoughts, feelings, and behaviors) of emotions and are introduced to self-monitoring to track how negative emotions impact their cannabis craving or use, and the cannabis diary to track frequency of cannabis use and the impact on emotions.

Therapist Our thoughts, feelings, and behaviors are all connected and all influence each other. When we experience negative affect, which can be sadness, anxiety, or even anger for example, we all have ways we react or respond to those feelings. For example, we might use our thoughts to suppress what we're feeling. We might physically remove ourselves from a situation to avoid feeling negatively. Or we might numb ourselves or distance ourselves emotionally so that we can get rid of the feeling. One way someone might accomplish all of these is to use a substance like cannabis which can be pretty effective at helping us get rid of unwanted thoughts, change or remove ourselves from a situation, or make us feel good so our emotions feel less intense.

Sylvia	That makes a lot of sense. When I first started using, it was for fun with friends but it had the added benefit of making my anxious thoughts go away and making me feel better.
Therapist	Exactly, cannabis use can temporarily make us feel better by affecting our thoughts, feelings, and behaviors. Can you think of time where this happened for you?
Sylvia	Yeah, I remember that a few weeks ago I had a big essay that was due for one of my classes and I was feeling pretty nervous about it. I started to have thoughts of "I'm dumb" and "I can't do this." I was feeling really overwhelmed and decided to hit my vape and almost immediately those thoughts went away and I cared a lot less about the paper. I decided to go out with my friends instead and felt much better.
Therapist	That's interesting, so cannabis made those thoughts and feelings go away, but it also seems like you stopped trying to work on the paper at all.
Sylvia	Yeah, I ended up waiting until the night it was due to start working on it. I tend to procrastinate a lot.
Therapist	Thanks for sharing this example, it highlights the next point I wanted to make which is that even though cannabis can make the negative feelings and thoughts go away, it doesn't actually take away the thing that made you stressed to begin with. No amount of cannabis is going to get you out of needing to write the paper.
Sylvia	Yeah, that's true, even though I felt better in the moment, I still had to do it eventually.
Therapist	From what you said earlier, it seems like when you did sit down to work on the paper it was pretty stressful.
Sylvia	It was. Probably even more stressful than when I tried to work on it ahead of time because I now had the time pressure. I also knew it wouldn't be as good as I wanted it to be because I didn't have time.
Therapist	Counterintuitively, using these short-term fixes, like cannabis use, can actually make us feel more stressed in the long-term. Additionally, withdrawal from cannabis and the effects of cannabis can lead us to experience even more negative emotions which sometimes leads us to think we need to use even more cannabis to get rid of those feelings. That's how we can get stuck needing more and more to feel better. The goal of this treatment is to interrupt this cycle by giving you skills to manage your negative emotions when they first appear and actively engage with what's stressing you out rather than avoid it.

Session 3

The goal of the third session is to introduce mindfulness as a strategy to increase acceptance and tolerance of negative emotions and uncomfortable sensations or cravings. The transdiagnostic mechanisms targeted in this session are experiential avoidance, suppression, and distress intolerance. Clients are provided psychoeducation on mindfulness as non-judgmental and present-focused and its application to increase tolerance of discomfort and reduce cannabis use as an avoidance strategy. Clients are guided through both a Body Scan exercise to increase mindful awareness of emotions and physical sensations, and an Urge Surfing exercise to reduce reactivity to cannabis cravings.

Therapist The first skill we're going to learn is mindfulness. Have you heard of mindfulness before?

Sylvia I think so. It's when you meditate, right?

Therapist Meditation can be a form of mindfulness. We can think of mindfulness as a big umbrella that activities like meditation can fall under. Mindfulness trains our minds to be more aware of our bodies and minds in the present moment. It is the practice of paying attention to ourselves and our experiences in a non-judgmental way. All of our emotions, even the positive ones, follow a similar arc. They come on pretty quickly—have you ever seen anyone start to laugh slowly?

Sylvia Hmm I guess not, they usually just burst out with laughter!

Therapist Exactly! All of our emotions come on with a high peak and then slowly start to fade. One of the things we're going to learn is that we can ride that wave of emotion. We don't have to do anything to make our negative emotions go away, they'll go away on their own with time. Negative emotions may be uncomfortable, but we don't need to do anything to get rid of them. And, as we talked about last week, trying to get rid of them in the short term can actually prolong them, sometimes literally like when you decided to put off that essay. Using cannabis, or any substance, to deal with our emotions can make it more difficult to tolerate negative feelings on our own and we can start to feel like we need cannabis whenever we start to feel a negative feeling.

Sylvia I definitely understand that, sometimes when I start to feel anxious, I start reaching for my weed pen without even thinking about it.

Therapist It can become really automatic! Mindfulness is a way for us to press pause and find some space between the negative emotion and what we may do automatically to try to fix the emotion so that we can have time to feel the emotion and let it pass.

Session 4

The fourth session introduces cognitive reappraisal as a skill to target unhelpful thoughts and misappraisals maintaining negative affect and cannabis use. The "Taking Perspective" handout guides clients to examine the evidence for and against their thoughts to more accurately estimate the likelihood of negative outcomes occurring and decatastrophize underestimations of their ability to cope with negative outcomes.

Therapist Sometimes when we experience a negative emotion, our thoughts can start to spiral. We might catastrophize, overestimate the likelihood that something bad might happen, and ignore the positive things that are happening. Do you do any of these?

Sylvia	Yeah definitely, I've always been a catastrophizer. Once one thing goes wrong, I can't help but think about all the other things that are going to go wrong.
Therapist	Can you give me an example?
Sylvia	The other day at work, I gave a customer the wrong order and my mind immediately jumped to "I'm getting fired" and then kept going from there.
Therapist	Where else did your mind go?
Sylvia	I started to think about all the other times I messed up and convinced myself that if I get fired, I'll never be able to find another job and I'll have to live with my parents forever and I'll be a failure.
Therapist	Because you made this one mistake, it means that you're a failure.
Sylvia	Yes.
Therapist	What did you do when your mind started down this track? Did you do anything to try to stop it?
Sylvia	I told my manager I was taking my break and went outside to hit my vape.
Therapist	How did you feel after you used cannabis in that moment?
Sylvia	My thoughts stopped racing, but I felt really aware of everything I did at work for the rest of the time. I started to feel like I was being watched and monitored and that made me feel anxious again.
Therapist	Cannabis helped stop the spiral but didn't take away the anxiety completely. It sounds like it even amplified how you were feeling.
Sylvia	Yeah, that happens sometimes.
Therapist	Thanks for sharing this example. Today, we're going to learn some skills that can help you take perspective in the moments when you find yourself catastrophizing. These skills can help us slow down our thinking, be less reactive, look at the bigger picture, and think more flexibly. In order to be able to use these skills, we have to first be mindful of what we're feeling and accept that we are feeling that way. Then, once we know what we're feeling, we can change our thoughts to change how we feel. Let's practice using the scenario you just described. What was the likelihood you would get fired according to your anxious self?
Sylvia	Oh, 100%.
Therapist	And how bad would it be if that did happen on a scale of 0–100?
Sylvia	I would say 90.
Therapist	Okay, so now we're going to look at the evidence for your thought "I'm going to get fired." Has that ever happened before?
Sylvia	Not to me, but one of my coworkers was fired recently.
Therapist	Were they fired for the same mistake you made?
Sylvia	No…they were always late and I think my manager had given them a few warnings.
Therapist	Okay so evidence for this thought: your coworker was fired recently after getting a few warnings. Any other evidence?
Sylvia	My manager can be pretty impulsive and I don't think she likes me.

Therapist	How do you know she doesn't like you?
Sylvia	She's made some passive aggressive comments about weed around me before. She also never asks me to help her with tasks, she always asks someone else.
Therapist	Alright, so another piece of evidence for the thought is that your manager doesn't ask you for help and has made negative comments around you. What about evidence against the thought?
Sylvia	Well, we have a whole protocol for termination. Even my coworker who was fired had been placed on probation beforehand.
Therapist	Okay, so it sounds like they knew ahead of time that they were at risk for getting fired. What else?
Sylvia	I've never been written up in the past and my last evaluation was positive overall.
Therapist	Anything else?
Sylvia	I guess my manager does give me extra shifts when I ask for them, so maybe she does like me.
Therapist	Okay, in our evidence against the thought category we have: there's a protocol that has to be followed before anyone can be fired, your most recent evaluation was positive, and your manager has been supportive of your working more in the past. Keeping these things in mind, what are some alternative outcomes in this situation?
Sylvia	When I think about it, even if my mistake was really bad the worst that would happen in that moment is I would get a warning and maybe placed on probation. I've also made similar mistakes in the past and haven't been fired.
Therapist	So another way of thinking about it is: If I made a fire-able mistake, I would be placed on probation first and given the opportunity to make up for it?
Sylvia	Yeah, exactly.
Therapist	Okay, let's imagine the worst thing you imagined comes true. You make one mistake and you get fired. How would you cope?
Sylvia	I guess I would feel pretty bad about myself, but I have been thinking about leaving this job anyway so I might apply to some of the other jobs I've found.
Therapist	You'd apply to other jobs, what else?
Sylvia	I would try to end on good terms and let my manager know that I understood what I did was a mistake.
Therapist	You would try to repair the relationship with your manager.
Sylvia	Yeah, I think that would help me feel like I wasn't leaving them with a bad impression of me.
Therapist	If a friend were in a similar position, what would you say to them?
Sylvia	I would tell them that if their manager was that quick to fire people, it probably isn't the best place for them to be working anyway.
Therapist	Anything else?

Sylvia	I'd also let them know that even though this really bad thing happened, they'll find another job and it doesn't change how I feel about them.
Therapist	You sound like you'd have a lot of compassion for them.
Sylvia	Yeah, I would.
Therapist	Okay so let's zoom out, now that we've talked about the evidence for and against the thought, identified some alternative outcomes, brainstormed ways you would cope, and considered how you would respond to a friend in a similar situation, how likely is it that you would get fired in this situation?
Sylvia	I would say 30%.
Therapist	Okay, and how bad would it be if it did happen, 0–100?
Sylvia	Probably a 50.
Therapist	And if you had to come up with a new thought about this situation what would it be?
Sylvia	I made a mistake and even though it feels bad, my manager would still have to follow a process in order to fire me and I would be given an opportunity to try again. Even if I did get fired, I would be able to find another job and I don't have to leave on bad terms.

Session 5

Session five is the final skill lesson of AMT and targets avoidance and negative urgency by teaching clients how to problem solve stressors that lead to negative affect and cannabis use. The "Taking Action" form guides clients to identify specific problems, brainstorm potential solutions, weigh the pros and cons and develop an action plan with manageable goals. A secondary goal of this session is to review each of the skills for managing negative affect and introduce the "Choosing my Response" handout to help clients determine which skill to use when faced with negative affect to reduce cannabis use.

Therapist	So far, we've learned how to use mindfulness and thought challenging to help us when we feel negative emotions. Today, we're going to learn about problem solving. This skill is a way for us to use our behavior to address the situation or trigger directly, instead of avoiding it. Problem solving is especially helpful when there is a concrete issue to address. There are 4 steps to problem solving: identifying the problem, brainstorming, weighing pros and cons, and developing an action plan with small, manageable goals. Can you think of a problem that you'd like to work on today?
Sylvia	I know that last time we talked about me being worried I'm going to get fired, but I'm actually really unhappy at my job.
Therapist	Tell me more.
Sylvia	Even though it works with my schedule now, I don't see myself working here long term and there aren't many opportunities to get a raise. It's also pretty stressful, my manager is pretty moody and it doesn't really feel like I'm part of a team. I feel really on edge whenever I'm at work.

Therapist Okay, so the problem is you're unhappy at work because of the environment and because you don't have many opportunities to get promoted. What are some things you could do?

Sylvia I mean, right now I just try not to think about it. But, I have started looking into other jobs.

Therapist Alright, so one thing you could do is look for other jobs. What else?

Sylvia I guess I could talk to my coworkers and see if they feel the same way.

Therapist Okay, what else could you do?

Sylvia I could also talk to my manager about how I've been feeling.

Therapist Anything else? We're just brainstorming, so the ideas don't have to all be realistic.

Sylvia Okay, in that case, I could just stop showing up to work.

Therapist Now that we have our list, we're going to evaluate how much time and effort it would take to implement the solution, the cost of the solution, any negative consequences to others the solution might cause, and whether we need help from others.

Sylvia Finding a new job would require a lot of time and effort, and I'm not sure I can do that right now. It also is expensive in the sense that I would probably have to miss work to interview. I don't think I would need help from anyone else, and I don't think it would really affect anyone else.

Therapist Great, what about talking to your coworkers?

Sylvia That would be pretty low effort and require less of my time. I can't think of any costs, but it might make my coworkers not feel good either and my manager might be upset if she knew we were talking about her. I also would need my coworkers to be available and willing to talk in order for this options to be helpful.

Therapist What about talking with your manager?

Sylvia That would require some effort, but not a lot of time. I can't think of any costs for this one either and I don't think it would affect others quite as much. I would need my manager to be able to implement this solution.

Therapist And lastly, what if you just stopped going to work?

Sylvia That would definitely not require effort from me. Even though I wouldn't have to use my time working, I would probably spend a lot of time worrying about what my coworkers and managers are thinking and if they're mad at me. I also would lose money because I'm not working. My coworkers and manager would have more work to do and they'd probably be pretty upset that I just ghosted them. I wouldn't need any help from others though.

Therapist Now that we have evaluated each solution, what seems like the best solution?

Sylvia Talking to my manager, for sure.

Therapist Okay, so let's think about an action plan. What do you need to do in order to talk to your manager about how you're feeling.

Sylvia I think it would be helpful to spend some time thinking about what I want to say to her and reflecting on how I'm feeling.

Therapist You might try to use mindfulness here to tune into your thoughts and emotions.

Sylvia Yeah, and then I think it would be helpful to write down the main things I want to tell her.

Therapist Okay, and then what would you need to do.

Sylvia I would need to let her know that I want to talk to her and ask to find a time to do that.

Therapist Any other steps?

Sylvia I think that's it!

Therapist Great, how do you feel about this plan?

Sylvia It's scary, but I think I can do it.

Therapist It is scary to tell someone, especially a manager, how we're feeling. But, it can be worth it if it helps us solve our problem. We can use all of the skills we talked about together to solve a problem, we can first use mindfulness to tune into how we're feeling and help us identify the problem. We can look at our thoughts and challenge any that might be keeping us stuck or preventing us from taking action. Then, we can use problem solving to address the challenge head on.

Sessions 6–12

The remaining sessions (sessions 6–12) focus on designing and practicing exposures to the situations and stimuli that often lead to cannabis use. Exposures target avoidance, negative urgency, distress intolerance, and cognitive misappraisals. During session 6, clients are given the rationale for exposures and create their Distress List of avoided and distressing stimuli (i.e., bodily sensations, images, and situations) that lead to cannabis use. To create their Distress List, clients complete an interoceptive "Sensation Assessment" to identify feared bodily sensations and use the "Identifying Distressing Images" form to identify feared images for imaginal exposures. They also identify a list of distressing situations that leads to cannabis cravings or use. Lastly, clients design their first between-session exposure practice using the "Setting up a Facing Distressing Situations" form. The goal of the first exposure is to practice remaining abstinent in a distressing context without any pre-exposure coping.

Therapist Now that we've reviewed each of the skills and you've had a chance to practice them, we're going to put them to the test using exposure. Have you heard of exposure before?

Sylvia No, I don't think so.

Therapist Exposure practices are exercises we can do to purposefully bring on negative emotions so that we can 1) learn that we can tolerate those negative feelings and 2) use our skills, not cannabis, to cope. By repeatedly experiencing negative emotions and not using cannabis to cope, we give ourselves the chance to learn that these negative feelings are

	temporary, harmless, and tolerable, which will ultimately make us less afraid and avoidant of them in the future. There are lots of ways to do exposure practices because there are lots of ways to feel negative emotions. We're going to practice exposing ourselves to negative physical sensations, negative experiences, and negative thoughts/images.
Sylvia	This sounds really difficult.
Therapist	It is, and that's the point, we want you to believe you can experience and tolerate difficult things and we can't do that unless you have the experience of surviving those difficult things.

The remaining sessions (7–12) continue exposure exercises both in- and between-sessions to help clients learn that they can tolerate distress without using cannabis. Specifically, exposures highlight that feared outcomes often do not occur, and if they do occur, they can be handled. Clients also practice their new affect management skills in the context of coping with distress, as well as to manage cannabis cravings.

Therapist	Alright, now that we've discussed what exposures are, it's time to design an exposure practice. Let's start by having you think of something that feels difficult to do without using cannabis.
Sylvia	Oh yeah, I think it's impossible for me to get out of bed if I don't hit my weed pen first.
Therapist	Why is that?
Sylvia	Well, my mind will become so flooded with worries that I won't be able to get my day started and I'll spend all day in bed.
Therapist	So your fear is that without cannabis, you won't be able to get started and you'll spend all day in bed. That sounds like a great exposure to practice for homework this week. Is there anything that's similar that we can do together? It could be anything that makes you feel like you need cannabis in order to start.
Sylvia	I guess I've been avoiding starting my final paper. I usually hit my weed pen to calm my nerves and help me think of a topic. I'm less critical of what I write.
Therapist	Great, let's do an exposure around that. So, the fear is: if I don't use cannabis, I won't be able to start my paper. How can we test that out?
Sylvia	I could try writing my paper.
Therapist	Okay, let's make that more specific, how much would you need to write in order to test out this fear?
Sylvia	Well, when I don't use first, I usually give up after 10 minutes of trying to write.
Therapist	Would a good test be to set a 10 minute timer and try to write the first 5 sentences of your essay?
Sylvia	If I could do that, that would be a miracle. I don't think it's going to happen though.
Therapist	Let's find out. What's your anxiety rating, 0–100, right now?
Sylvia	A 70.

Therapist	And how likely is it that you won't be able to write the first 5 sentences of your essay without using cannabis, 0–100?
Sylvia	100.
Therapist	Okay, let's do it. I'm going to set a timer, and you can go ahead and get started.

After each exposure practice, clients consolidate their new learning by discussing the discrepancies between their pre-exposure predictions and the actual outcomes of the exposure, with an emphasis on recognizing their ability to tolerate distress and resist urges to use cannabis.

Therapist	Time's up! On a scale of 0–100 where is your anxiety right now?
Sylvia	A 30.
Therapist	Okay, and how would you rate the most anxious your felt during those 10 minutes?
Sylvia	Right after you said I could start, my heart started pounding. I was definitely at a 90.
Therapist	Did what you were worried about happen? Were you able to write the 5 sentences without using cannabis?
Sylvia	Yes, I took a few moments when we got started to be mindful and acknowledge I was feeling nervous and craving a hit. Then I just told myself to start writing whatever came to mind. When you said time was up, I'd actually finished the paragraph.
Therapist	Wow, so you wrote more than you expected!
Sylvia	I did, but I don't think it's very good.
Therapist	Let's stay focused on the outcome we decided to test at the beginning. We decided to see whether you could write anything, not whether it was "high quality" writing. Keeping that in mind, did your feared outcome come true?
Sylvia	I guess not.
Therapist	And how do you know?
Sylvia	Well, I have at least 7 sentences written.
Therapist	Did you learn anything from doing this exposure exercise?
Sylvia	Yeah, I learned that even if my anxiety is really intense when I sit down to write, it does go away as I get going. It was like the more words I wrote down, the more my anxiety decreased. I also noticed that my craving for cannabis went away by the time the 10 minutes were up.
Therapist	It sounds like you learned that getting started is an effective way to get started, and you can get started even when you're feeling anxious. You also learned that the craving can go away as you start working.
Sylvia	Definitely.
Therapist	Okay, last piece: if you were to do this exact exposure practice again, how anxious would you be, 0–100?
Sylvia	Maybe a 50.
Therapist	Okay, and what's the likelihood you wouldn't be able to do the task?
Sylvia	Like a 10.

Therapist That's really different from where you started! When you do more of these practices, you'll have times like today where your anxiety goes down. But you also might have times where you don't experience any changes, and that's okay. The goal is to keep trying. The research shows us that the reduction in fear comes from the cumulative learning that happens when we keep trying these exercises.

During the final session, in addition to completing an in-session exposure and consolidating new learning, clients review skills and concepts learned in therapy and their progress towards treatment goals. Feedback on the process of treatment is elicited and clients are encouraged to share the skills they have found most helpful and identify ongoing areas for skills practice. Therapists provide clients with feedback by identifying strengths, reviewing progress in reducing cannabis use and highlighting changes in negative affect and maladaptive responding to negative affect. Lastly, clients and therapists collaboratively identify and problem solve future potential stressors and discuss the skills the client can use to cope and remain abstinent in negative affect-inducing contexts.

Case Summary

As demonstrated in the case example, building skills to replace maladaptive responses to negative affect helped Sylvia learn to confront and manage the situations that contributed to her anxiety while simultaneously reducing reliance on cannabis use and building tolerance to cannabis cravings. By increasing mindfulness, Sylvia learned how to observe her emotions and sensations without immediately reacting to them or trying to suppress them. She also learned to challenge cognitive misappraisals that overestimated the likelihood of situations going wrong in her life and underestimated her ability to cope with those situations, especially without using cannabis first. She also learned problem solving strategies to approach difficult situations and address problems head on, rather than experientially avoiding through cannabis use and behaviorally avoiding through procrastination, thus letting her problems, and her negative emotions, exacerbate with time. Lastly, exposures helped Sylvia practice all of the skills she learned in the first half of treatment by purposefully confronting uncomfortable thoughts, feelings, and situations to test out her beliefs about the situations and her own ability to cope, and build her tolerance of distress.

The transdiagnostic theoretical model of AMT conceptualizes both ED and SUD as symptoms of the same underlying problematic processes. As such, it helps clients understand their emotional distress and substance use not as two distinct issues, but rather the consequences of unhelpful responses to distress. Skillful and effective delivery of the psychoeducation for the theoretical model of AMT to increase client buy-in and engagement is integral to the success of AMT, particularly given that many of the interventions are uncomfortable or challenging for clients to implement. Helping clients understand the role that their reactions play in maintaining their substance use and distress allows them to recognize their agency to enact change and reduce the hold that SUD and emotional distress have over their quality of life.

Special Considerations

The skills-based nature of AMT has some potential pitfalls that therapists should be mindful of so that they can provide culturally responsive care. The goal of the toolbox approach of AMT is to give clients a wide array of skills to select from and to empower them to choose the skills that work best for them to manage difficult situations or feelings. When presenting each skill, therapists need to make sure clients understand more than just the broad rationale for using the skill. Role plays and in-session practices are some of the built in features of AMT to help clients experience the individualized application of each skill in real time with their therapist. Exposure practices are a core component of AMT and may present some challenges for therapists. If not delivered in a culturally responsive way, exposure practices can reinforce client-therapist power dynamics that may interfere with the effectiveness of the exercises, particularly when working with clients with marginalized identities. Therapists should remember that willingness to do exposure practices comes from a strong therapeutic alliance and trust between client and therapist.

The transdiagnostic approach to treatment of ED allows therapists to adopt a personalized model of psychotherapy that incorporates culture and identity into clinical care. A key component of AMT is the functional assessment, which focuses on *how* the target mechanisms and processes show up in each client's life. Culturally responsive implementation of AMT involves tailoring the skills to the needs of each client, focusing on empowering the client, helping clients identify conscious processes that can be articulated and accessed, utilizing outcome and process assessment that incorporates the client's perspective, and leveraging naturally occurring strengths for each client throughout treatment.

Conclusion

Recovery from SUD is challenging in part because most treatments focus on the symptoms of the SUD and not the emotional context and function of the use behavior. In contrast, AMT focuses on teaching skills to target the maladaptive emotional responses that maintain ED and co-occurring SUD, ultimately giving clients the tools they need to reduce their use and prevent SUD from worsening. Initial examination of this treatment provides evidence that AMT outperforms traditional CBT models on outcomes associated with the maintenance and exacerbation of cannabis use, indicating that targeting the shared mechanisms underlying substance use and emotional distress improves treatment outcomes. The efficacy of AMT in a CUD sample of young adults is promising for SUD more broadly, as the principles and components of this treatment are likely to be relevant for a variety of substances of dependence across the lifespan, and can be flexibly integrated in a variety of settings and with a variety of populations.

References

Aldao, A., & Nolen-Hoeksema, S. (2010). Specificity of cognitive emotion regulation strategies: A transdiagnostic examination. *Behaviour Research and Therapy, 48*(10), 974–983.

Baker, R., Holloway, J., Thomas, P. W., Thomas, S., & Owens, M. (2004). Emotional processing and panic. *Behaviour Research and Therapy, 42*(11), 1271–1287.

Barlow, D. H., Sauer-Zavala, S., Carl, J. R., Bullis, J. R., & Ellard, K. K. (2014). The nature, diagnosis, and treatment of neuroticism back to the future. *Clinical Psychological Science, 2*(3), 344–365.

Brown, T. A., & Barlow, D. H. (2009). A proposal for a dimensional classification system based on the shared features of the DSM-IV anxiety and mood disorders: Implications for assessment and treatment. *Psychological Assessment, 21*(3), 256.

Buckner, J. D., Keough, M. E., & Schmidt, N. B. (2007). Problematic alcohol and cannabis use among young adults: The roles of depression and discomfort and distress tolerance. *Addictive Behaviors, 32*(9), 1957–1963.

Burns, L., Teesson, M., & O'Neill, K. (2005). The impact of comorbid anxiety and depression on alcohol treatment outcomes. *Addiction, 100*(6), 787–796.

Cuthbert, B. N. (2014). The RDoC framework: Facilitating transition from ICD/DSM to dimensional approaches that integrate neuroscience and psychopathology. *World Psychiatry: Official Journal of the World Psychiatric Association (WPA), 13*(1), 28–35.

Howell, A. N., Leyro, T. M., Hogan, J., Buckner, J. D., & Zvolensky, M. J. (2010). Anxiety sensitivity, distress tolerance, and discomfort intolerance in relation to coping and conformity motives for alcohol use and alcohol use problems among young adult drinkers. *Addictive Behaviors, 35*(12), 1144–1147.

Johnston, L. D., O'Malley, P. M., & Bachman, J. G. (2000). Monitoring the future national results on adolescent drug use: Overview of key findings, 1999. U. S. Department of Health and Human Services. Bethesda, Maryland.

Kushner, M. G., Abrams, K., Thuras, P., Hanson, K. L., Brekke, M., & Sletten, S. (2005). A follow-up study of anxiety disorder and alcohol dependence in comorbid alcoholism treatment patients. *Alcoholism: Experimental and Clinical Research, 29*, 1432–1443.

Magidson, J. F., Liu, S. M., Lejuez, C. W., & Blanco, C. (2012). Comparison of the course of substance use disorders among individuals with and without generalized anxiety disorder in a nationally representative sample. *Journal of Psychiatric Research, 46*(5), 659–666.

McGee, R., Williams, S., Poulton, R., & Moffitt, T. (2000). A longitudinal study of cannabis use and mental health from adolescence to early adulthood. *Addiction, 95*(4), 491–503.

Roemer, L., Salters, K., Raffa, S. D., & Orsillo, S. M. (2005). Fear and avoidance of internal experiences in GAD: Preliminary tests of a conceptual model. *Cognitive Therapy and Research, 29*(1), 71–88.

Sauer-Zavala, S., Boswell, J. F., Gallagher, M. W., Bentley, K. H., Ametaj, A., & Barlow, D. H. (2012). The role of negative affectivity and negative reactivity to emotions in predicting outcomes in the unified protocol for the transdiagnostic treatment of emotional disorders. *Behaviour Research and Therapy, 50*(9), 551–557.

Sauer-Zavala, S., Gutner, C. A., Farchione, T. J., Boettcher, H. T., Bullis, J. R., & Barlow, D. H. (2017). Current definitions of "transdiagnostic" in treatment development: A search for consensus. *Behavior Therapy, 48*(1), 128–138.

Substance Abuse and Mental Health Services Administration. (2014). *Results from the 2013 National Survey on Drug Use and Health: Summary of national findings* (NSDUH Series H-48, HHS Publication No. (SMA) 14-4863). Substance Abuse and Mental Health Services Administration.

Wittchen, H. U., Fröhlich, C., Behrendt, S., Günther, A., Rehm, J., Zimmermann, P., et al. (2007). Cannabis use and cannabis use disorders and their relationship to mental disorders: A 10-year prospective-longitudinal community study in adolescents. *Drug and Alcohol Dependence, 88*, S60–S70.

Wolitzky-Taylor, K., Bobova, L., Zinbarg, R. E., Mineka, S., & Craske, M. G. (2012). Longitudinal investigation of the impact of anxiety and mood disorders in adolescence on subsequent substance use disorder onset and vice versa. *Addictive Behaviors, 37*(8), 982–985.

Wolitzky-Taylor, K., Guillot, C. R., Pang, R. D., Kirkpatrick, M. G., Zvolensky, M. J., Buckner, J. D., & Leventhal, A. M. (2015). Examination of anxiety sensitivity and distress tolerance as transdiagnostic mechanisms linking multiple anxiety pathologies to alcohol use problems in adolescents. *Alcoholism: Clinical and Experimental Research, 39*(3), 532–539.

Wolitzky Taylor, K., McBeth, J., Guillot, C. R., Stone, M. D., Kirkpatrick, M. G., Zvolensky, M. J., & Leventhal, A. M. (2016). Transdiagnostic processes linking anxiety symptoms and substance use problems among adolescents. *Journal of Addictive Diseases, 35, 266–277.*

Wolitzky-Taylor, K., Glasner, S., Tanner, A., Ghahremani, D. G., & London, E. D. (2022). Targeting maladaptive reactivity to negative affect in emerging adults with cannabis use disorder: A preliminary test and proof of concept. *Behaviour Research and Therapy, 150*, 104032.

Chapter 7
Smoking Cessation and Anxiety Sensitivity

Brooke Y. Redmond, Justin M. Shepherd, and Michael J. Zvolensky

Tobacco Use

Over 28 million adults in the United States (US) currently smoke cigarettes (Cornelius et al., 2023). Smoking is related to numerous chronic health conditions, including cardiovascular disease, pulmonary disease, and cancer (Centers for Disease Control and Prevention, 2020). Given the high prevalence of smoking and associated negative health-related consequences, it is not surprising that cigarette smoking remains the leading cause of preventable morbidity and mortality in the United States, accounting for approximately 443,000 deaths each year (Centers for Disease Control and Prevention, 2022).

Tobacco Use and Mental Health

Individuals with elevated mental health conditions who smoke cigarettes are among the most vulnerable in terms of difficulty quitting smoking (Garey et al., 2020a). Mental health conditions are highly comorbid with smoking (Lipari & Van Horn,

B. Y. Redmond · J. M. Shepherd
Department of Psychology, University of Houston, Houston, TX, USA

M. J. Zvolensky (✉)
Department of Psychology, University of Houston, Houston, TX, USA

Department of Behavioral Science, The University of Texas MD Anderson Cancer Center, Houston, TX, USA

HEALTH Institute, University of Houston, Houston, TX, USA
e-mail: mjzvolen@central.uh.edu

K. Wolitzky-Taylor (ed.), *Treating Comorbid Substance Use and Emotional Disorders*, CBT: Science Into Practice, https://doi.org/10.1007/978-3-031-62971-6_7

2017) and increase risk of smoking cessation failure (Garey et al., 2020b; Kalkhoran et al., 2019), and individuals with mental health conditions who smoke cigarettes have disproportionately high rates of tobacco-related disease and death (Callaghan et al., 2014; Goodwin et al., 2014). As such, individuals with mental health conditions are recognized as a smoking-related health disparities group (Kalkhoran et al., 2019; Williams et al., 2013).

Risk Factor for Mental Health Conditions and Smoking Behavior

Anxiety sensitivity An integrative, theory-driven approach to address the heterogeneity of mental health conditions associated with cigarette smoking is to focus on transdiagnostic processes that underpin both mental health conditions and smoking behavior (Zvolensky & Leventhal, 2016). Anxiety sensitivity (AS) is a relatively stable, but malleable factor (Taylor, 1999) defined as the extent to which individuals believe anxiety and anxiety-related sensations (e.g., racing heart) have harmful personal consequences (McNally, 2002; Reiss et al., 1986). The global AS construct encompasses lower-order factors related to fears of physical, mental, and social experiences (Zinbarg et al., 1997). According to expectancy theory, AS serves to amplify anxious and fearful responding to evocative stimuli (Reiss, 1991). Theoretically, individuals higher in AS are more likely to be frightened of harmless heart palpitations because they believe these sensations will lead to feared outcomes (e.g., cardiac arrest), whereas individuals lower in AS do not fear these sensations because they believe them to be benign.

AS and smoking There are interrelated, but distinct, lines of independently replicated studies that have documented the role of AS in a multitude of smoking maintenance and relapse processes (Leventhal & Zvolensky, 2015; Otto et al., 2016; Redmond et al., 2023). Notably, within these studies the effects of AS for smoking processes were not explained by severity of tobacco dependence, gender, trait-like tendencies to experience negative affect states (e.g., neuroticism), or other types of substance use problems (e.g., alcohol; Leventhal & Zvolensky, 2015). For example, prior work has found that AS is related to negative affect reduction motives and expectancies (Farris et al., 2015a, b; Langdon et al., 2018). AS is also related to the tendency to smoke in an inflexible manner and greater smoking-related avoidance (Langdon et al., 2018). Other empirical work has demonstrated that AS is associated with the tendency to perceive quitting as more difficult (Langdon et al., 2016), expectations of smoking deprivation to be personally threatening (Farris et al., 2015b; Guillot et al., 2016), more problems when attempting to quit (Redmond et al., 2023), and perceived barriers for cessation (Langdon et al., 2018; Redmond et al., 2023). Importantly, many of these findings have been replicated among diverse groups of individuals who smoke. For instance, among Latinx persons who smoke, AS is related to more severe levels of cigarette dependence, problems experienced during prior quit attempts, and perceived barriers for smoking cessation (Zvolensky et al., 2019) as well as expectancies pertaining to the positive and negative consequences of smoking (Shepherd et al., 2020) and acute abstinence (Zvolensky et al., 2023). Other related work conducted among Black/African American individuals who smoke has shown that AS is related to smoking motives (Garey et al., 2023) and increased severity of withdrawal symptoms (Kelly et al., 2020).

AS Reduction Program for Smoking

We have developed an integrated treatment protocol for targeting AS among individuals who smoke, informed by an integrated theoretical model of their relation. This theoretically derived intervention program integrates AS reduction cognitive-behavioral therapeutic strategies with evidence-based smoking cessation counseling strategies. This program, termed the AS Reduction Program for Smoking (ASRP-S), is structured around the theoretically relevant cognitive risk factor, AS. By structuring the intervention around AS, the program is expected to simultaneously improve mental health and smoking behavior. The program focuses on three elements: (1) psychoeducational provision of an integrated therapeutic rationale, (2) decreasing emotional sensitivity and reactivity to anxiety, bodily cues, and nicotine withdrawal via cognitive-behavioral methods, and (3) specialized smoking-oriented psychoeducation and relapse prevention. See Table 7.1 for an overview of these elements.

Element one: Integrated therapeutic rationale Persons with high AS are likely to believe that smoking helps them manage and/or cope with negative affect and do not understand that smoking may promote or exacerbate mental health problems. To address this, the current treatment emphasizes the importance of providing clients with a thorough psychoeducational rationale for targeting smoking and AS. One aspect of this discussion needs to address targeting these behaviors concurrently because of their negative bi-directional relationship and compounded impact on one's health. This rationale is particularly important because it provides a foundation for the treatment to not only focus on proven strategies for smoking cessation, but also on helping the individual learn and practice strategies to better manage interpreting, coping, and tolerating emergent withdrawal symptoms and anxiety symptoms. Specifically, we introduce the concepts of fear of anxiety and smoking as a maladaptive way of coping with anxiety-related distress. We pay attention to highlighting the process of the forward-feeding anxiety cycle, whereby catastrophic thinking and AS can lead to both subjective threat evaluations and heightened attention to threatening stimuli, resulting in a greater risk for panic attacks as well as the exacerbation of interoceptive states like withdrawal symptoms. We also indicate that such reactions may sensitize a person to the interoceptive and environmental

Table 7.1 Treatment elements and associated components

Element	Components
1. *Integrated therapeutic rationale*	How smoking promotes or exacerbate mental health problems
	Rationale for targeting AS and smoking together
	Fear of anxiety, catastrophic thinking, and smoking are maladaptive coping mechanisms
	2–3 sessions focused on AS exclusively, but embedded throughout the whole treatment
2. *Decreasing AS* via *cognitive-behavioral methods*	Decrease emotional sensitivity and reactivity to interceptive stimuli
	Help individuals who smoke learn a sense of tolerance, control, and safety when experiencing anxiety symptoms
	Interoceptive exposure, cognitive restructuring, and acceptance strategies
	Clinical practice guidelines from *Treating Tobacco Use and Dependence*
1.3. *Specialized smoking-oriented psychoeducation and relapse prevention*	Provide positive reinforcement and social support for quitting
	Discuss past quit experiences
	Set a quit date
	Self-monitoring program for smoking and coping behaviors
	Identify high-risk smoking situations
	Discuss abstinence violation effect
	Teach adaptive coping strategies
	Enlist social support for quitting
	Remove all tobacco from environment

cues that signal such distress in the future, leading to smoking as a way of coping. Finally, we articulate that targeting AS and modifying it via thinking (cognitive) and exposure (behavioral) exercises is important to enhance *both* smoking cessation outcomes and mental health. We emphasize that practicing cognitive-behavioral exercises both in and out of session is an important element of the intervention that directly contributes to each individual's ultimate success.

Element two: Decreasing AS via cognitive-behavioral methods The second core element involves using empirically derived cognitive-behavioral strategies developed for AS to decrease emotional sensitivity and reactivity to interoceptive stimuli. Importantly, exposure exercises are adapted to target interoceptive cues across varying intensities of nicotine withdrawal (elicited via deprivation from smoking for various time periods). This intervention component is aimed to help individuals who smoke learn (or relearn) a sense of tolerance, control, and safety in the presence of anxiety-related sensations: a task presumably accomplished through helping individuals directly experience sensations in a controlled fashion, where emotionally corrective outcomes are facilitated, rather than in the naturally occurring context where catastrophic misinterpretation of these symptoms may occur (e.g., during cessation or smoking abstinence).

Accordingly, we integrate (1) interoceptive exposure with (2) corrective information about anxiety and cognitive interventions designed to teach clients alternatives to catastrophic misinterpretations of the sensations and their feared consequences ("I will lose control"), as well as (3) continued use of situational exposure. Specifically, we use cognitive restructuring aimed at targeting the elimination of catastrophic beliefs about the meaning and consequences of anxiety sensations and symptoms of withdrawal. In addition to cognitive restructuring strategies, acceptance-based strategies are employed to foster increased tolerance for anxiety and related sensations. Specially, patients are encouraged to observe, describe, and express their emotional reactions to bodily sensations and nicotine deprived states. Furthermore, we systematically employ interoceptive exposure to extinguish fears of aversive internal sensations, with specific preparation for sensations that would be experienced as part of smoking discontinuation (withdrawal). Clients are explicitly taught that the goal of such therapeutic work is not to attempt the impossible task of eliminating anxiety or emotion-laden withdrawal sensations, but rather to ensure that these internal cues are not interpreted fearfully, escalating bothersome sensations into debilitating anxiety. Exposure to somatic and other interoceptive symptoms in advance of cessation theoretically should help ensure that clients have practice with an alternative model of symptom management well before the characteristic symptoms of smoking discontinuation are encountered.

Interoceptive exposure is described, demonstrated, and practiced in session and individuals are encouraged to practice the exercises outside of session (as part of assigned between session work). The importance of varying practice contexts to facilitate the "unlearning" of fear responses across settings is emphasized as a rationale for frequently practicing exercises out of session. Three interoceptive exposure exercises (e.g., head rolling, voluntary hyperventilation, and chair spinning) are typically completed each session, which is generally feasible within the given time constraints. For example, dizziness is induced by a head-rolling exercise in which clients gently swing their heads around in circles with their eyes closed for 1 minute. The repeated use of such exercises provides adaptation to the sensations (habituation) and reduces the probability that such sensations will trigger anxiety in future circumstances. While performing these exercises, we draw a clear connection between aversive anxiety-related states and somatic changes and discuss such experiences in the context of changing smoking behavior (e.g., during a cessation attempt). For example, patients are encouraged to mindfully attend to the experience of bodily sensations when reducing cigarette consumption or trying to abstain from smoking and recognize the impact of such experiences in terms of motivation to smoke. Once the client can identify and isolate bodily sensations, they are coached to modify their cognitive reactions to these sensations by reframing them in more adaptive ways and accepting them as "normal" reactions.

As the client progresses through the interoceptive exposure exercises, we increase exposure intensity by incorporating periods of smoking deprivation into the interoceptive exposure exercises. By adapting existing exposure-based interventions to withdrawal symptoms, it may be possible to decrease withdrawal symptoms, a primary factor in poor cessation outcomes. Clients are asked to practice at least one self-exposure per day out of session along with monitoring their performance using an exposure monitoring data recording card. It also is emphasized to individuals that these exercises are useful in terms of maintaining treatment goals and relapse prevention.

Element three: Specialized smoking-oriented psychoeducation and relapse prevention The final element of the treatment program provides evidence-based information for altering smoking behavior that is specifically designed for a population vulnerable to anxiety. We base our discussion generally on clinical practice guidelines from the U.S. Department of Health and Human Services, *Treating Tobacco Use and Dependence* (Fiore et al., 2008). This component includes a variety of information, representing nine separate aspects. First, we provide positive reinforcement and social support for quitting. For example, therapists are instructed to congratulate clients for deciding to quit smoking, review the positive health consequences of quitting, and express their willingness to help the client succeed. Second, we discuss past quit experiences. These past quit attempts are reviewed to identify what strategies contributed to success and what factors hindered previous attempts. Third, we work with the client to set a quit date. This quit date occurs only after the client has demonstrated progress in interoceptive exposure exercises in and outside of session (i.e., successfully and regularly completing between session work). Here, it is important to have observed progress both for the exposure exercises in withdrawal and non-withdrawal states. Fourth, we initiate a formal self-monitoring program for smoking and other (alternative) coping behaviors (e.g., physical exercise). Specifically, clients track each cigarette they smoke through their quit date and note situational cues for smoking as well as alternative strategies that they could have used instead of smoking.

Fifth, we work with the client to identify idiographic high-risk situations for smoking. The focus of this topic is to anticipate situations that likely will place them at risk for relapse and plan how to handle such situations ahead of time (without smoking). Sixth, we present and discuss the abstinence violation effect (Marlatt & Gordon, 1985). Namely, clients are prepared for the possibility of lapsing and given strategies for coping with the potential negative emotional reactions to lapsing. For example, clients are encouraged to identify and alter maladaptive thinking patterns about lapsing (e.g., altering thoughts such as "I might as well give up because I just had a cigarette" to "I just smoked, but this is not an excuse to alter my longer-term effort of changing my smoking behavior").

Seventh, we help clients identify and develop skills to support adaptive coping strategies. Due to the unique psychological concerns of individuals with high AS, these coping strategies often reflect three key aspects of self- and emotion-regulation. The first pertains to coping behaviors that would alter negative emotional experiences in the short-term, particularly anxiety. The second pertains to longer-term health-oriented lifestyle behaviors such as physical exercise. Therapists assist the client in developing behavioral and cognitive strategies for coping with emotionally salient events in the short-term and help develop plans for evoking longer-term health-oriented change. Third, therapists help each client identify specific high-risk situations for smoking and provide support to avoid them altogether. For example, therapists advise clients to avoid the use of alcohol or other substances to assist in smoking quit attempts or management of affect.

Eighth, we attempt to help clients enlist social support for quitting. Therapists advise clients to tell their friends and family about their quit date and discuss ways to increase social support during the quit attempt. For example, clients often are encouraged to share with friends and family that their "weak moments" tend to be related to dysregulated affect (e.g., worry, anxiety) and that they are trying to quit smoking by responding differently to such affective events. We believe this approach enhances the psychological environment for behavior change while explicitly recognizing the role of anxiety-specific processes in such behavior change. Clients also are encouraged, when applicable, to ask individuals who smoke in their household to avoid smoking in their presence. Finally, clients are encouraged to prepare for quitting by removing all tobacco products and related smoking accessories (e.g., lighters, ashtrays) from their environment. This strategy helps remove unnecessary risks for tobacco use prior to vulnerable time periods and acts as a "behavioral index" of commitment to change.

Illustrative Overview of Treatment

ASRP-S consists of four in-person, individually delivered 90-minute sessions. The treatment can easily be adapted for small groups by including group process issues (confidentiality, group guidelines, etc.) during the first session. ASRP-S is a prevention program; thus, all therapy sessions are presented prior to quit day/treatment session 4. Each session includes specific objectives (see Table 7.1), and between session work assignments. The structure consists of reviewing between session work and past session content, outlining and addressing current session objectives, assigning between session work, and previewing topics covered in the upcoming session. Clients are provided with a client binder during the first session to help guide their treatment. Below, we provide a practical clinical guide for implementing ASRP-S. This guide serves as a model for administering ASRP-S, but therapists should exercise clinical judgment when utilizing this manualized treatment. Indeed, the program was intentionally developed to be flexible and easily adapted to fit the unique needs of clients. There are several clinical tactics that therapists should incorporate into each session. To decrease redundancy, these tactics are not discussed in the guidelines for each session, but reviewed here. First, the overall goal and integrated nature of this treatment should be reiterated at each session. This will serve to reinforce the client's involvement in treatment and openness to new and different skills. Consistent with this approach, it will be necessary for therapists to revisit and link themes throughout treatment. Doing so will provide clients with a thorough, coherent understanding of the treatment as well as the function of different strategies and skills. As a result, clients may better assimilate treatment elements and have greater success. Second, the flexible nature of ASRP-S supports a client-centered, motivational interviewing directive. As such, therapists are to personalize the treatment to the client's unique experiences as much as possible. This will include drawing from the client's cigarette use history, past quit experiences, and specific anxiety-related symptoms and distress. In some instances, however, personalized examples may not be appropriate. Thus, when necessary, therapists may provide generic examples to help illustrate complex topics. Therapists should employ open-ended and reflective questioning to obtain information from clients and encourage clients to ask questions during treatment. To aid in guiding you through the session overview, we will provide a case formulation of a client that would be an ideal candidate for this protocol followed by example dialogue at the end of each session overview.

Case formulation Thomas is a 36-year-old Caucasian male who is interested in receiving treatment for smoking cessation. Thomas was referred to treatment by his primary care provider. Thomas began smoking cigarettes at the age of 20 and currently smokes about a pack per day. Thomas reported that he started smoking socially in college and now smokes out of habit and to manage his stress. Thomas is currently motivated to quit smoking in order to improve his health. Thomas also experiences elevated AS; he is attuned to his bodily sensations and fearful of what his symptoms may indicate, particularly regarding his health. Importantly, Thomas has a number of strengths, including a strong social support system. In terms of limitations, Thomas engages in social drinking which may interfere with treatment gains. Thomas' reported history, clinical interview, and self-report measures indicates he experiences elevated AS and a history of smoking behavior in response to stress/anxiety. Treatment should include a focus on simultaneously assessing smoking cessation in the context of elevated anxiety symptoms.

Session 1 The introduction session consists of obtaining informed consent, therapist introduction, and an overview of the treatment. To begin, the therapist orients the client to the goal-oriented nature of the treatment and the overall structure of program, including time commitment, confidentiality, and assignments. It is critical that the therapist stresses the importance of treatment attendance and participation during treatment as well as outside of treatment. During this session, the therapist should provide reinforcement and empathetic support for client's decision to quit and emphasize that the goal of this treatment is to assist with smoking abstinence. This is achieved by candidly discussing the potential difficulties associated with smoking (i.e., stress, withdrawal) and pitting them against client's goals and values for improved physical and mental health.

The therapist presents the need to address specific mental health risk factors in the context of smoking cessation. Specifically, AS is introduced as a targetable, malleable risk factor for quit failure and emotional distress that may complicate quit success. The client is informed of theoretical and empirical data for targeting AS in the context of smoking cessation treatment to assist with quit success. Subsequently, the integrated treatment goal is presented: to achieve smoking abstinence through integrating AS reduction with the most valid smoking cessation practices. Moreover, to assuage potential client resistance, the therapist should emphasize that this novel treatment contains activities that may be unfamiliar to the client. The therapist should encourage client to practice flexibility by suggesting that they be willing to try exercises and activities "outside of their comfort zone" or different from what they have tried in the past.

The therapist facilitates a discussion on cigarette use and history, including typical use and past quit attempts. With regards to past quit attempts, the therapist will want to obtain a thorough understanding of the client's quit history. Factors that assisted with the quit attempt, quit-related benefits, and factors that contributed to relapse should be discussed and summarized. Consistent with a motivational interviewing approach (Miller & Rollnick, 2012; Rollnick & Miller, 1995), reasons for smoking followed by reasons for quitting should be reviewed with each client. If appropriate, the therapist briefly introduces the paradoxical effects of withdrawal and the smoking cycle. This is followed by a discussion of barriers to smoking cessation.

The next part of this session presents a more in-depth explanation of smoking as a maladaptive coping mechanism for anxiety-related symptoms. The paradoxical effect of smoking is reviewed in further detail. Components covered should include the influence of cigarette use severity and dependence on withdrawal; the overlap between withdrawal and distress and other negative feelings; the relation between long-term smoking and increased aversive physical sensations as a consequence of poorer physical health; the misinterpretation of withdrawal and physical sensations as anxiety when they are actually consequences of cigarette use; and the use of cigarettes to alleviate misinterpreted experiences.

AS is then introduced as a factor related to both smoking and anxiety. The therapist should provide a formal, well-defined definition of AS and the catastrophizing nature of AS. It will be necessary for the therapist to ensure the client understands (a) the concept of AS, (b) the malleability of AS, and (c) the relation between AS and catastrophizing as it relates to the anxiety and smoking cycle. Specifically, the therapist should relate AS back to the paradoxical effect of smoking and emphasize the additive influence of elevated AS on the misinterpretation of nicotine-related withdrawal and aversive physical sensations. Psychoeducation on AS and smoking is followed by an explanation of and rationale for interoceptive exposures to target and subsequently treat AS. The client is then informed that interoceptive exposures will begin the following treatment session.

The last section of this session includes psychoeducation on smoking cessation medications, setting a quit date, and assignment of between session work. A rationale for including a quit smoking medication as an adjunct to therapy should be provided to each client. Over the counter quit smoking medications (nicotine replacement therapy [NRT] patches, NRT gum, NRT lozenge, etc.) can be purchased by the client directly. Other medications, including bupropion and varenicline, require a prescription and should be monitored by a physician. The therapist should educate their client on potential side effects of different medications and possible contraindications. Consultation with a caring physician is advised when applicable. The therapist and client should then identify the date of the fourth treatment session and schedule that as the quit day. As mentioned earlier in the chapter, the quit date depends on the client's progress; thus, the date should be adjusted as needed to best meet the client's needs. The pharmacotherapy agent selected will determine the appropriate time to initiate use, but use should commence either on or before the scheduled quit date. Lastly, the client is provided with cigarette consumption and mood monitoring forms to use over the next week. The therapist should provide a rationale for the importance of careful and thorough monitoring.

The client is then provided with quit smoking self-help materials and a client binder. The therapist should encourage the client to review the provided materials and ask questions at the following treatment session. At this stage, the therapist ensures the client's understanding of the material and invites any additional questions before concluding the session.

Session 1 Example Dialogue

Therapist	You mentioned you smoke cigarettes to help you cope with your stress and anxiety. You also mentioned when you have tried to quit smoking in the past, your stress and anxiety symptoms became worse, which led you to resume smoking.
Client	That is correct.
Therapist	The assessment you completed also indicated you have higher than average anxiety sensitivity. This means you may be particularly "tuned-in" to your bodily sensations and may have certain fears regarding what those symptoms may indicate. For example, you may have fears that a racing heart may be an indicator of a serious heart problem such as an indication of a heart attack.
Client	I think that is accurate. I tend to be very aware of my body. I think that is because I know smoking is bad for me so when I experience any physical symptoms, I think it might be something bad like the early signs of a disease which just stresses me out more.
Therapist	Exactly! Having these concerns leads you to focus more attention on your bodily symptoms. By increasing our hypervigilance to these symptoms, we are more likely to notice them which can subsequently increase the presence of them. Just like you said, being concerned about your symptoms brings on more stress and more stress may mean more bodily sensations. What do you typically do to cope in response?
Client	I usually smoke and that helps calm me down.

Therapist That is one way to cope with such stress, although as you will learn though the program, it is not helpful for you in the long term. That is because smoking will relieve your symptoms in the short term but in the long term, this repeated pattern of behavior will not only maintain your uncomfortable symptoms but it can actually make them worse over time. In order to disrupt this cycle, we will work on exercises to help you confront the uncomfortable sensations you are experiencing rather than avoid them through smoking.

Session 2 Between session work is reviewed at the beginning of the sessions. Barriers to completing the assignments should be addressed to prevent further difficulties and enhance effectiveness. After, the therapist outlines goals for the present session and reviews topics discussed at the previous session. Particular attention should be dedicated to revisiting smoking effects on the body, AS as a construct and a targetable risk factor, and the paradoxical effect of smoking.

Following the overview and review, exposure exercises are reintroduced. Similarities between physical sensations experienced during periods of anxiety and attempting to quit smoking are discussed. The therapist first explains that exposure exercises are intended to elicit uncomfortable physical sensations that mimic withdrawal symptoms experienced when attempting to quit and that these sensations, while uncomfortable, are not harmful. Interoceptive exposure exercises should be presented as a method to increase tolerance to uncomfortable sensations by purposefully inducing them in a controlled, safe environment. The therapist's goal is to ensure the client understands that it is the *interpretation* of these physical sensations that determines the client's response and experience, and that through repeated exposure and practice one can better understand and interpret the benign physical sensations that often accompany quitting smoking. Subsequently, a more accurate, appropriate interpretation of these sensations may positively impact their attempt to quit smoking.

Prior to introducing the exposure exercises, the therapist will want to explain the subjective units of distress (SUDs) metric and inform the client that they will be asked to give their distress rating after each exposure; this SUDs scale is a 0–10 Likert scale that is employed to determine the degree of distress (0 = none to 10 = extreme). The therapist should reiterate that the exposure exercises are not harmful and that they are intended to illicit physical sensations associated with quitting smoking such as dizziness, lightheadedness, shortness of breath, etc. Three example exercises include chair spinning, straw breathing, and hyperventilation. We typically start with one to two exposure exercises per session, each lasting for a few minutes. For each of these exercises, the therapist should demonstrate the exercise, then ask the client to engage in the exercise, and finally reinforce that the client to observe, describe, and express the sensations (this is accompanied by a distress rating). The therapist will want to emphasize that these sensations are *Normal* reactions to this behavior that are *OK* and we want to *Accept* them, even though they are uncomfortable (because they are not causing us harm and experiencing them in this fashion will help to make them less intense in the future, such as after quit day; NOA). After selecting the exercise that elicited a moderate amount of distress, have the client complete repeated trials until extinction has been reached. The client is shown how to monitor and track their exposure exercises.

Next, the client is taught strategies to identify thoughts, emotions, and behaviors. The therapist provides psychoeducation on the interconnectedness of these constructs and the importance of differentiating them, particularly in the context of quitting smoking. Considering the complexity of this topic, the therapist may want to offer examples for how to differentiate cognitions, emotions, and behaviors and their relatedness. The client should be encouraged to monitor and practice differentiating these three facets with an understanding that through repeated identification, one can begin to appreciate the impact of thoughts on emotions and behaviors and therefore appropriately adjust thoughts that might interfere with their quit success. Such work has the benefit to facilitate quit success. As a final aspect to this topic, the therapist will want to relate this skill back to the exposure exercises. Specifically, the therapist should communicate that skills to identify and change negative thoughts about one's ability to tolerate uncomfortable feelings and situations, whether general anxiety-related or quit-related, will be critical to their eventual success because it involves repeated exposure to these uncomfortable sensations and restructuring how one perceives and tolerates these sensations.

To further assist with smoking cessation, high-risk situations and social support warrant discussion in treatment. The therapist should work with the client to identify high-risk situations and develop a plan for how the client will respond to these situations. The therapist should provide a rationale for this exercise and ensure an appropriate, feasible plan is documented. In addition, the importance of social support during a quit attempt is discussed in this session. The key is for the client to understand that easily available cigarettes, often supported by individuals who smoke at social or other gatherings, significantly increase the likelihood of relapse.

For between session work, the client is asked to continue monitoring their smoking behavior as well as their mood and it's relation to smoking. This will provide a useful tool for the client to consider the interconnectedness among thoughts, emotions, and behaviors. In addition to the high-risk situations identified during session 2, the client should use time outside of the session to identify and plan for additional situations that might lead to smoking, and discuss their forthcoming quit attempt with friends and family. Additionally, the client is assigned to monitor and practice exposure exercises at least every other day for 15–20 minutes and record their exercises. The therapist will want to remind the client of the NOA acronym and encourage them to observe, describe, and express sensations as well as identify maladaptive thoughts they experience during their practice. The therapist ensures the client's understanding of the material, answers questions about the self-help materials, and invites any additional questions. The therapist also requests that the client arrive to the next session having abstained from cigarettes for at least 6-hours and explains that this will help the in-session exposure practices be more effective. Following this request and answering all questions, the therapist concludes the session.

Session 2 Example Dialogue

Therapist	As we discussed last week, the types of physical sensations people experience when trying to quit smoking are often very similar to the sensations experienced when people experience anxiety. That is, these sensations significantly overlap with each other, which is why this treatment is designed to target both types of symptoms simultaneously. These sensations may be uncomfortable, but they are not physically harmful to you. The goal of this program is to increase your tolerance or resilience to these uncomfortable sensations by experiencing these symptoms and not avoiding them through smoking. Do you have any questions before we begin?
Client	I do not.
Therapist	Great, let's begin! We are now going to practice exercises that are meant to elicit sensations that are often experienced during an attempt to quit smoking such as dizziness, light headedness, and shortness of breath. The first exercise will be spinning in a chair with your eyes open. Don't worry if you do not have a swivel chair, you can also spin standing up with your arms outstretched like this (*Therapist demonstrates exercise for client to see*). I would like you to take special notice of any sensations you are experiencing. When you start feeling sensations such as dizziness, I would like you to raise your hand. I will let you know when to stop. Are you ready to begin?
Client	Yes.
Therapist	Okay, let's get started.

(Client engages in exercise. Client raises their hand when they begin to feel sensations. Therapist has client continue for an additional 5–10 seconds beyond that point and then ends the exercise).

Therapist	You can now stop the exercise. Great job! I would like you to describe to me any sensations you felt.
Client	I definitely started to feel lightheaded and dizzy. I also felt a little bit nauseous.
Therapist	That is not surprising. These sensations are normal reactions to this behavior that are okay. Even though those sensations are uncomfortable, they are not harmful. Our goal is to continue to experience these sensations without responding to them with smoking. Experiencing these symptoms in the absence of smoking will help to make them less intense in the future, like after quit day.

Session 3 The focus of the third session is to practice interoceptive exposure exercises, develop adaptive coping strategies, and challenge maladaptive cognitions. This is the last session prior to the scheduled quit day; therefore, the therapist should take time to reflect the connection between the content of the current and previous

sessions and the scheduled quit attempt. At the beginning of the session, between session work is evaluated for completeness and new insights are discussed. Barriers to completing the assignments are addressed to prevent further difficulties and enhance effectiveness. After, the therapist outlines goals for the present session and reviews topics discussed at the previous session.

The first topic covered is the client's interoceptive exposure practice and monitoring. The therapist will want to gain an in-depth understanding of the client's experience with the exercises. Indeed, it will be important for the therapist and client to discuss the frequency and length of the practice, the length of smoking withdrawal before and after the practice, any noticeable changes in sensations, and how their thoughts about the sensations influenced their experience. Regarding cognitive interpretation of the sensations, the therapist and client should devote time to developing alternative thoughts that help decrease the intensity and impact of the exercises, if necessary.

Following discussion of the client's out of session practice, the client is instructed to practice two of the most anxiety provoking exercises in session. As before, the therapist first demonstrates the exercise. Then, the client practices the exercise, but is instructed to raise their hand when they feel sensations and continue the exercise for 5–10 seconds beyond that point. The therapist should reinforce the use of NOA and encourage the client to use these exercises as an opportunity to increase their resilience in preparation for possible withdrawal symptoms/sensations they may experience when they quit or reduce the number of cigarettes they smoke.

A brief review of the influence of cognitions on emotions and behavior is provided. Discussions should focus on how the client's thoughts during their out of session exposure practice impacted their anxiety. The therapist should emphasize the role of cognitive interpretation of symptoms on symptom severity and type. The goal is for the client to identify that changing their thoughts about the exercises and symptoms may lead to improvements in the severity of anxiety symptoms. The connection among cognitions, emotions, and behaviors should then be extended to smoking. In particular, the therapist and client should work together to identify maladaptive thoughts about smoking, discuss how such thoughts influence quit behavior, and generate alternative thoughts to aid cessation.

Next, the therapist and client revisit the importance of social support and planning for high-risk situations. The therapist will want to use the client's between session work related to social support as a way to broach this topic. Evocative questions regarding the client's experience talking to family and friends about quitting, and family and friends' reactions to discussions about quitting will help facilitate this discussion. The goal is to help the client understand the importance of and enlist social support when attempting to quit. Another important topic of discussion is high-risk situations and coping strategies. During this discussion, the therapist should elicit 1–2 additional high-risk situations and work with the client to document appropriate behavioral coping plans. The therapist also should use this opportunity to discuss the importance of making healthy lifestyle changes to reduce the impact of high-risk situations and encourage the client to consider short- and long-term lifestyle changes that will reduce the risk of a relapse.

The next section focuses on preparing one's environment for quitting. The client is instructed to remove all smoking paraphernalia from their home, car, and workplace. They should develop a plan for making cigarettes unavailable to them, activities to do instead of smoking, and tactics to manage stress without smoking. It is recommended that clients keep their schedules filled and busy during the first few weeks following quit day as this will support the quit attempt. The therapist and client should work together to develop a list of activities that the client will do prior to smoking during periods of intense cravings. The therapist should work with the client to document this information. For heavy smoking clients or clients with strong concern about cravings, the therapist may want to introduce fading wherein the client practices reducing their cigarette consumption prior to the scheduled quit date. Fading can be a helpful to attenuate craving intensity following the quit. To synthesize this information, the client receives a coping card that summarizes many of the discussed idea, including avoiding triggers, substitute behaviors, social support, mental coping, and stress reduction. The client is encouraged to create a personalized quit-smoking coping card that they can reference after quit day to help curb intense urges. The therapist should explain that waiting 5-minutes after the initial urge and referencing their coping card may significantly increase the chance of remaining abstinent.

The therapist should reinforce the client's commitment and preparedness to quit by highlighting specific knowledge and skills the client has to support their quit attempt. The therapist encourages the client to review the self-help materials information and practice the newly learned skills. Indeed, the client will want to continue monitoring their smoking and mood over the next week as well as continue practicing and challenging themselves with the exposure exercises at least every other day for 15–20 minutes; practices should be tracked. At least one set of exposure exercises should occur during a period of cigarette withdrawal. The therapist may also encourage the client to enlist additional support before the next appointment. Further, if the client opts to use NRT, the therapists should review proper use with the client.

At the end of the session, the therapist should answer any additional questions regarding the present session. Moreover, it is important that the therapist clearly outlines the agenda for the next week and state that it is the client's scheduled quit date. The client should be informed that the quit begins the morning of the day regardless of when the therapy appointment is scheduled; thus, the client should not use cigarettes, but practice their skills as soon as wakening the day of their quit. Finally, the therapist should take this time to recognize the difficulty in quitting smoking, congratulate the client on their accomplishments and commitment, and reinforce the client's ability to quit given their skills.

Session 3 Example Dialogue

Therapist	As we discussed last week, the way we think about and interpret things can have a profound impact on our feelings and behaviors. With quit day approaching next week, are you having any unhelpful thoughts related to quitting smoking?
Client	Yeah, as quit day is getting closer, I am definitely having more of those.
Therapist	What are some of those thoughts?
Client	I have been having the thought, "I don't know how I am going to be able to handle something stressful without having a cigarette."
Therapist	How do you think thoughts like that impact your feelings and behaviors?
Client	It contributes to anxiety about the whole process and reluctance to engage in quitting smoking.
Therapist	What are some other ways to interpret the situation?
Client	I could tell myself that I have never prepared to quit smoking like I am now.
Therapist	Great idea! What are some other things you could counter with?
Client	Smoking makes me feel better in the short term but in the long term it makes me feel worse.
Therapist	These are all great counter thoughts. I encourage you to continue to challenge your thoughts throughout this process using the forms we provided you.

Session 4 Prior to reviewing between session work, client compliance is evaluated. Specifically, the therapist assesses if the client has abstained from smoking, removed smoking paraphernalia from their home, car, and workplace, and used the quit smoking medication appropriately, if applicable. Following this, the between session work is checked for completeness. Difficulties completing the assignments are addressed. After, the therapist outlines goals for the present session and briefly reviews topics discussed at the previous session.

The client's current withdrawal symptoms/urges and current anxiety level are assessed using SUDs ratings. The therapist and client review the client's anxiety monitoring and discuss its relation to smoking and smoking urges. This provides an opportunity to focus on specific interpretations and meanings of nicotine cravings and/or anxiety. If the client is struggling with resisting smoking when experiencing uncomfortable sensations, the therapist should assist with providing corrective feedback and emphasize NOA. As needed, address maladaptive smoking-related cognitions with the client (e.g., future-oriented concerns about inability to get through cravings—emphasize present mindfulness). The therapist should work with the client to derive additional strategies to refrain from smoking. The therapist should introduce a form to track their cravings. In session, the therapist should confirm that the client explicitly recognizes the link between withdrawal, distress/anxiety, and urge to smoke. The therapist should review anxiety psychoeducation and the role of maladaptive cognitions, as needed. The therapist should work with the client to relate present experiences to exposure exercises while emphasizing behavior and thought change. Therapists should remind clients that symptoms are opportunities to increase tolerance.

As a next step, common barriers to maintaining abstinence and relapse prevention are reviewed. The therapist should emphasize the importance of preemptively developing a strategy and plan for how to cope with urges and high-risk situations, and identify the maladaptive belief that smoking will help reduce anxiety/stress as a risk factor for relapse. The therapist should also highlight additional factors to consider, including social support, staying focused on short-term quit goals, and openness to experience withdrawal symptoms rather than avoidance.

The therapist and client should then thoroughly review the client's between session work on high-risk situations, coping card development, and lifestyle changes. Therapists should reiterate how each of these facets contributes to quit success and failure. Any important final discussion points or suggestions regarding this area, including developing a plan for lapse and the importance of staying busy, should be discussed. Additionally, the therapist should re-emphasize the importance of enlisting social support prior to quit day and as needed, problem-solve with those who are still reluctant to do so.

Following, the therapist reviews smoking cessation benefits and the positive impact of smoking cessation on health. Attention should be directed to both the short- and long-term benefits of quitting. To encourage sustained abstinence, the client should be provided with a sample relapse prevention plan. Both the client's abstinence plan and the sample relapse prevention plan should be discussed in detail. Any concerns or questions should be thoroughly addressed to prevent relapse.

Prior to concluding the session, the therapist should highlight the important aspect of the treatment program. Specifically, the therapist should review the harmful consequences of smoking including increasing the risk of developing problems with anxiety. The therapist should review the rationale for reducing AS to facilitate quit success. The therapist should emphasize the importance of continuing to monitor anxiety in relationship to smoking urges and review skills learned in treatment that will help the client manage stress adaptively, including alternative coping strategies. The therapist should also reiterate the importance of practicing skills learned in treatment outside of treatment for the skill to become "second nature" and elicit the client's personalized feedback on the program. Finally, the therapist should build self-efficacy by congratulating the client and provide words of encouragement moving forward.

Session 4 Example Dialogue

Therapist Congratulations on quitting smoking! I wanted to talk a bit about any withdrawal symptoms you may be experiencing as well as urges to smoke and how you would rate them from 0 to 10 in terms of distress.

Client	Thank you! I have been experiencing increased irritability. I also notice overall, I feel more restless. I would say my irritability is a 6 and restlessness is at a 7. In terms of urge to smoke, that is an 8 out of 10.
Therapist	What about your feelings of anxiety, how would you rate those in terms of distress from 0–100?
Client	My anxiety is at about a 70.
Therapist	Thank you for providing that information. That is not surprising that your experiencing withdrawal symptoms and that your anxiety levels are elevated. It is also not surprising that you are experiencing increased urges to smoke. In the past, you have used smoking as a way to cope with uncomfortable feelings and sensations and your body is still learning that these symptoms are normal, harmless, and expected. By not smoking in response to your symptoms and urges, your body is also learning how to tolerate these symptoms and that they do not need to be avoided via smoking.
Client	It is definitely a learning process and I know it will take time.
Therapist	Absolutely. The more you practice the acceptance of these sensations, the greater tolerance your body will develop. Also, continuing to engage in the interoceptive exercises will also help your body become more comfortable with these sensations.

Status of Efficacy

The ASRP-S program has been developed in a theoretically driven manner and is supported indirectly by a relatively large body of empirical literature. Existing work has evaluated the treatment, in various formats (Zvolensky et al., 2014, 2018). The results of such work generally suggest reducing AS improves mental health and smoking behavior. A critical next step for this work will be to explore the generalizability of the ongoing, novel research to diverse populations most prone to chronic tobacco-related disease.

Summary

The present chapter focused on one transdiagnostic approach to addressing smoking cessation through an integrated AS and smoking treatment, ASRP-S. ASRP-S can be completed over a period of four in-person sessions aimed to target a number of cognitive and behavioral facets known to be associated with tobacco use. Clinicians should exercise their clinical judgment when administering ASRP-S to provide a personalized and flexible treatment approach that best addresses client needs.

Acknowledgment Research reported in this publication was supported by the National Institute on Minority Health and Health Disparities (NIMHD) of the National Institutes of Health (NIH) to the University of Houston under Award Number U54MD015946. The content is solely the responsibility of the authors and does not necessarily represent the official views of the National Institutes of Health.

References

Callaghan, R. C., Veldhuizen, S., Jeysingh, T., Orlan, C., Graham, C., Kakouris, G., Remington, G., & Gatley, J. (2014). Patterns of tobacco-related mortality among individuals diagnosed with schizophrenia, bipolar disorder, or depression. *Journal of Psychiatric Research, 48*(1), 102–110. https://doi.org/10.1016/j.jpsychires.2013.09.014

Centers for Disease Control and Prevention. (2020). *Smoking & tobacco use home: Health effects.* https://www.cdc.gov/tobacco/basic_information/health_effects/index.htm#:~:text=Smoking%20causes%20cancer%2C%20heart%20disease,immune%20system%2C%20including%20rheumatoid%20arthritis

Centers for Disease Control and Prevention. (2022). *Diseases and death.* https://www.cdc.gov/tobacco/data_statistics/fact_sheets/fast_facts/diseases-and-death.html

Cornelius, M. E., Loretan, C. G., Jamal, A., Davis Lynn, B. C., Mayer, M., Alcantara, I. C., & Neff, L. (2023). Tobacco product use among adults – United States, 2021. *MMWR. Morbidity and Mortality Weekly Report, 72*(18), 475–483. https://doi.org/10.15585/mmwr.mm7218a1

Farris, S. G., Leventhal, A. M., Schmidt, N. B., & Zvolensky, M. J. (2015a). Anxiety sensitivity and pre-cessation smoking processes: testing the independent and combined mediating effects of negative affect-reduction expectancies and motives. *Journal of Studies on Alcohol and Drugs, 76*(2), 317–325.

Farris, S. G., Paulus, D. J., Gonzalez, A., Mahaffey, B. L., Bromet, E. J., Luft, B. J., Kotov, R., & Zvolensky, M. J. (2015b). Anxiety sensitivity mediates the association between post-traumatic stress symptom severity and interoceptive threat-related smoking abstinence expectancies among World Trade Center disaster-exposed smokers. *Addictive Behaviors, 51*, 204–210. https://doi.org/10.1016/j.addbeh.2015.07.031

Fiore, M. C., Jaen, C. R., Baker, T., Bailey, W., Benowitz, N., Curry, S., Dorfman, S., Froelicher, E., Goldstein, M., & Healton, C. (2008). *Treating tobacco use and dependence: 2008 update.* US Department of Health and Human Services.

Garey, L., Olofsson, H., Garza, T., Rogers, A. H., Kauffman, B. Y., & Zvolensky, M. J. (2020a). Directional effects of anxiety and depressive disorders with substance use: A review of recent prospective research. *Current Addiction Reports, 7*, 344–355.

Garey, L., Olofsson, H., Garza, T., Shepherd, J. M., Smit, T., & Zvolensky, M. J. (2020b). The role of anxiety in smoking onset, severity, and cessation-related outcomes: A review of recent literature. *Current Psychiatry Reports, 22*(8), 38. https://doi.org/10.1007/s11920-020-01160-5

Garey, L., Senger, A. R., Smit, T., Nizio, P., Matoska, C. T., Kauffman, B., Businelle, M. S., Gallagher, M. W., & Zvolensky, M. J. (2023). Anxiety sensitivity and reasons for smoking among Black smokers. *Addictive Behaviors, 139*, 107593. https://doi.org/10.1016/j.addbeh.2022.107593

Goodwin, R. D., Wall, M. M., Choo, T., Galea, S., Horowitz, J., Nomura, Y., Zvolensky, M. J., & Hasin, D. S. (2014). Changes in the prevalence of mood and anxiety disorders among male and female current smokers in the United States: 1990–2001. *Annals of Epidemiology, 24*(7), 493–497. https://doi.org/10.1016/j.annepidem.2014.01.014

Guillot, C. R., Leventhal, A. M., Raines, A. M., Zvolensky, M. J., & Schmidt, N. B. (2016). Anxiety sensitivity facets in relation to tobacco use, abstinence-related problems, and cognitions in treatment-seeking smokers. *Addictive Behaviors, 56*, 30–35.

Kalkhoran, S., Thorndike, A. N., Rigotti, N. A., Fung, V., & Baggett, T. P. (2019). Cigarette smoking and quitting-related factors among US adult health center patients with serious mental illness. *Journal of General Internal Medicine, 34*(6), 986–991. https://doi.org/10.1007/s11606-019-04857-3

Kelly, M. E., Guillot, C. R., Quinn, E. N., Lucke, H. R., Bello, M. S., Pang, R. D., & Leventhal, A. M. (2020). Anxiety sensitivity in relation to cigarette smoking and other substance use in African American smokers. *Psychology of Addictive Behaviors, 34*(6), 669–679. https://doi.org/10.1037/adb0000573

Langdon, K. J., Farris, S. G., Hogan, J. B. D., Grover, K. W., & Zvolensky, M. J. (2016). Anxiety sensitivity in relation to quit day dropout among adult daily smokers recruited to participate in a self-guided cessation attempt. *Addictive Behaviors, 58*, 12–15.

Langdon, K. J., Bakhshaie, J., Lopez, A., Tavakoli, N., Garey, L., Raines, A. M., Kauffman, B. Y., Schmidt, N. B., & Zvolensky, M. J. (2018). Anxiety sensitivity physical and cognitive concerns in relation to smoking-oriented cognition: An examination among treatment-seeking adults who smoke. *Journal of Addiction Medicine, 12*(3), 212–219. https://doi.org/10.1097/adm.0000000000000389

Leventhal, A. M., & Zvolensky, M. J. (2015). Anxiety, depression, and cigarette smoking: A transdiagnostic vulnerability framework to understanding emotion–smoking comorbidity. *Psychological Bulletin, 141*(1), 176.

Lipari, R. N., & Van Horn, S. (2017). Smoking and mental illness among adults in the United States. In *The CBHSQ report* (p. 1). Substance Abuse and Mental Health Services Administration (US). [Record #57 is using a reference type undefined in this output style.].

Marlatt, G. A., & Gordon, J. R. (Eds) (1985). Relapse prevention: maintenance strategies in the treatment of addictive behaviors (New York, Guilford Press).

McNally, R. J. (2002). Anxiety sensitivity and panic disorder. *Biological Psychiatry, 52*(10), 938–946.

Miller, W. R., & Rollnick, S. (2012). *Motivational interviewing: Helping people change*. Guilford Press.

Otto, M. W., Eastman, A., Lo, S., Hearon, B. A., Bickel, W. K., Zvolensky, M., Smits, J. A., & Doan, S. N. (2016). Anxiety sensitivity and working memory capacity: Risk factors and targets for health behavior promotion. *Clinical Psychology Review, 49*, 67–78.

Redmond, B. Y., Salwa, A., Bizier, A., & Zvolensky, M. J. (2023). Evaluating distress tolerance and anxiety sensitivity as simultaneous and concurrent transdiagnostic risk factors for smoking quit problems and perceived barriers for cessation. *Cognitive Therapy and Research, 47*(5), 1–7.

Reiss, S. (1991). Expectancy model of fear, anxiety, and panic. *Clinical Psychology Review, 11*(2), 141–153.

Reiss, S., Peterson, R. A., Gursky, D. M., & McNally, R. J. (1986). Anxiety sensitivity, anxiety frequency and the prediction of fearfulness. *Behaviour Research and Therapy, 24*(1), 1–8.

Rollnick, S., & Miller, W. R. (1995). What is motivational interviewing? *Behavioural and Cognitive Psychotherapy, 23*(4), 325–334.

Shepherd, J. M., Bakhshaie, J., Nizio, P., Garey, L., Viana, A. G., & Zvolensky, M. J. (2020). Anxiety symptoms and smoking outcome expectancies among Spanish-speaking Latinx adult smokers: Exploring the role of anxiety sensitivity. *Journal of Ethnicity in Substance Abuse, 21*(5), 1–21. https://doi.org/10.1080/15332640.2020.1759476

Taylor, S. (1999). *Anxiety sensitivity: Theory, research, and treatment of the fear of anxiety*. Lawrence Erlbaum Associates Publishers.

Williams, J. M., Steinberg, M. L., Griffiths, K. G., & Cooperman, N. (2013). Smokers with behavioral health comorbidity should be designated a tobacco use disparity group. *American Journal of Public Health, 103*(9), 1549–1555. https://doi.org/10.2105/ajph.2013.301232

Zinbarg, R. E., Barlow, D. H., & Brown, T. A. (1997). Hierarchical structure and general factor saturation of the Anxiety Sensitivity Index: Evidence and implications. *Psychological Assessment, 9*(3), 277.

Zvolensky, M. J., & Leventhal, A. M. (2016). Affect and health behavior Co-occurrence: The emerging roles of transdiagnostic factors and sociocultural factors. *Behavior Modification, 40*(1–2), 3–6. https://doi.org/10.1177/0145445515627307

Zvolensky, M. J., Bogiaizian, D., Salazar, P. L., Farris, S. G., & Bakhshaie, J. (2014). An anxiety sensitivity reduction smoking-cessation program for spanish-speaking smokers. *Cognitive and Behavioral Practice, 21*(3), 350–363. https://doi.org/10.1016/j.cbpra.2013.10.005

Zvolensky, M. J., Garey, L., Allan, N. P., Farris, S. G., Raines, A. M., Smits, J. A. J., Kauffman, B. Y., Manning, K., & Schmidt, N. B. (2018). Effects of anxiety sensitivity reduction on smoking abstinence: An analysis from a panic prevention program. *Journal of Consulting and Clinical Psychology, 86*(5), 474–485. https://doi.org/10.1037/ccp0000288

Zvolensky, M. J., Bakhshaie, J., Shepherd, J. M., Garey, L., Peraza, N., Viana, A. G., Brown, J. T., & Brown, R. A. (2019). Anxiety sensitivity and smoking outcome expectancies among Spanish-speaking Latinx adult smokers. *Experimental and Clinical Psychopharmacology, 27*(6), 569–577. https://doi.org/10.1037/pha0000270

Zvolensky, M. J., Shepherd, J. M., Clausen, B. K., Garey, L., Kauffman, B. Y., Viana, A. G., Heggeness, L. F., Bizier, A., Zappi, C., & Reitzel, L. R. (2023). Smoking abstinence expectancies among Latinx smokers: An initial test and evaluation of individual difference factors. *Cognitive Therapy and Research, 47*, 269–281. https://doi.org/10.1007/s10608-023-10351-2

Chapter 8
Third Wave Behavioral Treatment for Comorbid SUD and Emotional Disorders

Antoine Lebeaut, Shelby J. McGrew, Angela L. Slotts, and Anka A. Vujanovic

Overview

Substance use disorders (SUD) are highly prevalent among adults in the United States (U.S.; Grant et al., 2015, 2016). It is estimated that approximately 17% of the U.S. population (46.3 million people) over the age of 12 met *Diagnostic and Statistical Manual of Mental Disorders, Fifth Edition* (*DSM-5*; American Psychiatric Association, 2013) criteria for a SUD in the past year, including 29.5 million people who met diagnostic criteria for alcohol use disorder (AUD) and 24 million people who met diagnostic criteria for other (non-alcohol) SUD (e.g., cannabis, opioid, and/or stimulant) (SAMHSA, 2021). And while the rate of substance use has stabilized over the past decade, particularly among adolescents (NIDA, 2013, 2022), the public health impact of both substance use and SUD has remained significant (Roberts et al., 2021). Indeed, the prevalence of SUD is associated with increased morbidity and mortality due to substance overdose, substance-related health consequences (e.g., lung cancer, heart and/or liver disease, stroke, and higher suicide risk; Aldridge et al., 2018; Mack et al., 2017). Relatedly, substantial economic costs in health care, rehabilitative services, and labor (e.g., reduced productivity or increased absenteeism) are related to SUD and substance use (Lo et al., 2020). As such, it is

A. Lebeaut
Department of Psychology, University of Houston, Houston, TX, USA

S. J. McGrew · A. A. Vujanovic (✉)
Department of Psychological and Brain Sciences, Texas A&M University, College Station, TX, USA
e-mail: avujanovic@tamu.edu

A. L. Slotts
Department of Family and Community Medicine, The University of Texas Health Science Center at Houston, Houston, TX, USA

K. Wolitzky-Taylor (ed.), *Treating Comorbid Substance Use and Emotional Disorders*, CBT: Science Into Practice, https://doi.org/10.1007/978-3-031-62971-6_8

critical to understand the underlying phenomenology of SUD to inform primary, secondary, and tertiary prevention efforts and treatment among substance using populations.

Emotional disorders (e.g., anxiety-related disorders, depressive disorders, trauma- and stressor-related disorders) frequently co-occur with SUD (Grant et al., 2016) and are thus highly clinically relevant to understanding the risk and maintenance factors associated with the development and onset of SUD. Epidemiologic research suggests that the 12-month prevalence rates of SUD in U.S. adults with an anxiety-related or mood disorder range from 15% to 20%, respectively (Grant et al., 2004) with even higher rates (46%) among those with post-traumatic stress disorder (PTSD; Pietrzak et al., 2011). Similarly, the 12-month prevalence rates of an anxiety-related or mood disorder in U.S. adults with a SUD range from 12% to 26%, respectively (Grant et al., 2004). Moreover, the co-occurrence of PTSD and SUD is well-established across distinct populations, including the general population (Blanco et al., 2013), military veterans (Smith & Cottler, 2018), and first responders (Bonumwezi et al., 2022).

Various theoretical models may explain SUD comorbidity/emotional disorder. For instance, the "common factors" model posits that shared etiological and maintenance factors across both SUD and emotional disorders, such as maladaptive cognitions/behaviors, genetic predisposition, environmental conditions (e.g., domestic violence), and/or personality traits, may help explain the comorbidity (Stohler & Rössler, 2005). However, the most widely studied theory for this elevated comorbidity rate is the self-medication hypothesis, a causal model that posits that individuals with elevated mood, anxiety, and/or trauma-related symptoms may be more likely to engage in substance use to cope with the negative emotional states associated with emotional disorders (Hawn et al., 2020; Khantzian, 1997). That is, the substance (e.g., alcohol, cannabis, opioids) temporarily alleviates symptoms and distress, and as a result, serves a strong short-term negative reinforcer and fuels a negative reinforcement model of substance use (Baker et al., 2004). While many factors are related to treatment-seeking behaviors, including stigma, the perceived need for treatment, and the availability of treatment facilities (Blanco et al., 2015), the co-occurrence of SUD and emotional disorders poses unique implications for treatment and may inform the low treatment-seeking rates typically found among substance-using populations (Witkiewitz et al., 2022).

Available interventions for SUD and SUD/emotional disorders vary in their approach, structure/format (e.g., intensive outpatient programs, residential treatment), and efficacy. Traditional approaches to SUD treatment include medication-assisted therapies (e.g., methadone maintenance treatment), mutual-aid and self-help groups (e.g., Alcoholics Anonymous), cognitive behavioral therapy (CBT), motivation interviewing, and contingency management (Witkiewitz et al., 2022). Current guidelines underscore the value and efficacy of simultaneously treating these co-occurring conditions concurrently or integratively (Minkoff, 2001).

Considering the well-established efficacy of CBT for SUD (McHugh et al., 2010) as well as for numerous emotional disorders (Lorenzo-Luaces et al., 2021), integrative CBT approaches that simultaneously treat both disorders have been developed and tested (Kelly & Daley, 2013). Such CBT approaches utilize manualized protocols to identify (via functional analysis) and explicitly target maladaptive cognitions and behaviors. For instance, integrative CBT for SUD and major depressive disorder (MDD) may include a functional analysis of the associations between dysfunctional cognitive appraisal/beliefs and substance use, psychoeducation, thought-challenging exercises, and harm-reduction techniques (Vujanovic et al., 2017). This may in turn lead to improvements in self-efficacy, alterations of maladaptive, negative cognitions, and promote healthy coping-related behaviors. While integrative CBT has garnered empirical support (Kelly & Daley, 2013), access to evidence-based treatment remains low and there is a continued need to improve current approaches (Han et al., 2017). Furthermore, the lack of well-controlled randomized controlled trials (RCT) on integrative CBT, coupled with the relative diversity of approaches (e.g., settings, formats, duration, and populations and substances studied), limits their scope and generalizability (Vujanovic et al., 2017). Thus, there is a critical need to improve extant treatments for SUD/emotional disorders and to develop novel, evidence-based intervention approaches.

Third wave interventions for SUD/emotional disorders, which are commonly conceptualized to include Acceptance and Commitment Therapy (ACT; Hayes et al., 2012), mindfulness-based interventions (MBI), Dialectical Behavioral Therapy[1] (DBT; Linehan, 1993), Metacognitive Therapy (Wells, 2011), and other transdiagnostic approaches (e.g., Unified Protocol; Barlow et al., 2011), offer an alternative approach to traditional CBT treatment strategies. Building on the previous iterations (e.g., "waves") of CBT, comprised of behavior therapy (e.g., behavior modification via analysis and conditioning), cognitive therapy (e.g., identification and alterations in maladaptive thoughts and cognitive schemas), and integrative cognitive and behavioral approaches (e.g., traditional CBT), third wave interventions employ a process-based approach to the treatment of mental disorders (Hayes, 2004; Hayes & Hofmann, 2017). Constructs such as acceptance, mindfulness, metacognitions, personal values, psychological flexibility (each further described below), and relationships are readily incorporated in treatments that focus on the context, processes, and functions associated with a person's internal experiences and how they may relate to these experiences (Hayes, 2004). Third wave approaches emphasize context- and process-based therapeutic strategies, such as metaphors, mindfulness-based exercises, and behavioral actions, that serve to complement and improve, rather than replace, traditional CBT (Hayes et al., 2006). As such, these treatment strategies are uniquely equipped to address features and mechanisms associated with SUD and emotional disorders, including experiential avoidance, emotional regulation difficutlies, subtance-related urges/cravings, and dysfunctional congitiosn and behaviors (Hayes, 2004).

[1] DBT was originally conceptualized as a behavior therapy (Linehan, 1993) and was developed well before other interventions conceptualized as "third wave", such as ACT and the Unified Protocol. However, DBT explicitly integrates and clinically focuses on transdiagnostic factors (e.g., mindfulness, distress tolerance, and emotion regulation); and thus, it was later conceptualized as a third wave approach.

Aims

Accordingly, the scope and goal of this chapter is to provide an overview and discussion of empirically supported third wave interventions for the treatment of comorbid SUD and emotion disorders. Specifically, we will (1) synthesize the current research supporting their use and highlight important areas for growth, (2) discuss pertinent conceptual and theoretical underpinnings for specific treatment strategies and relevant mechanisms of change, and (3) describe two case formulations related to the treatment of SUD/emotion disorders in clinical settings. Finally, we will provide additional information on the implementation of third wave approaches, discuss notable limitations, and offer suggestions for future directions to better inform prevention and treatment approaches using third wave treatment strategies.

Clinical Research

There is a growing body of literature examining third wave interventions for the treatment of SUD/emotional disorders. ACT and other third wave treatments emphasize identification of the core principles and processes that underlie various mental health conditions. Additionally, such intervention strategies seek to address the purpose of problematic thoughts and emotions by demonstrating new ways of relating to them. Thus, these approaches underscore patients' ability to change the way they associate with and understand their own internal experiences. As third wave interventions seek to address a variety of presenting issues, they are considered transdiagnostic in nature (Hayes & Hofmann, 2017) and represent a promising avenue for integrative treatments.

ACT has gained recent empirical attention for treatment of comorbid SUD and emotional disorders, with much of the clinical research investigating its efficacy for co-occurring PTSD and SUD. ACT-based treatment has demonstrated promising outcomes for the treatment of PTSD/AUD (Berghoff & Tull, 2019; Hermann et al., 2016; Vujanovic et al., 2017). Moreover, among incarcerated women with posttraumatic stress and SUD broadly, ACT may be more effective than traditional CBT for reduction of drug use and improvement of mental health symptoms (Lanza et al., 2014). ACT has also been used for treatment of MDD and AUD and while these studies were small in nature, their positive results suggest promising potential for the efficacy of ACT in targeting co-occurring MDD and SUD (Petersen & Zettle, 2009; Thekiso et al., 2015). Further, a web-based ACT smoking cessation treatment has demonstrated efficacy for increasing quit rates and lowering depressive symptoms among smokers with depressive symptoms (Jones et al., 2015). Indeed, this work highlights the potential for ACT as an integrative treatment for comorbid SUD/emotional disorders.

MBI overlap with ACT, emphasizing the processes involved in thinking and feeling. MBI commonly intend to encourage (a) present-focused awareness and (b) nonjudgmental acceptance of internal experiences (e.g., thoughts, emotions, bodily sensations). For example, Valenstein-Mah et al. (2019) tested the feasibility and acceptability of a specific MBI, loving-kindness meditation, among college students ($N = 75$) with co-occurring PTSD and problem drinking. This meditation is commonly used in MBI and involves practicing kindness towards oneself and others. And while the loving-kindness MBI was found to be helpful by participants, there were no significant differences between the loving-kindness MBI and referral to treatment-as-usual on PTSD symptoms, alcohol outcomes, or state mindfulness (Valenstein-Mah et al., 2019). Other clinical research has examined the use of MBI for co-occurring PTSD and SUD, with Fortuna and Vallejo (2015) developing Mindfulness-Based Cognitive Therapy for Adolescent PTSD and SUD. Preliminary work using this MBI demonstrated improvements in PTSD and depression symptoms, as well as reduction in cannabis use (Fortuna et al., 2018). With regard to co-occurring depression and SUD, mindfulness-based relapse prevention (MBRP; Bowen et al., 2014) may be one promising treatment option. MBRP was developed to improve substance use urges following SUD treatment (Bowen et al., 2014). Among a sample of 74 adults with comorbid MDD and SUD, MBRP was associated with decreased anxiety and depression symptoms, as well as cravings (Zemestani & Ottaviani, 2016). MBRP has also been found to reduce negative affect, impairment, and stimulant use among adults with co-occurring SUD and anxiety and mood conditions (Glasner-Edwards et al., 2017).

DBT is a cognitive-behavioral intervention that was originally developed for use among individuals with borderline personality disorder (BPD); this treatment involves targeting skills such as emotion regulation (i.e., the capacity to modulate emotional reactions when faced with psychological stressors; Gratz & Roemer, 2004), mindfulness (i.e., purposeful awareness of and focus to the present moment and the nonjudgmental acceptance of adverse emotional states; Baer et al., 2006), distress tolerance (i.e., the capacity to endure adverse physical and/or psychological states; Leyro et al., 2010), and interpersonal effectiveness (i.e., the ability to effectively interact with others, maintain relationships, and preserve self-respect (Linehan, 1993). While DBT was originally conceptualized as a behavior therapy (Linehan, 1993), its integration of mindfulness and other transdiagnostic factors (e.g., distress tolerance and emotion regulation) led to its clinical conceptualization as a third wave approach, although it was developed decades ahead of other interventions conceptualized as "third wave". While BPD is outside of the scope of the present chapter, we will highlight clinical research that has adapted DBT for use among individuals with emotional disorders and SUD. Meta-analytic work has revealed that DBT is an effective treatment for individuals with SUD (Haktanir & Callender, 2020). Further, though originally developed in the context of BPD, skills taught in DBT may be efficacious for treating emotional conditions, more broadly, including post-traumatic stress (Benfer et al., 2021), treatment-resistant depression (Harley et al., 2008), and generalized anxiety disorder (Afshari & Hasani, 2020). As such, DBT has been utilized as a treatment for both SUD and emotional disorders;

however, there is a relative paucity of work examining DBT as an integrative treatment for the co-occurrence of these conditions.

Description of Strategies

Third wave treatment strategies rely on distinct mechanisms of change that may be unique to each approach (see Fig. 8.1). However, while third wave interventions are discrete and differ in their foundational approach to treatment, they tend to have shared, common mechanisms of change. For example, "psychological flexibility", the ability to attend to the present moment and adjust to difficult circumstances using relevant context and values, is an important component of third wave interventions as inflexibility is thought to underlie psychopathology. Indeed, psychological flexibility is considered a mechanism of change in ACT (Hayes et al., 2012), as well as other third wave interventions, including DBT (Linehan, 1993). Accordingly, the following description of mechanisms of change is not meant to be an exhaustive

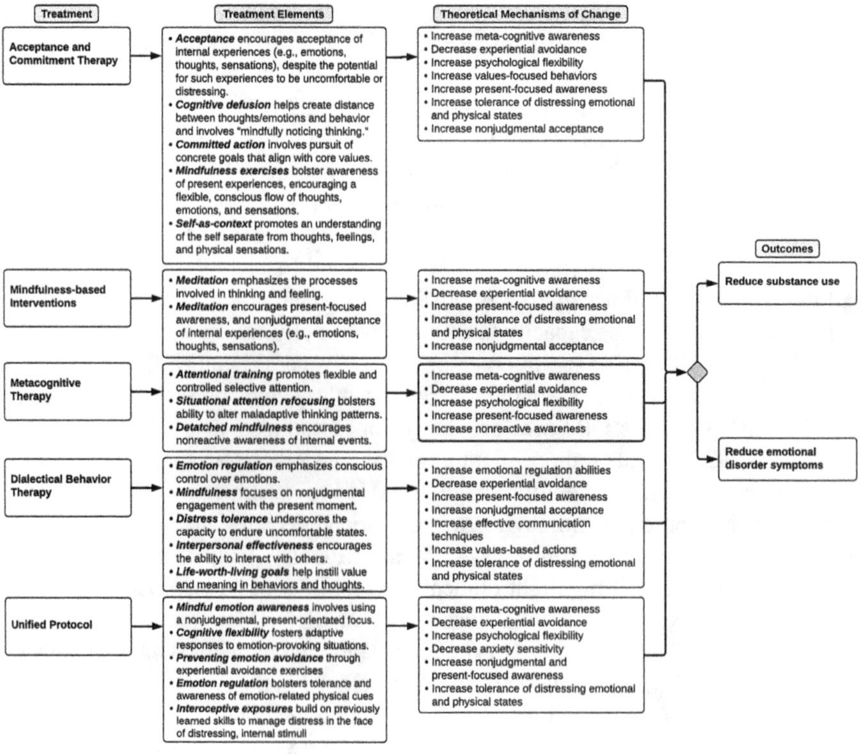

Fig. 8.1 Third wave interventions for co-occurring emotional disorders and substance use disorders

list, but rather, to offer a review of pertinent mechanisms and underscores their distinct and shared relations with third wave approaches.

"Acceptance" is a construct that spans third wave interventions and promotes psychological flexibility. Within ACT, MBI, and DBT frameworks, this skill focuses on acceptance of internal experiences (e.g., emotions, thoughts, sensations). Specific techniques seek to aid patients with acceptance, rather than avoidance of, internal experiences that may be distressing or uncomfortable. According to Hayes et al. (2012), acceptance is an active behavior, rather than a passive one. Intentional acceptance of internal experiences (e.g., thoughts, memories, and/or emotions) can allow for a state of interest, curiosity, and observation of these experiences that may be typically avoided (Hayes et al., 2012). As such, acceptance skills emphasize patients' capacity for the experiencing of such states, rather than encouraging active efforts to change them.

The self-medication model posits that substances are often used to cope with uncomfortable or distressing internal states (Khantzian, 1997). Through acceptance-based techniques that are present in third wave interventions, patients may be empowered to experience unpleasant thoughts and feelings rather than actively work to suppress them by using substances. Further, patients may be encouraged to notice their thoughts, feelings, and cravings for substances as finite experiences that will pass as one way of promoting nonjudgmental acceptance. Acknowledgement that these experiences are fleeting through techniques such as "urge surfing" substance-related cravings may help patients learn to respond in ways that coincide with their long-term values and objectives, rather than in an "automatic", maladaptive manner (e.g., substance use; Bowen et al., 2020). This approach can be found across third wave therapies, including ACT, DBT, MBI (e.g., MBRP), metacognitive therapy, and transdiagnostic therapies.

"Cognitive defusion" is another core process involved in psychological flexibility (Hayes et al., 2012). This technique may be conceptualized as "mindfully noticing thinking" (Hayes et al., 2012). Cognitive defusion is intended to help patients notice their thoughts from a distance as a way of creating space between thought/emotion and behavior, with the overarching goal of increasing psychological flexibility. As an example, one technique involves watching thoughts as if they were written on leaves floating down a stream. Another technique includes labeling thoughts as "thoughts" when practicing metacognitive awareness to create an internal "buffer" between oneself and the thoughts. Cognitive defusion may be used to help patients distance themselves from thoughts or emotions related to substance use. When fused with thoughts or feelings, patients may find themselves "buying into" these experiences and treating them as factual information, rather than practicing nonjudgmental acceptance. For example, patients with co-occurring SUD and emotional conditions may have thoughts that in order to gain relief from emotional symptoms, they must use substances. Thus, this skill may give patients the "mental space" to defuse from their maladaptive conditions and engage in adaptive techniques that may provide relief, such as behavioral activation strategies. And while the terminology is distinctly ACT-based, the concept of cognitive defusion can be found in DBT and across MBI approaches as well.

"Committed action" or "life-worth-living goals" also promote psychological flexibility. These actions/goals may be conceptualized as an individual's ability to engage in behavior that is steered by their personal values and goals, despite encountering unhelpful thoughts, feelings, or sensations. Indeed, committed action encourages patients to identify and commit to concrete goals that help them live in accordance with their core values (Hayes et al., 2012). Similarly, life-worth-living goals can serve to help and motivate individuals to transform problematic behaviors (Linehan, 1993). Thus, the focus of committed action and life-worth-living goals is behavioral change, whereas acceptance and defusion are more cognitive in nature; however, each strategy may be used in conjunction to promote psychological flexibility. For instance, in SUD/emotional disorder interventions, committed action can involve identification of behaviors that are in-line with values and discussion of implementation of such behaviors, which run contrary to avoidance behaviors such as substance use (Hermann et al., 2016). Furthermore, integrative treatment can bolster the willingness to experience uncomfortable states to support committed action (Hermann et al., 2016).

Mindfulness exercises have been incorporated into various third wave intervention modalities. Baer and Krietemeyer (2006) posit that mindfulness includes present-focused awareness, nonjudging of inner experiences, and nonreactivity to inner experiences. Higher levels of mindfulness allow for awareness of and adaptive responses to present experiences, as mindfulness encourages a flexible, conscious flow of thoughts. Accordingly, mindfulness is another component of third wave behavioral treatments that bolsters psychological flexibility.

Higher levels of mindfulness are related to lower levels of mental health symptoms, such as PTSD, anxiety, and depression (Bajaj et al., 2016; Vujanovic et al., 2020). Further, mindfulness techniques have been efficacious for the reduction of substance use severity (Zgierska et al., 2009). According to the negative reinforcement model, avoidance of negative affect is one motivation for substance use (Baker et al., 2004). Individuals with higher levels of mindfulness may be more aware of internal and physical states related to negative affect and substance use withdrawal. This mindful awareness may allow for conscious efforts to respond to such states in a way that aligns with long-term goals and values. As such, individuals with higher levels of mindfulness may be less likely to use substances as a way of avoiding uncomfortable internal and somatic states characteristic of emotional disorders.

Lastly, "self-as-context", or "detached mindfulness" when considering a meta-cognitive therapy framework, is often referred to as the "noticing self" and another psychological flexibility-promoting technique that may be used in third wave interventions for SUD/emotional disorders. Similar to other techniques, self-as-context is geared towards bolstering a present-focused understanding of one's conscious experience. Hayes et al. (2012) posits that self-as-context undermines attachment to the "fused" self, or certain narratives about the self in the service of promoting connection to a self, based on the "I/here/now". As such, Hayes et al. (2012) indicates that self-as-context techniques may help patients adopt a new perspective of the self, such that they are able to view inner experiences as unique and separate from consciousness, which in turn, can empower them to conceptualize their inner world as nonthreatening.

Within the lens of SUD/emotional disorders, self-as-context or detached mindfulness may be a promising technique for addressing to co-occurrence of these conditions. Although work on self-as-context as a mechanism of change among dual diagnosis patients appears to be limited, some work has investigated the role of self-stigma, a related concept that can be characterized by shame and evaluative thoughts tied to identification with a stigmatized group (Corrigan & Rao, 2012). Self-stigma may act as a barrier to engagement with behaviors, such as treatment-seeking, that align with individuals' core values and long-term goals. Research shows that self-stigma is high among individuals using substances and with serious mental illness; self-stigma is associated with delays in treatment-seeking and lower quality of life and self-esteem (Link et al., 2002). Third wave interventions, such as ACT, have been shown to reduce self-stigma among substance users (Luoma et al., 2008). More research in this area is warranted to examine associations between self-stigma and self-as-context, as well as the efficacy of self-as-context in particular as a mechanism of change for SUD/emotional disorders.

Case Formulation

Mental health professionals may be interested in using third wave interventions as a treatment approach for a patient presenting with SUD comorbidity/emotional disorder. While limited manualized protocols exist for targeting SUD/emotional disorder comorbidities with third wave interventions, the extant literature underscores the malleability of these interventions to address dynamic and complex case presentations. Accordingly, below are two case formulations/vignettes that are meant to (1) highlight this flexibility for two third wave interventions: ACT and MBRP, (2) provide recommendations on how to implement ACT and MBRP with patients diagnosed with SUD/emotional disorder, and (3) provide sample dialogue between a therapist and their patient for certain steps. It is important to note that a full description of ACT and MBRP approaches are beyond the scope of this chapter. For full-length accounts of ACT and MBRP, please see Hayes et al. (2012) and Bowen et al. (2020) respectively.

ACT for Generalized Anxiety Disorder (GAD) with AUD

Case Introduction and Brief History Laura was a 22-year-old female referred by a family member to a community mental health center. Laura was a senior at a college in the neighboring state but had recently and unexpectedly taken a leave of absence from school and returned home. At the time of the intake, Laura was living at home with her parents and was working part-time at a local restaurant. She typically spent her days at home and would stay out late after her evening shift. Laura, the oldest of two siblings, had always felt she had to be a role model for her brothers and sister; however, when she presented for treatment, she described herself as a failure.

Presenting Complaints Laura reported that while she tended to be slightly nervous student, she experienced overwhelming worry and anxiety during this particular semester. She was struggling to complete job applications and was falling behind on coursework and studying. Laura stated she believed she was "broken" and frequently experienced disturbed sleep, relentless worry, fatigue, and restlessness. Laura also indicated she engaged in heavy alcohol use most nights of the week, consuming 6–8 drinks per night after her work shift.

Assessment Laura was assessed using a semi-structured diagnostic interview. Laura endorsed symptoms consistent with full diagnostic criteria for GAD and severe AUD. Laura was also asked to complete questionnaires that would help measure her current GAD symptoms, quantify the frequency and quantity of her alcohol use, and the severity of her alcohol-related cravings/urges (see Fig. 8.2). Additionally, Laura also completed questionnaires to assess her levels of experiential avoidance, thought suppression, and the frequency of negative self-statements prior to the start of treatment (see Fig. 8.2).

Case Conceptualization Utilizing an ACT framework, it was hypothesized that the severity of Laura's GAD and AUD was greatly influenced by severe experiential avoidance. That is, Laura had utilized avoidance as a coping mechanism to manage her severe worry. When confronted with anxious thoughts about her life after college and her ability to pass her exams and complete challenging coursework, Laura attempted to cope by not thinking or talking about her stress and eventually by using alcohol to "numb" her distress. Laura found the alcohol use to be a useful short-term

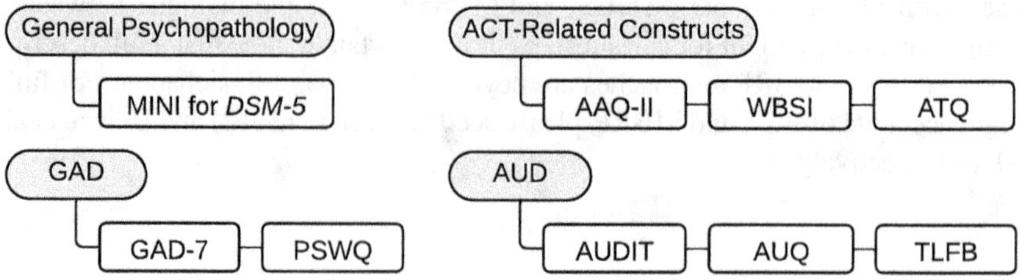

Fig. 8.2 GAD Generalized anxiety disorder, AUD Alcohol use disorder, MINI for *DSM-5* Mini-International Neuropsychiatric Interview for *DSM-5* (Sheehan et al., 1998), GAD-7 Generalized Anxiety Disorder-7 (Spitzer et al., 2006), PSWQ Penn State Worry Questionnaire (Meyer et al., 1990), AAQ-II Acceptance and Action Questionnaire-II (Bond et al., 2011), WBSI White Bear Suppression Inventory (Wegner & Zanakos, 1994), ATQ Automatic Thoughts Questionnaire (Hollon & Kendall, 1980), AUDIT Alcohol Use Disorders Identification Test (Babor et al., 1992), AUQ Alcohol Urge Questionnaire (Bohn et al., 1995), TLFB Timeline Follow Back Method for Alcohol (Sobell & Sobell, 1992)

strategy to provide immediate symptom relief, which solidified her avoidant coping in response to GAD symptoms. As a result, Laura's GAD symptoms were exacerbated, as the chronic avoidance interfered with cognitive-emotional processing, and this in turn intensified the alcohol use.

Introduction to Treatment and Psychoeducation ACT is a time-limited, transdiagnostic, CBT-oriented treatment that underscores the balance of accepting unwanted and distressing internal experiences with committed action towards living a life rich with value and meaning (Hayes et al., 2012). It addresses current psychological inflexibility by explicitly targeting six core interrelated processes, including (1) mindfulness, (2) nonjudgmental acceptance of psychological experiences, (3) cognitive defusion, (4) self-as-context, (5) identifying values, and (6) committed action in service of these values (Hayes et al., 2012). For Laura, the beginning of treatment included an introduction to the ACT framework, psychoeducation on the interaction between GAD and AUD, a comprehensive assessment of her values in life and goals in therapy, and an examination of potential internal and external barriers to achieving these goals. Here is an example of what value-setting/assessment looked like for Laura and her therapist:

Laura	Ever since the start of my senior year, I just don't feel like myself anymore.
Therapist	What is your mind telling you now? What thoughts come up as you say you 'don't feel like yourself.'
Laura	I feel lost and broken.
Therapist	Those are powerful thoughts, powerful words—"lost and broken." If you go with those thoughts and let them tell you what to do, where does that lead you?
Laura	It leads me to isolating and drinking most of the time.
Therapist	How does isolating and drinking impact the things in your life that are most important to you?
Laura	Well, I'm not as connected with my family and I'm not working on my education in order to get a better job.
Therapist	So, it sounds like thoughts like "lost and broken" are leading to some behaviors that are not aligned with your values. Would you be willing to try to let go of that judgment to see yourself in a different way?
Laura	I want to change, but I'm scared and anxious I'm going to keep falling behind.
Therapist	You want to change AND you're scared. Can you hold both of those at the same time? Can you feel scared and move toward family and friends or school?
Laura	I don't know. I want to be close to my family and friends again. I want to go to back to college. These things are important to me.
Therapist	Those are important values. Does doing what you have been doing help you get closer or further away from those values of reconnecting with loved ones and pursuing your education?

Laura	Further away. I'm just in a hole by myself right now.
Therapist	So, to reconnect, to go back to college, to live a valued life again, you would need to venture out of the hole, even if it's scary—even if it happens in small steps.

For patients with AUD/GAD in ACT and as demonstrated above, it may be especially important to differentiate between working towards a goal (e.g., something that can be crossed off a list) and identifying a value. For example, a patient may want to "stop drinking" (i.e., a goal); thus, it may be helpful to redirect the dialogue by inquiring about what that goal is in service of or what would be meaningful or important about working on that specific goal, while also keeping harm-reduction approaches in mind. It may be the case that this patient values independence, and their use of substances (i.e., a dependance) is diametrically opposed to this value. For a patient who is new to ACT or therapy generally, it is helpful to approach psychoeducation in a collaborative and individualized manner by using simplified terms (i.e., avoiding jargon), incorporating relevant ACT-related metaphor, visual aids, and handouts, and to encourage feedback and active learning via check-ins and probing for questions, comments, and/or confusion.

In-Session and Out-of-Session Exercises Identifying a patient's values is an essential step in ACT and serves as a compass for the patient and therapist as other core principles, such as defusion, acceptance, being present, and self-as-context, are targeted. Accordingly, connecting values to actions and acting in the direction of one's values (i.e., committed action) can serve to reinforce these behaviors and promote compliance in therapy. For Laura, exercises and metaphors that targeted experiential avoidance were prioritized given its role on both the intensity of her GAD symptoms as well as her alcohol use. Specifically, exercises that promoted cognitive defusion and self-as-context (e.g., the observing self), were utilized and are presented in the following dialogue:

Therapist	Have you ever noticed that distressing thoughts can appear out of nowhere and we buy right into them? What's a distressing or unhelpful thought you may be having right now?
Laura	I'm damaged.
Therapist	Ok, so let's take a step back from that thought and say to yourself "I'm noticing that I'm having a thought about being damaged."
Laura	I'm noticing that I'm having a thought about being damaged.
Therapist	Do you notice the difference?
Laura	Yes, it feels further away.
Therapist	Great. It's not about feeling better or getting rid of the thought, but to create separation between us and our unhelpful thoughts so we don't get stuck. We also start to view ourselves as a "self" separate from our thoughts.
Laura	Can you give me another example?

Therapist Absolutely, imagine you're in front of a river and you see leaves and sticks floating down stream. You don't have to dive into the river, you can simply watch from the riverbank. In other words, as thoughts float into view, you can notice them and see them pass by, but you don't have to be in the water with them.

Laura So, I can see and notice my thoughts and can also avoid getting soaked.

Therapist Exactly!

Laura was also asked to practice this exercise outside of session and to engage with it creatively by coming up with her own cognitive defusion metaphors, in order to increase her psychological flexibility and reduce experiential avoidance. She was also instructed to apply this exercise to her frequently and intrusive alcohol-related cravings. A helpful method to increase out-of-session practice for patients is to assess potential barriers that may interfere with completing the exercises and troubleshoot these barriers in advance.

Course of Treatment and Consolidation of Therapy In tandem with measurement-based assessment, a therapist using ACT should periodically check-in with their patient to evaluate their progress, identify barriers to change, garner feedback, and highlight mastered skills and area for growth. For Laura's treatment, these check-ins led to the discovery of additional problematic behaviors and cognitions that fueled the vicious cycle of GAD and AUD, such as a strong desire to change or control her negative internal experiences, which were further addressed via experiential exercises and incorporating acceptance linked to her own values. The skills and tools used and learned in ACT are flexible and process-based (e.g., cognitive defusion mindfulness, self-as context, mindfulness exercises, and committed action), which allows for their continued use as goals and values may change both in treatment and after treatment consolidation. Thus, considering that both the intensity of Laura's GAD and AUD symptoms reduced to within manageable limits and functionality substantially improved, she and her therapist made plans for consolidation of services. Moreover, follow-up appointments were scheduled to serve as "booster" sessions to revisit ACT skills and exercises.

MBRP for MDD with SUD

Brief Case Introduction and History Leo was a 36-year-old male, referred by his primary care physician to an outpatient psychological services clinic. Leo was a father to two children and had been married to his wife for 10 years. Leo was laid off from his job as a manager for a small logistics company due to a change of company ownership.

Presenting Complaints When he presented for his intake appointment, Leo reported that he had felt depressed and unmotivated since losing his job 6 months ago and reported increased alcohol and cannabis use. When probed, Leo stated that he felt as if he failed his family, despite their financial and emotional support during this time, and he was unsure how to cope with his distress in a healthy manner. He indicated that he had experienced brief episodes of depressed mood during difficult periods in adolescence, but reported this was "the worst and longest one" he had experienced. Accordingly, Leo was interested in starting psychotherapy.

Assessment Leo was assessed using a semi-structured diagnostic interview to rule-out other diagnoses and confirm presenting diagnoses. It was concluded that Leo met full diagnostic criteria for MDD comorbid with SUD (alcohol and cannabis). Leo was also instructed to complete questionnaires that would measure the severity of his depressive symptoms and the frequency and quantity of substance use (see Fig. 8.3). Moreover, Leo was instructed to complete MBRP-related questionnaires that would assess his levels of trait and state mindfulness and experiential avoidance prior to the start of treatment (see Fig. 8.3).

Case Conceptualization Considering an MBRP framework, it was hypothesized that Leo's MDD and SUD may be impacted by multiple factors, including a reduced ability to cope with negative emotional states (e.g., depressed mood) and internal experiences (e.g., cravings) that precipitate substance use, low acceptance and tolerance of these emotional states and internal experiences, and an increased sense of urgency to ease distress via substance use. Coupled with external factors, such as sudden job loss, Leo increased his substance use to cope with the uncertainty and feelings of failure. Therefore, Leo has difficulty managing and tolerating his current emotional state, which is exacerbated by his frequent use of alcohol and cannabis to temporarily alleviate discomfort.

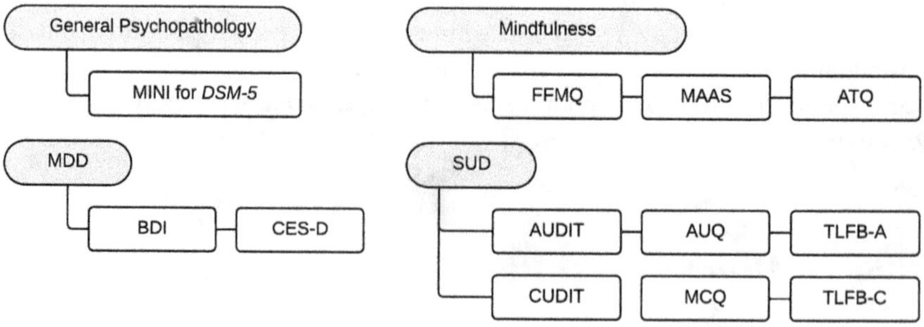

Fig. 8.3 MDD Major depressive disorder, SUD Substance use disorder, MINI for *DSM-5* Mini-International Neuropsychiatric Interview for *DSM-5* (Sheehan et al., 1998), BDI Beck Depression Inventory (Beck et al., 1961), CES-D Center for Epidemiological Studies-Depression Scale (Lewinsohn et al., 1997), FFMQ Five Facet Mindfulness Questionnaire (Baer et al., 2006), MAAS Mindful Attention Awareness Scale (Brown & Ryan, 2003), ATQ Automatic Thoughts Questionnaire (Hollon & Kendall, 1980), AUDIT Alcohol Use Disorders Identification Test (Babor et al., 1992), AUQ Alcohol Urge Questionnaire (Bohn et al., 1995), TLFB Timeline Follow Back Method for Alcohol (Sobell & Sobell, 1992), CUDIT Cannabis Use Disorders Identification Test (Adamson & Sellman, 2003), MCQ Marijuana Craving Questionnaire (Heishman et al., 2001), TLFB Timeline Follow Back Method for Cannabis (Sobell & Sobell, 1992)

Introduction to Treatment and Psychoeducation MBRP is a transdiagnostic, time-limited third wave intervention that explicitly integrates evidence-based practices found in MBI and Relapse Prevention to reduce the severity of substance use, comorbid mood symptoms, and likelihood of relapse (Bowen et al., 2014; Zemestani & Ottaviani, 2016). MBRP incorporates formal and informal techniques, such as sitting and body scan mediations, diaphragmatic breathing exercises, and mindfulness in daily activities, that promote increased exposure to and awareness of internal, private experiences that can trigger substance use. Additionally, comprehensive psychoeducation on the utility of mindfulness in daily life and in high-risk situations and the role of automatic thinking (i.e., auto-pilot) on relapse, a relapse chain analysis, and collaborative assessment of a patient's current triggers for SUD and cravings are all provided throughout the course of treatment. For Leo, an important initial step was helping him not only be aware of his substance use triggers, but also understand how they be related to is depressive symptoms. Here is an example of what this step looked like for Leo and his therapist:

Therapist	So, you said there was time in the past week when you ended up drinking and smoking much more than you usually do. What happened before that?
Leo	My wife had asked me how my job applications have been going. I've been really trying to submit them, but I also feel dread and stressed when I do it, so I don't do it as much as I should.
Therapist	And when she asked you, what emotions did you feel?
Leo	I felt guilty and ashamed because I hadn't worked on any.
Therapist	Did you feel any physical sensations too?
Leo	I think I remember hearing my heartbeat in my ears. It was beating so fast.
Therapist	And what thoughts popped in your head during that moment?
Leo	I thought to myself, 'I can't do this' and 'I'm too pathetic.'
Therapist	Then what happened? What did you do?
Leo	I stormed off and went on a bender. I feel anxious just thinking about it right now.
Therapist	Let's sit with that anxiety together for a moment. Would you be willing to sit with that feeling and breathe through it with me?

It is important to explicate a chain of events with the patient in order to identify and promote awareness of triggers, particularly when they occur in high-risk situations or coincide with negative emotional states and thoughts. Indeed, for the therapist and Leo, understanding the factors that increase his feelings of dread and stress and the frequency of his problematic thoughts (i.e., "I can't do this"; "I'm too pathetic") was the first step in improving Leo's ability to be nonjudgment and nonreactive to this internal, private experiences.

In-Session and Out-of-Session Exercises MBRP incorporates numerous formal and informal exercises to be used for in-session and out-of-session practice. For a patient who is new to mindfulness, it may be helpful to provide additional psychoeducation using simplified definitions of mindfulness and visually based metaphors. For example, the introduction of "urge (wave) surging" (i.e., visualizing oneself surfing on a wave that represents their urge to use and feeling it rise to its peak and then slowly subside on its own) may serve as a powerful metaphor and visualization exercise to facilitate the management of urges. This can be coupled with the introduction of being fully aware of the present urge, acknowledging how they may be feeling in that particular moment, practicing nonjudgement, and noticing the ebb and flow of the urge. Exercises that help patients further engage in mindfulness and reduce psychological and physiological tension, such as "box breathing" may be incorporated as well. Here is an example of what this looked like for Leo and his therapist:

Therapist	I'd like to introduce you to a breathing technique called "box breathing" that might help you be more aware of the present moment and improve your ability to cope with stress. This type of exercise can also make you more aware of your cravings and urges to use alcohol or cannabis and help you better manage them in the moment. Would you like to give it a try?
Leo	Sure, I'd be willing to try. What is box breathing?
Therapist	Box breathing is a simple mindfulness-based technique that involves consciously and purposefully regulating your breath to calm your thoughts and body. Let's try it together. First, find a comfortable sitting position. Now, inhale deeply through your nose to a count of four and then hold your breath for another count of four [*Therapist demonstrates, and Leo follows*].
Therapist	Great job. Now, exhale slowly and completely through your mouth for another count of four *[Therapist demonstrates, and Leo follows]*.
Therapist	The last step is to complete the box by holding your breath again for a count of four *[Therapist demonstrates, and Leo follows]*.
Therapist	Way to stick with it! We just completed one cycle of box breathing. You can repeat this as many times as you like until you feel more grounded and relaxed. It's an excellent, portable tool that you can use when you're feeling overwhelmed or have a strong urge/craving to use.

Leo was also instructed to practice this exercise outside of session and to engage with it even when he was not feeling overwhelmed or craving alcohol or cannabis in order to further master the skill. While many patients are readily able to complete this exercise, it is important to assess potential barriers that may interfere with completing it, such as medical contraindications (e.g., breathing difficulty) and troubleshoot these barriers in advance.

Course of Treatment and Consolidation of Therapy MBRP is administered using a manualized, session-by-session protocol and therefore, the course of treatment can be highly structured and time-limited. The central goal is twofold: (1) improve the patient's ability to be aware of their triggers and cravings and how they are both impacted by their mood, (2) develop a mastery of mindfulness-based exercises that promote (a) nonjudgmental, purposeful awareness of the present moment and (b) nonreactivity to ongoing stressors, urges/cravings, and negative, unhelpful thoughts. For Leo, once this central goal was achieved, the course of treatment pivoted to improving positive maintenance factors, including addressing self-care, -efficacy, and -compassion as well as enhancing social support. These factors helped Leo take advantage of the resources at his disposable, such as his close-knit family, and use them as an ongoing source of support during his treatment and recovery. Moreover, follow-up appointments were scheduled to serve as "booster" sessions to revisit MBRP skills and exercises.

Future Directions

There is strong theoretical support for the use of third wave interventions for the treatment of co-occurring emotional disorders and SUD. Third wave treatments share many notable strengths that go beyond those of found in traditional CBT (Hayes et al., 2006), particularly when treating complex symptom presentations that are common for individuals with substance-related comorbidities. Indeed, these interventions are highly adaptable due to their context- and process-based frameworks and integration of transdiagnostic treatment targets, such acceptance, mindfulness, metacognitions, behavioral values-based action, and psychological flexibility, which can be uniquely useful to tackling the myriad of symptoms associated with comorbid SUD/emotional disorders (Hayes, 2004; Hayes & Hofmann, 2017).

However, empirical support is limited and varies across disorders and treatment modalities. For instance, there is a growing body of literature supporting the use of third wave approaches for MDD/SUD (Roos et al., 2020; Vujanovic et al., 2017) and PTSD/SUD (Vujanovic & Back, 2019). Conversely, intervention development research examining the efficacy of ACT, MBI, DBT, and metacognitive therapy in the treatment of various psychiatric conditions, such as anxiety-related disorders, comorbid with SUD is wanting. Moreover, integrative third wave therapies are lacking for SUD/emotional disorder comorbidities, which is unfortunate given the challenge faced by clinicians on how to prioritize and integrate various treatment components from evidence-based practices, especially for SUD (Back et al., 2009).

The developing use and applicability of third wave interventions for various psychiatric conditions, including emotional disorders comorbid with SUD, has the potential to advance current approaches to mental health services for this difficult-to-treat population and address pertinent barriers to care. And considering the shared cognitive-affective factors that underlie and maintain these conditions, the integration of empirically supported transdiagnostic elements, such as values-based behavioral actions, distress tolerance skills, and mindfulness, hold great clinical significance and promise. Thus, there is a critical need for future research to not only examine the efficacy of existing third wave approaches among populations with comorbid conditions, but also expand towards further developing integrative, third wave interventions.

References

Adamson, S. J., & Sellman, J. D. (2003). A prototype screening instrument for cannabis use disorder: The Cannabis Use Disorders Identification Test (CUDIT) in an alcohol-dependent clinical sample. *Drug and Alcohol Review, 22*(3), 309–315. https://doi.org/10.1080/0959523031000154454

Afshari, B., & Hasani, J. (2020). Study of dialectical behavior therapy versus cognitive behavior therapy on emotion regulation and mindfulness in patients with generalized anxiety disorder. *Journal of Contemporary Psychotherapy, 50*(4), 305–312. https://doi.org/10.1007/s10879-020-09461-9

Aldridge, R. W., Story, A., Hwang, S. W., Nordentoft, M., Luchenski, S. A., Hartwell, G., Tweed, E. J., Lewer, D., Vittal Katikireddi, S., & Hayward, A. C. (2018). Morbidity and mortality in homeless individuals, prisoners, sex workers, and individuals with substance use disorders in high-income countries: A systematic review and meta-analysis. *Lancet, 391*(10117), 241–250. https://doi.org/10.1016/S0140-6736(17)31869-X

American Psychiatric Association. (2013). *Diagnostic and statistical manual of mental disorders* (5th ed.). Author.

Babor, T. F., De La Fuente, J., Saunders, J., & Grant, M. (1992). *AUDIT: The alcohol use disorders identification test: Guidelines for use in primary health care*. World Health Organization.

Back, S. E., Waldrop, A. E., & Brady, K. T. (2009). Treatment challenges associated with comorbid substance use and posttraumatic stress disorder: Clinicians' perspectives. *American Journal on Addictions, 18*(1), 15–20. https://doi.org/10.1080/10550490802545141

Baer, R. A., & Krietemeyer, J. (2006). Overview of mindfulness- and acceptance-based treatment approaches. In *Mindfulness-based treatment approaches: Clinician's guide to evidence base and applications* (pp. 3–27). Elsevier Academic Press. https://doi.org/10.1016/B978-012088519-0/50002-2

Baer, R. A., Smith, G. T., Hopkins, J., Krietemeyer, J., & Toney, L. (2006). Using self-report assessment methods to explore facets of mindfulness. *Assessment, 13*(1), 27–45. https://doi.org/10.1177/1073191105283504

Bajaj, B., Robins, R. W., & Pande, N. (2016). Mediating role of self-esteem on the relationship between mindfulness, anxiety, and depression. *Personality and Individual Differences, 96*, 127–131. https://doi.org/10.1016/j.paid.2016.02.085

Baker, T. B., Piper, M. E., McCarthy, D. E., Majeskie, M. R., & Fiore, M. C. (2004). Addiction motivation reformulated: An affective processing model of negative reinforcement. *Psychological Review, 111*(1), 33–51. https://doi.org/10.1037/0033-295x.111.1.33

Barlow, D. H., Farchione, T. J., Fairholme, C. P., Ellard, K. K., Boisseau, C. L., Allen, L. B., & Ehrenreich-May, J. (2011). *Unified protocol for transdiagnostic treatment of emotional disorders: Therapist guide*. Oxford University Press.

Beck, A. T., Ward, C. H., Mendelson, M., Mock, J., & Erbaugh, J. (1961). An inventory for measuring depression. *Archives of General Psychiatry, 4*, 561–571.

Benfer, N., Spitzer, E. G., & Bardeen, J. R. (2021). Efficacy of third wave cognitive behavioral therapies in the treatment of posttraumatic stress: A meta-analytic study. *Journal of Anxiety Disorders, 78*, 102360. https://doi.org/10.1016/j.janxdis.2021.102360

Berghoff, C. R., & Tull, M. T. (2019). Third-wave behavioral therapies for the co-occurrence of PTSD and substance use disorders. In A. A. Vujanovic & S. E. Back (Eds.), *Posttraumatic stress and substance use disorders: A comprehensive clinical handbook*. Routledge. https://doi.org/10.4324/9781315442648

Blanco, C., Xu, Y., Brady, K., Perez-Fuentes, G., Okuda, M., & Wang, S. (2013). Comorbidity of posttraumatic stress disorder with alcohol dependence among US adults: Results from national epidemiological survey on alcohol and related conditions. *Drug and Alcohol Dependence, 132*(3), 630–638. https://doi.org/10.1016/j.drugalcdep.2013.04.016

Blanco, C., Iza, M., Rodriguez-Fernandez, J. M., Baca-Garcia, E., Wang, S., & Olfson, M. (2015). Probability and predictors of treatment-seeking for substance use disorders in the U.S. *Drug and Alcohol Dependence, 149*, 136–144. https://doi.org/10.1016/j.drugalcdep.2015.01.031

Bohn, M. J., Krahn, D. D., & Staehler, B. A. (1995). Development and initial validation of a measure of drinking urges in abstinent alcoholics. *Alcoholism, Clinical and Experimental Research, 19*(3), 600–606. https://doi.org/10.1111/j.1530-0277.1995.tb01554.x

Bond, F. W., Hayes, S. C., Baer, R. A., Carpenter, K. M., Guenole, N., Orcutt, H. K., Waltz, T., & Zettle, R. D. (2011). Preliminary psychometric properties of the acceptance and action questionnaire-II: A revised measure of psychological inflexibility and experiential avoidance. *Behavior Therapy, 42*(4), 676–688. https://doi.org/10.1016/j.beth.2011.03.007

Bonumwezi, J. L., Tramutola, D., Lawrence, J., Kobezak, H. M., & Lowe, S. R. (2022). Posttraumatic stress disorder symptoms, work-related trauma exposure, and substance use in first responders. *Drug and Alcohol Dependence, 237*, 109439. https://doi.org/10.1016/j.drugalcdep.2022.109439

Bowen, S., Witkiewitz, K., Clifasefi, S. L., Grow, J., Chawla, N., Hsu, S. H., Carroll, H. A., Harrop, E., Collins, S. E., Lustyk, M. K., & Larimer, M. E. (2014). Relative efficacy of mindfulness-based relapse prevention, standard relapse prevention, and treatment as usual for substance use disorders: A randomized clinical trial. *JAMA Psychiatry, 71*(5), 547–556. https://doi.org/10.1001/jamapsychiatry.2013.4546

Bowen, S., Chawla, N., Grow, J., & Marlatt, A. (2020). *Mindfulness-based relapse prevention for addictive behaviors* (2nd ed.). Guilford Press.

Brown, K. W., & Ryan, R. M. (2003). The benefits of being present: Mindfulness and its role in psychological well-being. *Journal of Personality and Social Psychology, 84*(4), 822–848. https://doi.org/10.1037/0022-3514.84.4.822

Corrigan, P. W., & Rao, D. (2012). On the self-stigma of mental illness: Stages, disclosure, and strategies for change. *Canadian Journal of Psychiatry, 57*(8), 464–469. https://doi.org/10.1177/070674371205700804

Fortuna, L. R., & Vallejo, Z. (2015). Treating co-occurring adolescent PTSD and addiction: Mindfulness-based cognitive therapy for adolescents with trauma and substance-abuse disorders. In *Treating co-occurring adolescent PTSD and addiction: Mindfulness-based cognitive therapy for adolescents with trauma and substance-abuse disorders*. New Harbinger Publications.

Fortuna, L. R., Porche, M. V., & Padilla, A. (2018). A treatment development study of a cognitive and mindfulness-based therapy for adolescents with co-occurring post-traumatic stress and substance use disorder. *Psychology and Psychotherapy, 91*(1), 42–62. https://doi.org/10.1111/papt.12143

Glasner-Edwards, S., Mooney, L. J., Ang, A., Garneau, H. C., Hartwell, E., Brecht, M. L., & Rawson, R. A. (2017). Mindfulness based relapse prevention for stimulant dependent adults: A pilot randomized clinical trial. *Mindfulness (N Y), 8*(1), 126–135. https://doi.org/10.1007/s12671-016-0586-9

Grant, B. F., Stinson, F. S., Dawson, D. A., Chou, S. P., Dufour, M. C., Compton, W., Pickering, R. P., & Kaplan, K. (2004). Prevalence and co-occurrence of substance use disorders and independent mood and anxiety disorders: Results from the national epidemiologic survey on alcohol and related conditions. *Archives of General Psychiatry, 61*(8), 807–816. https://doi.org/10.1001/archpsyc.61.8.807

Grant, B. F., Goldstein, R. B., Saha, T. D., Chou, S. P., Jung, J., Zhang, H., Pickering, R. P., Ruan, W. J., Smith, S. M., Huang, B., & Hasin, D. S. (2015). Epidemiology of DSM-5 alcohol use disorder: Results from the national epidemiologic survey on alcohol and related conditions III. *JAMA Psychiatry, 72*(8), 757–766. https://doi.org/10.1001/jamapsychiatry.2015.0584

Grant, B. F., Saha, T. D., Ruan, W. J., Goldstein, R. B., Chou, S. P., Jung, J., Zhang, H., Smith, S. M., Pickering, R. P., Huang, B., & Hasin, D. S. (2016). Epidemiology of DSM-5 drug use disorder: Results from the national epidemiologic survey on alcohol and related conditions-III. *JAMA Psychiatry, 73*(1), 39–47. https://doi.org/10.1001/jamapsychiatry.2015.2132

Gratz, K. L., & Roemer, L. (2004). Multidimensional assessment of emotion regulation and dysregulation: Development, factor structure, and initial validation of the difficulties in emotion regulation scale. *Journal of Psychopathology and Behavioral Assessment, 26*, 41–54. https://doi.org/10.1007/s10862-008-9102-4

Haktanir, A., & Callender, K. A. (2020). Meta-analysis of dialectical behavior therapy (DBT) for treating substance use. *College of Education Faculty Research and Publications, 4*, 74–87. https://epublications.marquette.edu/edu_fac/598
Han, B., Compton, W. M., Blanco, C., & Colpe, L. J. (2017). Prevalence, treatment, and unmet treatment needs of US adults with mental health and substance use disorders. *Health Affairs (Millwood), 36*(10), 1739–1747. https://doi.org/10.1377/hlthaff.2017.0584
Harley, R., Sprich, S., Safren, S., Jacobo, M., & Fava, M. (2008). Adaptation of dialectical behavior therapy skills training group for treatment-resistant depression. *The Journal of Nervous and Mental Disease, 196*(2), 136–143. https://doi.org/10.1097/NMD.0b013e318162aa3f
Hawn, S. E., Cusack, S. E., & Amstadter, A. B. (2020). A systematic review of the self-medication hypothesis in the context of posttraumatic stress disorder and comorbid problematic alcohol use. *Journal of Traumatic Stress*. https://doi.org/10.1002/jts.22521
Hayes, S. C. (2004). Acceptance and commitment therapy, relational frame theory, and the third wave of behavioral and cognitive therapies. *Behavior Therapy, 35*(4), 639–665. https://doi.org/10.1016/S0005-7894(04)80013-3
Hayes, S. C., & Hofmann, S. G. (2017). The third wave of cognitive behavioral therapy and the rise of process-based care. *World Psychiatry, 16*(3), 245–246. https://doi.org/10.1002/wps.20442
Hayes, S. C., Luoma, J. B., Bond, F. W., Masuda, A., & Lillis, J. (2006). Acceptance and commitment therapy: Model, processes and outcomes. *Behaviour Research and Therapy, 44*(1), 1–25. https://doi.org/10.1016/j.brat.2005.06.006
Hayes, S. C., Strosahl, K. D., & Wilson, K. G. (2012). *Acceptance and commitment therapy: The process and practice of mindful change* (2nd ed.). Guilford Press.
Heishman, S. J., Singleton, E. G., & Liguori, A. (2001). Marijuana craving questionnaire: Development and initial validation of a self-report instrument. *Addiction, 96*(7), 1023–1034. https://doi.org/10.1046/j.1360-0443.2001.967102312.x
Hermann, B. A., Meyer, E. C., Schnurr, P. P., Batten, S. V., & Walser, R. D. (2016). Acceptance and commitment therapy for co-occurring PTSD and substance use: A manual development study. *Journal of Contextual Behavioral Science, 5*(4), 225–234. https://doi.org/10.1016/j.jcbs.2016.07.001
Hollon, S. D., & Kendall, P. C. (1980). Cognitive self-statements in depression: Development of an automatic thoughts questionnaire. *Cognitive Therapy and Research, 4*(4), 383–395.
Jones, H. A., Heffner, J. L., Mercer, L., Wyszynski, C. M., Vilardaga, R., & Bricker, J. B. (2015). Web-based acceptance and commitment therapy smoking cessation treatment for smokers with depressive symptoms. *Journal of Dual Diagnosis, 11*(1), 56–62. https://doi.org/10.1080/15504263.2014.992588
Kelly, T. M., & Daley, D. C. (2013). Integrated treatment of substance use and psychiatric disorders. *Social Work in Public Health, 28*(3–4), 388–406. https://doi.org/10.1080/19371918.2013.774673
Khantzian, E. J. (1997). The self-medication hypothesis of substance use disorders: A reconsideration and recent applications. *Harvard Review of Psychiatry, 4*(5), 231–244. https://doi.org/10.3109/10673229709030550
Lanza, P. V., García, P. F., Lamelas, F. R., & González-Menéndez, A. (2014). Acceptance and commitment therapy versus cognitive behavioral therapy in the treatment of substance use disorder with incarcerated women. *Journal of Clinical Psychology, 70*(7), 644–657. https://doi.org/10.1002/jclp.22060
Lewinsohn, P. M., Seeley, J. R., Roberts, R. E., & Allen, N. B. (1997). Center for Epidemiological Studies-Depression Scale (CES-D) as a screening instrument for depression among community-residing older adults. *Psychology and Aging, 12*, 277–287.
Leyro, T. M., Zvolensky, M. J., & Bernstein, A. (2010). Distress tolerance and psychopathological symptoms and disorders: A review of the empirical literature among adults. *Psychological Bulletin, 136*(4), 576–600. https://doi.org/10.1037/a0019712
Linehan, M. M. (1993). *Cognitive-behavioral treatment of borderline personality disorder*. Guilford Press.

Link, B. G., Struening, E. L., Neese-Todd, S., Asmussen, S., & Phelan, J. C. (2002). On describing and seeking to change the experience of stigma. *Psychiatric Rehabilitation Skills, 6*(2), 201–231. https://doi.org/10.1080/10973430208408433

Lo, T. W., Yeung, J. W. K., & Tam, C. H. L. (2020). Substance abuse and public health: A multilevel perspective and multiple responses. *International Journal of Environmental Research and Public Health, 17*(7). https://doi.org/10.3390/ijerph17072610

Lorenzo-Luaces, L., Lemmens, L. H. J. M., Keefe, J. R., Cuijpers, P., & Bockting, C. L. H. (2021). The efficacy of cognitive behavioral therapy for emotional disorders. In A. Wenzel (Ed.), *Handbook of cognitive behavioral therapy: Overview and approaches* (pp. 51–89). American Psychological Association. https://doi.org/10.1037/0000218-003

Luoma, J. B., Kohlenberg, B. S., Hayes, S. C., Bunting, K., & Rye, A. K. (2008). Reducing self-stigma in substance abuse through acceptance and commitment therapy: Model, manual development, and pilot outcomes. *Addiction Research and Theory, 16*(2), 149–165. https://doi.org/10.1080/16066350701850295

Mack, K. A., Jones, C. M., & Ballesteros, M. F. (2017). Illicit drug use, illicit drug use disorders, and drug overdose deaths in metropolitan and nonmetropolitan areas-United States. *Morbidity and Moratlity Weekly Report - Centers for Disease Control and Prevention, Issue*. https://doi.org/10.15585/mmwr.ss6619a1

McHugh, R. K., Hearon, B. A., & Otto, M. W. (2010). Cognitive behavioral therapy for substance use disorders. *The Psychiatric Clinics of North America, 33*(3), 511–525. https://doi.org/10.1016/j.psc.2010.04.012

Meyer, T. J., Miller, M. L., Metzger, R. L., & Borkovec, T. D. (1990). Development and validation of the penn state worry questionnaire. *Behavior Research and Therapy, 28*, 487–495.

Minkoff, K. (2001). Developing standards of care for individuals with co-occurring psychiatric and substance use disorders. *Psychiatric Services, 52*(5), 597–599. https://doi.org/10.1176/appi.ps.52.5.597

NIDA. (2013). *Drug facts: National wide trends*. https://nida.nih.gov/sites/default/files/drugfacts_nationtrends_6_15.pdf

NIDA. (2022, 12/15/2022). *Most reported substance use among adolescents held steady in 2022*. https://nida.nih.gov/news-events/news-releases/2022/12/most-reported-substance-use-among-adolescents-held-steady-in-2022

Petersen, C. L., & Zettle, R. D. (2009). Treating inpatients with comorbid depression and alcohol use disorders: A comparison of acceptance and commitment therapy versus treatment as usual. *The Psychological Record, 59*, 521–536.

Pietrzak, R. H., Goldstein, R. B., Southwick, S. M., & Grant, B. F. (2011). Prevalence and Axis I comorbidity of full and partial posttraumatic stress disorder in the United States: Results from Wave 2 of the National Epidemiologic Survey on Alcohol and Related Conditions. *Journal of Anxiety Disorders, 25*(3), 456–465. https://doi.org/10.1016/j.janxdis.2010.11.010

Roberts, A., Rogers, J., Mason, R., Siriwardena, A. N., Hogue, T., Whitley, G. A., & Law, G. R. (2021). Alcohol and other substance use during the COVID-19 pandemic: A systematic review. *Drug and Alcohol Dependence, 229*(Pt A), 109150. https://doi.org/10.1016/j.drugalcdep.2021.109150

Roos, C., Bowen, S., & Witkiewitz, K. (2020). Approach coping and substance use outcomes following mindfulness-based relapse prevention among individuals with negative affect symptomatology. *Mindfulness (N Y), 11*(10), 2397–2410. https://doi.org/10.1007/s12671-020-01456-w

SAMHSA. (2021). *National Survey on Drug Use and Health (NSDUH)*. https://www.samhsa.gov/data/release/2021-national-survey-drug-use-and-health-nsduh-releases

Sheehan, D. V., Lecrubier, Y., Sheehan, K. H., Amorim, P., Janavs, J., Weiller, E., Hergueta, T., Baker, R., & Dunbar, G. C. (1998). The mini-international neuropsychiatric interview (M.I.N.I.): The development and validation of a structured diagnostic psychiatric interview for DSM-IV and ICD-10. *Journal of Clinical Psychiatry, 59*(Suppl 20), 22–33;quiz 34-57.

Smith, N. D. L., & Cottler, L. B. (2018). The epidemiology of post-traumatic stress disorder and alcohol use disorder. *Alcohol Research: Current Reviews, 39*(2), 113–120. https://pubmed.ncbi.nlm.nih.gov/31198651, https://www.ncbi.nlm.nih.gov/pmc/articles/PMC6561398/

Sobell, L. C., & Sobell, M. B. (1992). Timeline follow-back: A technique for assessing self-reported alcohol consumption. In *Measuring alcohol consumption: Psychosocial and biochemical methods* (pp. 41–72). Humana Press. https://doi.org/10.1007/978-1-4612-0357-5_3

Spitzer, R. L., Kroenke, K., Williams, J. B., & Löwe, B. (2006). A brief measure for assessing generalized anxiety disorder: The GAD-7. *Archives of Internal Medicine, 166*(10), 1092–1097. https://doi.org/10.1001/archinte.166.10.1092

Stohler, R., & Rössler, W. (2005). *Forward*. Karger Medical and Scientific Publishers.

Thekiso, T. B., Murphy, P., Milnes, J., Lambe, K., Curtin, A., & Farren, C. K. (2015). Acceptance and commitment therapy in the treatment of alcohol use disorder and comorbid affective disorder: A pilot matched control trial. *Behavior Therapy, 46*(6), 717–728. https://doi.org/10.1016/j.beth.2015.05.005

Valenstein-Mah, H., Simpson, T. L., Bowen, S., Enkema, M. C., Bird, E. R., Cho, H. I., & Larimer, M. E. (2019). Feasibility pilot of a brief mindfulness intervention for college students with posttraumatic stress symptoms and problem drinking. *Mindfulness (N Y), 10*(7), 1255–1268.

Vujanovic, A. A., & Back, S. E. (2019). *Posttraumatic stress and substance use disorders: A comprehensive clinical handbook* (1st ed.). Routledge. https://doi.org/10.4324/9781315442648

Vujanovic, A. A., Meyer, T. D., Heads, A. M., Stotts, A. L., Villarreal, Y. R., & Schmitz, J. M. (2017). Cognitive-behavioral therapies for depression and substance use disorders: An overview of traditional, third-wave, and transdiagnostic approaches. *The American Journal of Drug and Alcohol Abuse, 43*(4), 402–415. https://doi.org/10.1080/00952990.2016.1199697

Vujanovic, A. A., Smith, L. J., Green, C., Lane, S. D., & Schmitz, J. M. (2020). Mindfulness as a predictor of cognitive-behavioral therapy outcomes in inner-city adults with posttraumatic stress and substance dependence. *Addictive Behaviors, 104*, 106283. https://doi.org/10.1016/j.addbeh.2019.106283

Wegner, D. M., & Zanakos, S. (1994). Chronic thought suppression. *Journal of Personality, 62*, 615–640.

Wells, A. (2011). *Metacognitive therapy for anxiety and depression*. Guilford Press.

Witkiewitz, K., Pfund, R. A., & Tucker, J. A. (2022). Mechanisms of behavior change in substance use disorder with and without formal treatment. *Annual Review of Clinical Psychology, 18*, 497–525. https://doi.org/10.1146/annurev-clinpsy-072720-014802

Zemestani, M., & Ottaviani, C. (2016). Effectiveness of mindfulness-based relapse prevention for co-occurring substance use and depression disorders. *Mindfulness (N Y), 7*(6), 1347–1355. https://doi.org/10.1007/s12671-016-0576-y

Zgierska, A., Rabago, D., Chawla, N., Kushner, K., Koehler, R., & Marlatt, A. (2009). Mindfulness meditation for substance use disorders: A systematic review. *Substance Abuse, 30*(4), 266–294. https://doi.org/10.1080/08897070903250019

Chapter 9
Cognitive-Behavioral Therapy for Co-occurring Anxiety and Opioid Use Disorder in People with Chronic Pain

R. Kathryn McHugh, Allen J. Bailey, and Miryam Yusufov

Chronic pain affects an estimated one in five adults in the United States and approximately 7% of adults experience "high-impact" chronic pain, characterized by significant functional impact (Rikard et al., 2023). Chronic pain is even more common in certain groups, including people with opioid use disorder (OUD) and people with anxiety disorders (Demyttenaere et al., 2007; Hser et al., 2017). Accordingly, chronic pain is often a consideration in the treatment of co-occurring anxiety disorders and OUD. This chapter will provide an overview of this co-occurrence and considerations in the application of cognitive-behavioral therapy (CBT) to the treatment of these conditions.

Epidemiology and Pathways to Co-occurrence

Both chronic pain and anxiety disorders are highly prevalent in people with OUD. An estimated 30% to more than 60% of people with OUD have chronic pain (Blanco et al., 2016; Hser et al., 2017) and over 60% have a lifetime anxiety disorder (Conway et al., 2006). Although reliable estimates of the prevalence of these three conditions together are not available, these data suggest that both anxiety disorders

R. K. McHugh (✉)
Division of Alcohol, Drugs and Addiction, McLean Hospital, Belmont, MA, USA
e-mail: kmchugh@mclean.harvard.edu

A. J. Bailey
Department of Psychiatry, Harvard Medical School, Belmont, MA, USA

M. Yusufov
Department of Psychosocial Oncology and Palliative Care, Dana-Farber Cancer Institute, Boston, MA, USA

K. Wolitzky-Taylor (ed.), *Treating Comorbid Substance Use and Emotional Disorders*, CBT: Science Into Practice, https://doi.org/10.1007/978-3-031-62971-6_9

and chronic pain are more common than not in people with OUD, and likely often co-occur.

The co-occurrence among anxiety, OUD, and chronic pain involves a multi-directional interplay of risk factors and symptoms. The likelihood of medical exposure to opioids via prescription is elevated in both people with chronic pain and people with psychiatric disorders. For example, people with psychiatric disorders are more than twice as likely to be prescribed opioids than those without psychiatric disorders (Davis et al., 2017; Sullivan et al., 2006). Once exposed to opioids (medicinally or otherwise), psychiatric disorders are associated with an increased likelihood of opioid misuse and OUD (Cochran et al., 2014; Hassan et al., 2017). Among people with chronic pain, psychiatric symptoms in general—and anxiety symptoms in particular—appear to increase risk for the misuse of opioid medications (Martel et al., 2020; McHugh et al., 2019; Rogers et al., 2019). Opioid misuse is also prospectively associated with the onset of anxiety disorders, suggesting that this is not a unidirectional association (Katz et al., 2013; Martins et al., 2012).

This co-occurrence may be attributable, at least in part, to shared risk factors for developing these disorders, such as exposure to childhood trauma (Taghian et al., 2021). At a functional level, opioids have stress relieving properties and thus are often used to relieve negative affective states, as well as to provide analgesia (Han et al., 2017; Weiss et al., 2014). Consistent with this, opioid craving appears to mediate the association between negative affective states and opioid misuse (Martel et al., 2014). In other words, negative affect may increase the motivational state for opioids to achieve relief of both anxiety and pain, thereby leading to potential misuse. Furthermore, OUD is associated with an array of consequences, many of which can increase risk for anxiety disorder onset (e.g., exposure to chronic stress, heightened stress reactivity) and potential for the development of pain-related conditions (e.g., opioid hyperalgesia, risk for injury).

Once these three conditions co-occur, symptom interplay may serve to further maintain each condition. For example, opioids are highly negatively reinforcing in the context of pain and anxiety, maintaining continued use to mitigate these states. Anxious avoidance and anxiety-related cognitive biases (e.g., catastrophizing) exacerbate pain, and fear of pain may worsen anxiety symptoms. Withdrawal from opioids also can result in exacerbations of pain and anxiety, further fueling this cycle (Alford et al., 2006). This complex entanglement of risk factors and symptom interplay introduces a clinical picture that benefits from integrating treatment elements to address all disorders concurrently.

Treatment Efficacy

At this time, there are no evidence-based behavioral or pharmacological treatment protocols specifically design to address anxiety and OUD in people with chronic pain; however, some evidence for outcomes in this population can be gleaned from secondary analyses of OUD treatment trials. The current gold standard for the treatment of OUD is medication—consisting of either full or partial agonists (methadone, buprenorphine) or antagonists (naltrexone) of the mu opioid receptor (Committee on Medication-Assisted Treatment for Opioid Use Disorder, 2019). Medication for OUD (MOUD) is associated with large reductions in opioid use, reduction of overdose risk and improvement in functioning, and it has been shown to be similarly effective for the treatment of OUD in people with and without chronic pain (Dreifuss et al., 2013; Ilgen et al., 2006). In other words, a lack of access to treatment for chronic pain should not preclude or delay the receipt of MOUD. Nonetheless, MOUD alone is unlikely to adequately address pain or anxiety. Although opioid agonist (and partial agonist) maintenance therapies have analgesic effects, the pain-relieving properties of these medications are not prolonged and thus additional interventions are generally needed to manage pain in this population (Alford et al., 2006). Similarly, there is some evidence that people with psychiatric conditions (such as posttraumatic stress disorder) benefit from the addition of behavioral therapy to MOUD, whereas MOUD alone may be sufficient for many people without these conditions (McHugh et al., 2021).

The role of medication treatment for anxiety and pain, however, is more complex. Medications with indication for the treatment of anxiety (e.g., benzodiazepines) and treatment of pain (e.g., opioids, muscle relaxants) may be contraindicated in many people with OUD, due to risks of medication interaction, overdose or misuse. For example, the risks and benefits of the use of benzodiazepines in people with OUD continue to be debated, and the paucity of research in this area precludes evidence-based clinical guidance on prescribing practices (DuPont, 2017; Park, 2017; Saitz, 2017). These complexities with respect to medication highlight the critical importance of behavioral therapies in working with this population.

Cognitive-behavioral approaches may be particularly well-suited for treating co-occurring anxiety and OUD in people with chronic pain, given evidence for their efficacy for substance use disorders (Magill et al., 2019), anxiety disorders (Hofmann & Smits, 2008) and chronic pain, individually (Dixon et al., 2007; Hoffman et al., 2007). Existing CBT protocols for these conditions share many features and can target maintaining factors, such as cognitive distortions (catastrophizing), anxiety sensitivity, anhedonia, and maladaptive coping that are common to OUD, anxiety disorders, and chronic pain.

Taken together, the co-occurrence of anxiety and OUD in people with chronic pain is common and introduces significant clinical complexity. Common vulnerability and maintaining mechanisms—and potential limitations of medications—make CBT a highly promising treatment for this co-occurrence. Of note, there is not a current evidence base or specific treatment that is targeted to these three conditions. Accordingly, in this chapter, we seek to leverage existing knowledge in the treatment of each of these conditions individually to provide guidance on the application of treatment. Nonetheless, further research will be essential to understanding the optimal treatment for this population.

Implementing CBT for Co-occurring Anxiety and OUD in People with Chronic Pain

In this section, we provide a description of principles for integrating CBT for anxiety and OUD in people with chronic pain. It is important to note that for the treatment of these co-occurring and sometimes chronic conditions, CBT is often only one component of the overall treatment plan. The management of chronic pain and OUD often requires an interdisciplinary treatment team, including medication management for OUD as well as multimodal management of chronic pain from primary care or relevant subspeciality care (e.g., pain medicine). Communication with other members of the treatment team can offer opportunity to assess engagement and compliance and to leverage behavioral strategies to support medication adherence or other barriers to engagement in treatment (e.g., motivational barriers).

Getting Started

The primary objectives for the early sessions of treatment include providing education and establishing treatment goals. Nonetheless, at this stage, it may also be valuable to consider opportunities for a "quick win"—or a brief, simple intervention component that might afford some level of change for the patient in the short-term. Achieving a "quick win" can help the patient to build a sense of self-efficacy and hope about the potential benefit of engaging in treatment. Some targets to consider at this stage include basic stress management skills (e.g., breathing exercises, progressive muscle relaxation), simple behavioral interventions for sleep (e.g., reducing light exposure prior to bed, introducing a consistent bed and wake time), or behavioral skills for medication management. Opportunities for a "quick win" often emerge during assessment or early treatment sessions and indications for potential targets can include notable skills deficits (e.g., lack of identifiable adaptive stress management strategies) or symptoms for which simple, discrete behavioral interventions may offer benefit (e.g., poor pre-sleep routine, lack of schedule for taking medication).

When working with individuals with OUD, education on overdose is an essential component of treatment and should be done both at the first meeting and re-evaluated throughout the treatment episode. Important domains for discussion include adherence to prescribed MOUD, access to overdose rescue (e.g., naloxone), presence of risk reduction behaviors (e.g., avoidance of using opioids alone), and knowledge about overdose risks. In light of the ever-evolving drug supply, providers working with this population should make every effort to ensure that they remain informed of the current, local landscape of overdose risks and drug supply concerns to provide accurate information to patients. Consultation with addiction specialists or specialist organizations is essential for people who are not regularly working with this population.

Emphasis on the interplay of symptoms and/or the presence of common maintaining features for all disorders is a cornerstone of most co-occurring disorder or transdiagnostic treatments. Accordingly, psychoeducation may focus on establishing an integrated picture of the disorder that considers how symptoms and behavioral responses to symptoms influence each other. Although disorder-specific education (e.g., education on social anxiety) can be used based on the individual's specific diagnostic presentation, two general domains of education can apply broadly to these conditions: (1) the three-component model of emotion, and (2) the role of escape and avoidance behaviors in the maintenance of disorder symptoms.

The three-component model is a flexible psychoeducational tool that can be adapted to the individual to support awareness and understanding of symptoms. This model of emotion defines the three components of any emotional state as cognition, physical sensations, and behaviors. Although typically used as a tool to describe emotions, this can be extended to the experience of pain and drug craving to provide a simple, unifying model. This model also can serve as an opportunity to introduce CBT intervention components that specifically target each component (e.g., cognitive reappraisal for maladaptive cognition).

Escape and avoidance behaviors are core maintaining mechanisms of all three conditions, and typically serve to offer short-term relief, but at long-term cost. For this population, characterized often by maladaptive "quick fix" avoidance or escape behaviors, psychoeducation may focus on demonstrating the potential benefits of avoidance and escape behaviors (e.g., behavioral avoidance, opioid use) in the *short-term* for distress relief, but at the *long-term* costs of symptom maintenance and associated functional consequences. For example, when someone uses opioids to reduce anxiety, this may provide immediate relief, but worsens anxiety symptoms in the medium- to long-term and serves to perpetuate disorder consequences, such as inability to engage in valued relationships or roles. The desire for short-term relief is heightened by psychosocial and physical stress, which is associated with craving, withdrawal, pain, and anxiety. Accordingly, the ability to behave in a way that is consistent with long-term objectives can become exceptionally difficult during times of heightened symptoms. A major goal of CBT is to provide skills to enhance the ability to tolerate these symptoms without choosing a quick fix avoidance or escape behavior. Nonetheless, dedicating time to validating the challenge of selecting healthy behaviors in the context of high levels of distress can be highly valuable for building rapport.

Functional Analysis

Functional analysis is a core CBT tool that can serve as a bridge between education and intervention and helps to individualize treatment targets. Functional analysis is an essential CBT tool and may be particularly useful in the context of complex multi-disorder presentations because it allows for a consideration of how the different symptoms may precipitate each other. This can also be used regularly

Table 9.1 Functional analysis example

Trigger	Behavior	Short-term consequence	Long-term consequence
I woke up with severe low back pain	Stayed in bed, cancelled physical therapy appointment	I felt less anxiety, felt relief not having to leave the house	Felt down and lonely, pain did not improve
Friend offered me a benzodiazepine to help manage stress	Took the benzodiazepine	Felt less anxious	Felt shame for taking benzodiazepine, provided positive urine screen at my medication appointment
Doctor left me a message saying to call back to get my test results from my appointment	Deleted message with the number so I could not call back	Felt relief that I wouldn't hear bad news	More anxiety because I don't know if test results were OK or not

throughout treatment to inform ongoing assessment and intervention modifications.

An example functional analysis is presented in Table 9.1. This format entails assessment of the triggers (i.e., internal and external contexts) prior to the behavior, the behavior itself and both its short (proximal) and long-term (distal) consequences. This serves multiple purposes. First, it reinforces education demonstrating that most maladaptive behaviors are associated with proximal benefits, but distal costs. Second, this provides guidance for intervention points, including modifying triggers or building skills to better tolerate triggers without engaging in quick fix behaviors. Finally, it provides a tool for ongoing assessment of treatment progress to identify areas in which the patient may be struggling to make behavior changes.

When considering intervention based on functional analysis, targets can include the trigger and the behavior. If the trigger is something that can reasonably be modified, removed, or avoided, this provides an important intervention point. However, this is not always possible, in which case, modifying the behavior through building resilience or alternative responding to the trigger may be a more appropriate intervention. For example, if a pattern of difficulty declining offers of drugs emerges, intervention may entail modifying the trigger (e.g., ending unhealthy relationships, deleting and blocking phone numbers) and enhancing tolerance to the trigger (e.g., developing drug refusal skills, see more below). The decision about whether to modify the trigger, behavior, or both may depend on both feasibility of those changes and the patient's values. Deleting (and blocking) contact information of the person from whom drugs were purchased is a trigger-focused intervention. However, if that person is a valued relationship (e.g., a family member) or a relationship that may be difficult to avoid (e.g., a co-worker), removing these triggers may not be possible, at least initially.

Modifiable triggers may include people, places or things that can be removed from the patient's environment. For example, drug paraphernalia may be removed from the home to reduce the risk of cue-induced craving (a craving state precipitated by seeing a drug-use reminder). Such decisions to modify the environment should be made with thoughtful collaboration with the patient, and consideration of risk mitigation, such as ensuring that a supportive person is present when any drugs are removed from the environment. Other triggers may not be modifiable, or easily modifiable, such as anxiety states or environments or people who cannot be avoided. For people with chronic pain, additional challenges may include pain states as well as potential physical challenges or limitations (e.g., pain that may limit certain activities). In these circumstances, building new skills for managing triggers without engagement in maladaptive behaviors is the next step.

Skills Building: Coping Plans, Refusal Skills, and Avoidance of High-Risk Situations

Coping plans are a key component of CBT for substance use disorders that can apply across all three disorders. A coping plan establishes a set of strategies and approaches to managing stress that can be practiced and referenced by the patient. This plan may evolve over time as the individual either adds new skills or strategies or gathers evidence for the strategies most effective for them. Although many formats of coping plans exist, several core principles can guide this skill-building exercise. First, strategies should be clear, specific and reasonable. For example, a general coping skill such as "exercise" may be strengthened by considering details such as types of exercise that are accessible (and, for people with chronic pain, approved by medical providers), when and how often this might be used, and identifying strategies for removing or reducing barriers (e.g., identifying someone to exercise with). Second, greater variety can support application across the many contexts in which they may be needed. This may include variety in the difficulty of the skill (e.g., financial barriers, implementation barriers) as well as its applicability to different types and intensities of stress. Low barrier strategies, like basic breathing exercises, taking a walk, or 24-hour support resources are often an essential component of a plan to ensure that some strategies are accessible regardless of environment. Coping plans may further be enhanced by inclusion of both strategies for when stress occurs and also for *prior* to the onset of stress. Proactive coping—or coping strategies implemented regardless of stress level—can help to build resilience and ensure regular engagement in coping strategies. Proactive coping strategies may include activities like regular exercise, mindfulness or meditation, social contact, and engagement of positive affect.

Drug refusal skills are a central component of CBT for substance use disorders. Drug refusal can be challenging for people with social anxiety, particularly those with anxiety related to assertiveness. Accordingly, engaging in these skills may require integration of social anxiety interventions, such as exposure (see more below). Drug refusal skills training entails identifying situations in which someone may be offered a drug, identifying a response to the offer for drugs, and rehearsing this in a role play. Encouraging clear, direct refusal (e.g., "no," "I am not using opioids anymore.") is preferable to indirect or vague refusal ("Maybe later." "I can't today."). Engagement in drug refusal skills may raise discussions about whether to disclose the OUD or other conditions. Such discussions should be done in close collaboration with the patient and with consideration of the risks and benefits of disclosing their disorders to others. Once refusal statements have been identified, these can be role-played with the therapist to gain practice prior to encountering a need for refusal when drugs are available.

Navigating high-risk situations is another core CBT for substance use disorder skill. Although related to removal of triggers, high-risk situations are distinct in that these are substantial triggers that place people at high risk of symptom exacerbation and should be planned for in advance. With respect to OUD, this involves identifying situations that are risky for relapse to opioid use, such as places where the person previously obtained or used substances, highly stressful situations that might elicit strong drug craving, or exposure to people who are not supportive of recovery. Addressing high-risk situations in this population can be challenging because of the somewhat contradictory messages between avoidance of high-risk situations (consistent with CBT for OUD) and the approach orientation of treatments for anxiety. This is discussed more in the next section.

Exposure-Based Interventions

One challenge in the treatment of co-occurring OUD and anxiety is that although avoidance may be encouraged in some circumstances in OUD treatment, avoidance is almost universally discouraged in anxiety disorder treatment. For example, someone with OUD and social anxiety may benefit from avoiding certain high-risk social situations to reduce risk of opioid use but may want to approach social situations to improve anxiety symptoms. Two principles can be helpful in navigating this challenge. The first is that the degree of avoidance recommended may vary across the course of treatment, with more encouragement of avoidance early in recovery, shifting to a reduction in avoidance later in treatment. This is akin to focusing on trigger interventions early in treatment (avoiding risky situations and people) and on behavioral interventions later (building resilience to risky situations). The other principle distinguishing situations in which avoidance may be encouraged vs. discouraged is whether the situation is values related. For example, going to a self-help meeting may be a better social anxiety exposure than going to a bar or party. This is made more complex when situations may be risky, but consistent with values. For example, if attending family events is a trigger for anxiety, but family relationships are important to the patient, approach is indicated. In situations where substances are available at family events, careful management is needed to achieve the dual goals of managing OUD and anxiety.

Fear exposure is a key, active ingredient in CBT for anxiety disorders. Critically, a growing body of literature consistently supports the safety of fear exposure in people with substance use disorders (Back et al., 2019; Mills et al., 2012; Tripp et al., 2020). In other words, engaging in exposure does not appear to increase risk for relapse. Briefly, fear exposure entails repeated exposure to feared situations, sensations, thoughts or memories to support learning of safety in the context of these cues. Exposure begins with an in-depth functional assessment to identify (1) the contexts in which anxiety is triggered, (2) the predicted feared consequences in these situations, and (3) the behaviors and strategies used to reduce anxiety by avoiding or escaping from these situations (Abramowitz et al., 2019). Repeated avoidance or escape from anxiety triggering situations precludes learning experiences that would demonstrate the safety or tolerability of that given situation and can lead to increasing anxiety over time. Exposure therapy allows individuals to break this cycle of avoidance by systematically engaging with anxiety-producing stimuli without engaging in avoidance/escape strategies (i.e., "response prevention"). This provides opportunities for patients to learn that the feared outcome is either less likely or less severe than anticipated and that feelings of anxiety are manageable, regardless of the subjective intensity (Abramowitz et al., 2019). With these broad principles, exposure therapy can and should be applied flexibly in response to each patient's idiosyncratic presentation of anxiety, coping strategies, and life goals.

Several considerations are important for using exposure-based interventions in this co-occurring population. First, a typical fear exposure will entail regular assessment of anxiety or distress level (e.g., a 0–100 rating of subjective distress). For people with OUD, also assessing drug craving during exposure offers value for identifying and responding to the link between anxiety and substance use. Second, particularly early in treatment, exposure should be thoughtful with respect to high-risk situations and consider opioid-related risks (e.g., relapse, overdose) when constructing exposures for homework. Although presence of a supportive friend of family member may somewhat weaken the effect of an exposure, early exposure situations may benefit from the presence of a supportive other, should risk for opioid use be an acute concern. Third, potential contribution of exposure activities to pain symptoms should be considered. For example, interoceptive exposures—consisting of exposure to feared physical sensations association with anxiety—should be approached with awareness of potential pain exacerbations (e.g., use of neck rolling in someone with chronic neck pain). Consultation with the medical team may be beneficial in determining the optimal exercises in this population.

Cognitive Interventions

Catastrophic biases in thinking are common to all three conditions, and pain decatastrophizing is a core CBT intervention for chronic pain. Pain catastrophizing is the tendency to interpret pain as intolerable, uncontrollable and/or harmful and is associated with poor outcomes in people with chronic pain, including opioid medication misuse (Martel et al., 2020). Cognitions such as "this will never feel better" fuel pain-related anxiety, worsening pain interference. Intervention for catastrophizing includes a three-step process of identifying the thought, considering evidence for and against the thought, and modifying the thought. For example, if someone had the thought that "I can't handle this," they may identify past times when they have coped with similar pain, or confirm that previously the pain did not last forever, and they were able to get through it. This thought can then be replaced with an alternative coping thought, such as "I have made it through pain like this before" or "I can cope with this by calling a friend." These same principles may be applied to anxiety-related cognitions (e.g., "This feeling will never go away") or OUD-related cognitions (e.g., "People will always think I'm an addict").

Managing worry is another common challenge in this population. Although some worry-related thoughts can be managed using cognitive reappraisal as described above, worry may benefit from the addition of scheduled worry or stimulus control (McGowan & Behar, 2013). This entails attempting to restrict time worrying to reduce its pervasiveness throughout the day. Individuals identify a 15- to 30-minute block each day as their "worry time." During this time, the patient can engage in worry, and ideally conduct problem-solving, where possible (e.g., if someone was worrying about their health, they could engage in problem-solving related to seeking appropriate medical care or engaging in healthy behaviors). Outside of that time, when a worry thought emerges, the participant delays engaging with that thought until the worry time. Worry time should not be scheduled prior to bedtime to avoid interference with sleep, and ideally is scheduled at a time that allows for some significant shift in context after worry time (e.g., prior to planned exercise or other pleasant activity).

Acceptance-Based Strategies

Although CBT has a robust and impressive evidence base for these conditions, the integration of acceptance-based strategies may be particularly well-suited to address the unique concerns of patients with co-occurring OUD, anxiety disorders, and chronic pain. For example, Acceptance and Commitment Therapy (ACT) is an evidence-based intervention that uses six processes to encourage contact with avoided thoughts, feelings, memories, and physical sensations—such as pain or anxiety. The overarching goal of ACT is to increase psychological flexibility (the degree to which people act on values, rather than impulses, thoughts, and feelings), while decreasing experiential avoidance (i.e., attempts to avoid thoughts, feelings, memories, and physical sensations). In summary, given the goals of ACT—and the underlying mechanisms driving OUD (e.g., avoidance, response to cravings, etc.), ACT and other acceptance-based strategies, such as mindfulness, may be well-suited to address co-occurring OUD and anxiety issues by undermining experiential control and avoidance, while encouraging values-based behaviors.

The evidence base for applications of acceptance based strategies for individuals coping with OUD and anxiety is growing, with support for the treatment of substance use disorders (Lee et al., 2015; Luoma et al., 2012), including co-occurring OUD and chronic pain (Abid Azam et al., 2017; Dindo et al., 2018). Of note, these studies reported reductions in opioid use and improvements in mood and pain interference (Abid Azam et al., 2017), and that ACT resulted in increased pain acceptance and values-based behavior (Dindo et al., 2018). Taken together, the literature on acceptance-based strategies for chronic pain and opioid use suggests that targeting values-based behavior, goal-setting, and specific acceptance strategies jointly improve pain coping and decrease opioid use.

Acceptance-based strategies offer a wide range of tools that clinicians can use with individuals struggling with chronic pain and opioid use. First, acceptance-based strategies, such as ACT, strongly encourage values identification as an initial step in behavioral treatment. This is in large part because values serve as the blueprint and guideline by which patients set goals, make decisions, and navigate challenges. For example, patients struggling with chronic pain will often cite "spending time with family and friends" as a value. This is not surprising, given that chronic pain and opioid use can jointly foster avoidance, which in turn fuels anxiety. Therefore, a key intervention is to help patients identify their values through online or in-person "values card sort" exercises. Second, one of the treatment goals of ACT is to help patients identify which unpleasant internal experiences they are willing to accommodate to advance their values. For example, if a patient values spending time with family, they may articulate willingness to experiment with experiencing somatic symptoms of anxiety at a family gathering—so that in a sense, they are "paying for" their value with anxiety as the metaphorical currency. Third, it is important to note that acceptance-based strategies can include a wide range of tools that are otherwise known to CBT, including activity planning and exposures. Therefore, applying ACT means that other widely known, pre-existing tools can be utilized as long as there are no cognitive interventions (e.g., cognitive reframing/restructuring, identifying evidence, etc.) that are known to be inconsistent with acceptance-based strategies. For example, if a patient is assigned to attend a family gathering as a behavioral experiment for coping with anxiety and chronic pain as a form of exposure, it is still consistent with ACT principles. However, if a patient is asked to estimate the probability of experiencing anxiety at the family gathering, the intervention is no longer ACT-consistent as it includes cognitive modification and probability testing. In summary, while there are clinical tools specific to acceptance-based strategies, there remains content overlap with CBT that can be freely used with patients struggling with opioid use and anxiety in the context of chronic pain.

Examples of key acceptance-based tools for co-occurring anxiety and opioid use in chronic pain patients:

- Identifying and rank-ordering values.
- Setting values-based goals.
- Practicing brief mindfulness exercises, particularly ones suited to pain.
- Generate creative hopelessness (list of everything the patient has tried to cope with chronic pain, OUD, anxiety) to build motivation for acceptance-based approaches.

- Encouraging use of activity pacing within the broader framework of values.
- Defining and underscoring "acceptance" as a framework to make room for unpleasant internal experiences rather than "giving up," loving, or liking pain.
- Exposure exercises that are related to the patient's values.
- Encouraging delay and replacement behaviors for substances—and underscoring the connection between the delay/replacement behavior and patient-reported values.

Relapse Prevention

After individuals have experienced symptom remission and improved functioning through anxiety treatment, it is common to discuss relapse prevention strategies before treatment termination. It is important to discuss with patients that anxiety and worry are unavoidable aspects of the human condition. Therefore, it can be valuable to provide psychoeducation helping patients to distinguish between typical increases in anxiety due to life circumstance (e.g., starting a new job) versus increases in anxiety that may indicate a reemergence of pathological anxiety. In the former case, clinicians can teach CBT problem-solving skills to aid patients in addressing life stressors when it is identified that the experienced anxiety is not excessive given the life circumstances. Furthermore, it is important for clinicians to work with patients to identify early warning signs that would indicate the patient is on a path towards relapse. Early warning signs can include increased subjective worry or life stress, but also less obvious indications such as "feeling run-down," irritability, or sleep disturbances (Robichaud & Dugas, 2015). Patients should also be coached to identify the reemergence of safety behaviors and coping strategies previously used to manage anxiety, for example, a patient beginning to spend more time researching their possible symptoms within the context of health anxiety or increasing avoidance of situations that may trigger anxiety. Lastly, clinicians can discuss with patients, especially of higher severity, warning signs that would indicate when the patient may need to re-engage with treatment or seek out additional support. This information can be collated into a "Relapse Prevention Plan" to help summarize the above material in a clear and easy to reference format. In some cases, patients may also choose to set aside time each week for a "personal session" to review problem areas in their life and continue therapeutic work in a self-directed fashion (Robichaud & Dugas, 2015).

Relapse prevention for OUD similarly focuses on identifying warnings signs that might indicate an individual is at higher risk for relapse into problematic substance use. In particular, clinicians should help patients to identify early warning signs such as neglecting self-care activities (e.g., good sleep hygiene), increasing exposure to risky situations, or increased irritability, which patients may not always associate with increased risk for relapse. Clinicians and patients should also discuss the management of high-risk situations that may arise in the future, for example, having a major surgery that will require medication management of pain while in recovery from OUD (Carroll, 1998). Discussing hypothetical high-risk situations allows the clinician and patient to assess the patient's ability to flexibly apply skills learned in therapy when encountering novel situations. Patients should identify a set of emergency social supports and "safe places" where a patient can go if they are in crisis (Carroll, 1998). It may also be helpful to identify reliable distractors (e.g., going to the gym) to create an easily accessible resource for patients during times of emotional distress. These discussions can be used to create or update an existing "Relapse Prevention Plan" that the patient can refer to after treatment termination. Lastly and importantly, overdose prevention should be considered one of the primary goals of any coping and relapse prevention within the context of OUD. Clinicians should provide psychoeducation about how abstinence leads to decreased drug tolerance and consequently an increased risk for accidental overdose and review overdose prevention methods and emergency responses.

Relapse prevention plans in this population should also consider the course of the chronic pain condition and how that might influence symptoms of OUD and anxiety in the long-term. Acute exacerbations or worsening of pain conditions may be a risk for worsening of OUD or anxiety symptoms, or relapse among people in recovery. Acceptance-based strategies may be of particular importance for patients who are navigating long-term, chronic health conditions that will introduce limits on functioning. Increased isolation, reduction in activities in general, or reduction in engagement in health-promoting behaviors may all be signs of worsening course that may indicate the need to re-engage with CBT or other behavioral treatment.

Treatment Challenges

There are many factors that can complicate the application of and response to CBT for OUD and anxiety in people with chronic pain. Here, we highlight two: motivation for treatment and the influence of social determinants of health. Both CBT for anxiety and OUD require active participation and sustained motivation for the patient to obtain long-lasting success. In both cases, the patient must cope with short-term discomfort in the form of withdrawal symptoms/craving and increased anxiety in the hope of achieving greater symptom improvement. Given the difficulty of these treatments, it is expected that patients' motivation will fluctuate through the course of treatment. Therefore, the clinician should continually assess the patient's motivation level and discuss with the patient the importance of cultivating motivation and willingness in treatment. It may be helpful to discuss patient beliefs that might get in the way of engaging with treatment effectively. Many individuals who struggle with anxiety will report "positive beliefs" related to their worry, for example, believing that checking in on their children constantly helps to show caring and keep their child safe (Robichaud & Dugas, 2015). It can be important to target these beliefs to help the patient understand that such behaviors may not actually be beneficial. Relatedly, it is extremely important to make sure patients understand and "buy-in" to the value of exposure therapy. A poor understanding of the exposure framework may serve as a barrier to being motivated to engage in exposure treatment. Similarly, individuals with OUD may have beliefs about an inability to reduce opioid use (e.g., "I'm hopeless") that will make it difficult to engage in treatment. Clinicians should work to identify these unhelpful beliefs so they can be restructured in a way more conducive to treatment engagement.

In the face of ambivalence to change or treatment, motivational interviewing (MI) has been shown to be an effective method for strengthening intrinsic motivation for change, especially in the context of SUDs. Motivational interviewing is a set of principles that focuses on evoking motivation and commitment from an individual in the context of behavioral changes (Miller & Rollnik, 2012). MI focuses on collaboration between patients and clinicians and works to honor the autonomy of the patient. This stands in contrast, to the clinician making prescriptive statements from a powerful position as "the expert." This includes working to evoke both "change talk" and identifying personal motivating factors for behavior change for each patient (e.g., cutting down on opioid use to improve one's relationship with their romantic partner). MI has also been used as an adjunct intervention in the context of anxiety treatment to help reduce treatment dropout and increase willingness to engage in treatment (Marker & Norton, 2018). Crucially, MI is not meant to be seen as a "one and done" intervention, but more as a flexible set of principles that can be used in response to ever-changing levels of motivation or willingness to engage in treatment.

There is a growing call in the mental health field to integrate macro-level variables (e.g., socioeconomic status, geographic area) into our case conceptualization of patients. The World Health Organization (WHO) has highlighted the importance of "social determinants of health" which include all the factors related to where patients were "born, grow, work and age" (WHO Commission on Social Determinants of Health & World Health Organization, 2008). Mounting evidence has demonstrated that such socio-cultural factors serve as a driving factor in many health problems and the usefulness of interventions on these factors such as affordable housing and nutrition support in the context of mental health outcomes (Marmot & Allen, 2014). It is therefore crucially important for clinicians to include both a thorough assessment of possibly relevant socio-cultural characteristics and a thoughtful case conceptualization that integrates this information along with symptom presentation. Clinicians should be aware of how such social characteristics can have a direct and often negative impact on treatment outcome. For example, if a patient is preparing for anxiety treatment and learns at the end of the month their rent will double, the clinician must think deeply and collaborate with the patient to create a plan of action that accounts for this reality. Even if it is not the primary presenting issue for the patient at the time of the referral, becoming homeless or needing to abruptly relocate is very likely to disrupt any intervention no matter how well developed and implemented. Therefore, the therapist may need to shift, even just temporarily, into a role more focused on case management and problem-solving.

Case Examples

In this section, we provide two case examples to illustrate principles and techniques described throughout this chapter. These case examples represent composite presentations to illustrate principles and do not include information about specific, identifiable individuals.

Case Example 1: CBT-Based Approaches

Monica is a 25-year-old, single, White, Hispanic woman. She misused opioid analgesics occasionally as an adolescent at parties and was then introduced to heroin by a boyfriend at age 21. Her opioid use quickly escalated, and she soon developed an OUD. She had attempted to discontinue opioid use several times "on (her) own," but would relapse within 1–2 months during times of stress. She reported struggling with social anxiety since childhood, characterized by worry that she would be judged as "stupid" or "ugly" and a significant fear of assertiveness. This fear worsened at age 19 when she was in a car accident that resulted in scarring on her arm and leg, at which time she began to struggle with chronic pain. She was highly reticent to seek treatment for her OUD because she said she "wasn't a junkie;" however, after a nonfatal, unintentional overdose that required emergency intervention, she agreed to engage in outpatient MOUD and individual therapy.

Monica started on sublingual buprenorphine for OUD and her treatment goals were to "feel less anxiety and to have healthier relationships." When considering the role of opioid use and avoidance in relieving unwanted distress, Monica identified the fundamental role of avoiding social anxiety in her symptoms. Monica further identified that although stress precipitated relapse, that this always occurred in the context of someone else offering drugs.

Therapist (T) It looks like the combination of stress and then social pressure is very high risk for you. What do you think would happen if you did decline an offer to use?

Monica (M) I've never even considered that. I can't imagine saying no in that situation, I just say yes, almost as a default. I do that with everything, I can't pick a restaurant or what to watch on TV if someone else is there. I don't even think about what I might want because what if they thought that was stupid?

Drug refusal skills were then engaged, combined with social anxiety exposures given the interrelatedness of these symptoms. Importantly, due to the high-risk nature of an offer for drugs, this was done in a stepwise fashion. First, Monica and the therapist engaged in extensive role play in the session, with increasing difficulty over time. Then, Monica practiced refusal of non-preferred drugs (e.g., alcohol) at work and family events to reduce anxiety responses to the offer. During treatment, she did not encounter an offer for opioids, yet continued practice of refusal was encouraging to support preparedness for that possibility.

T So, how did it go turning down a drink this weekend?
M This weekend was actually OK. I was still really anxious leading up to it, but the aftermath was much easier.
T What do you mean by the aftermath?
M After I did refuse, I was able to stay out of my head. Normally I would just spin, wondering what the other person thought, if I seemed cold or rude, but that's getting easier with time.
T What do you think you are doing differently to stop that spinning?
M I'm just seeing that people don't actually care that much, they move on quickly, so I can to. It is really helpful to change the subject after I turn down the drink, so we can all just move on. After I said no, I suggested that we flag down our server to order appetizers, and everyone went along with it.

Additional exposures were also targeted to social anxiety symptoms. Given her concern about disclosing her OUD, Monica was not willing to engage in self-help groups to support her recovery or as social anxiety exposures. In-session exposures including making phone calls to make specific requests (e.g., changing appointment times) and other assertiveness role plays. Outside of session, Monica leveraged her job at a restaurant to practice assertiveness skills within an exposure framework. This included requests for breaks to help manage her chronic leg and back pain as well as declining excessive or unreasonable requests to take extra shifts with minimal notice.

Monica also reported frequent catastrophizing related to her pain, which caused significant distress as well as avoidance, particularly of enjoyable activities. Upon further evaluation and education of catastrophic thinking patterns, she was able to identify broader instances of catastrophizing, which had been present since childhood. Monica in general found the decatastrophizing interventions to be helpful but continued to struggle with long-term catastrophizing related to the potential course of her chronic pain and worry about worsening pain and disability with age.

Despite concerns about MOUD (e.g., dislike for the taste of sublingual buprenorphine, concern about stigma), Monica remained adherent to prescribed buprenorphine throughout treatment and reported minimal difficulty with craving or urges to use opioids. She was able to identify a number of high-risk situations (e.g., specific bars) and relationships, and chose to avoid these situations. She did not report use of any opioids during treatment but reported that she did not anticipate "staying on buprenorphine forever."

Overall, Monica reported improvement in the severity of her anxiety symptoms and significant reduction in avoidance, particularly of conflict and assertiveness. She significantly increased activity, which she found had no worsening impact of her pain; however, she continued to experience approximately monthly pain exacerbations that required some rest and additional medical management. She reported significant improvements in quality of life, which she attributed to her ability to continue to engage in valued activities even when experiencing pain or anxiety. As part of her relapse prevention plan, she identified the continued use of her coping plan, daily physical activity (e.g., walking) and taking her medication as key relapse prevention goals. She identified potential relapse risk markers as increases in avoidance, irritability, and urges to reach out to former drug-using partners as signs that she needed to re-engage in treatment.

Case Example 2: Application of Acceptance-Based Strategies

Sam is a 60-year-old White male with cancer-related pain, receiving concurrent chemotherapy and opioid therapy. He has a longstanding history of alcohol use disorder, which worsened in the context of his cancer diagnosis and treatment. Sam attributes his psychological suffering and avoidance to a combination of difficult chemotherapy side effects and feeling that he does not have much to do. Sam discussed his history and motivations for behavioral therapy.

Therapist (T)	You're dealing with a lot of medical and psychological challenges right now. It's not surprising that you've been drinking more than usual and requesting early refills on your opioids.
Sam (S)	I feel like I'm drowning for at least 5 days after each chemo cycle—and I drink and use my opioids to get through it.
Therapist	Chemotherapy side effects are incredibly challenging—no wonder you're trying to suppress them. What motivates you for behavioral treatment at this time?
Sam	I don't want to use substances the way I'm using them anymore. Yes, I'm in a lot of pain and discomfort, especially after chemo, but I don't want a battle with substances too.
Therapist	It sounds like you've got enough of a battle with the cancer, chemotherapy, and pain—you don't want to add a substance use battle to it.
Sam	Exactly. And I really need help with that.

At this stage in behavioral treatment, Sam is motivated for behavioral treatment to address substance use. Given Sam's clinical presentation, he may benefit from acceptance-based strategies, in order to undermine his experiential control.

Therapist	Tell me a little bit about what is important to you in your life… what do you want your life to be about?
Sam	Well, I love to do things around the house… like house projects. I like going on small road trips.
Therapist	So, you value travel, creativity, and productivity.
Sam	Exactly—and using alcohol and opioids doesn't really fit in there.

Given Sam's stated values and motivation for change, he and the therapist set the following tentative treatment plan: (1) values identification and motivation for behavior change; (2) encouraging self-monitoring of pain, patterns of feeling unwell post-chemotherapy, and use of alcohol and opioids; (3) practice setting one-values based goal, such as spending 1 hour working on a house project; (4) introduction to delay and replacement behaviors (e.g., replacing an alcoholic beverage with sparking water and delaying opioid use by an hour); and (5) overview of activity pacing and using values to encourage use of that skill.

While Sam continues to use more alcohol and opioids than he would like, his monitoring record demonstrates a substantial decline in substance use. Sam and his therapist worked to identify patterns of experiential avoidance (i.e., the opposite of acceptance) that move Sam away from engaging with his values. For example, Sam reported wishing his pain would go away so that he could build a deck off the back of his house. He lamented that in his current physical state he would not be able to take on such a physically demanding task and that he looks forward to when he will be able to. The therapist and Sam discussed that although these thoughts and feelings are completely understandable, investing large amounts of time fantasizing about different life circumstances (i.e., being pain and cancer free so he could build a deck) is a powerful experiential avoidance strategy. Crucially, such avoidance strategies tend to lead to inaction, as Sam is essentially "waiting" to live his life once his symptoms improve.

The therapist and Sam worked together to try a new perspective. In particular, Sam reoriented his attention to flexibly interacting with his values (i.e., creativity and productivity) and lessened his focus on achieving specific end goals (i.e., building a deck). In addition, he worked to improve at not getting "hooked" on thoughts that lead him away from his values (e.g., fantasizing about a life without pain). This allowed Sam to brainstorm a variety of activities that allow him to engage with his values of creativity and productivity (e.g., building a bird house) in the here and now. Part of Sam's new perspective also includes being prepared to experience physical discomfort, fatigue, and feelings of sadness as a "trade off" to engage with what is important to him. As a result, Sam reported feeling more connected with his values—and feels that he has gotten into a "routine" around his valued activities immediately post-chemotherapy. Sam also reported an increase in valued activities when he is not experiencing side effects. Lastly, he reported being able to unhook from thoughts and feelings that previously would have kept him inactive and from feeling able to engage with his values.

Summary and Discussion of Key Points

Addressing the co-occurrence of OUD, anxiety, and chronic pain presents significant challenges due to the complexity of the presentation. Nonetheless, the interaction among symptoms provides opportunities to target common maintaining mechanisms that can be responsive to cognitive-behavioral interventions (e.g., worry, cognitive distortions, behavioral avoidance). Several key take-home points include:

1. *Risk for disorder onset is not one-directional:* It is not unusual for providers and patients to attempt to discern the precipitating cause of current symptoms, such as identifying an anxiety disorder as the "cause" of the opioid use disorder. Although clues may be identified based on timing of disorder onset, from a cognitive-behavioral perspective, once developed, these disorders interact and can fuel each other. Accordingly, integrating treatment elements and treating these co-occurring conditions as a single entity can help to best approach the mechanisms that can be targeted to improve symptoms.
2. *OUD risk education is essential:* OUD is a disorder with tremendously high mortality, including via overdose. With the increasing lethality of the illicit drug supply, assessment and education related to overdose risks is essential in working with anyone with OUD. MOUD is clearly associated with reduced mortality and is the current standard of care for this population.
3. *Applying CBT requires consideration of conflicting goals:* Although many CBT techniques apply to all three conditions (e.g., cognitive reappraisal), when working with this population there are opportunities for potentially conflicting goals. An example of this includes the conflict between approach-based exposure techniques with opioid relapse risks or potential for pain exacerbations. These conflicts are manageable with consideration of the balance between patient values and treatment goals. Grading exposures for difficulty as treatment progresses can be one strategy for managing conflicting goals (e.g., starting exposures with a supportive other present, ensuring stability of MOUD adherence prior to difficult exposure). Nonetheless, it is of note that evidence to date strongly supports the safety of fear exposure in people with substance use disorders.
4. *Integration of acceptance-based strategies can offer benefits:* For patients with chronic pain and a history of substance use disorder, many report a value of keeping their sobriety intact even through advanced disease, such as cancer—which is why acceptance-based strategies can be useful. The integration of acceptance-based strategies may also be useful when considering the long-term impacts of chronic pain, that may require lifelong management.

In summary, OUD, anxiety, and chronic pain can be a debilitating combination of conditions. Multimodal treatment, including MOUD, medical pain management, and case management support can be essential components of treatment. Coordination among team members offers opportunity to support the whole patient and to strengthen each intervention. CBT may be helpful, for example, in supporting compliance with other interventions through use of behavioral and motivational strategies. More research is clearly needed to advance this area, nonetheless, CBT is a highly promising intervention for this population.

References

Abid Azam, M., Weinrib, A. Z., Montbriand, J., Burns, L. C., McMillan, K., Clarke, H., & Katz, J. (2017). Acceptance and commitment therapy to manage pain and opioid use after major surgery: Preliminary outcomes from the Toronto General Hospital Transitional Pain Service. *Canadian Journal of Pain, 1*(1), 37–49. https://doi.org/10.1080/24740527.2017.1325317

Abramowitz, J. S., Deacon, B. J., & Whiteside, S. P. (2019). *Exposure therapy for anxiety: Principles and practice*. Guilford Press.

Alford, D. P., Compton, P., & Samet, J. H. (2006). Acute pain management for patients receiving maintenance methadone or buprenorphine therapy. *Annals of Internal Medicine, 144*(2), 127–134. https://doi.org/10.7326/0003-4819-144-2-200601170-00010

Back, S. E., Killeen, T., Badour, C. L., Flanagan, J. C., Allan, N. P., Ana, E. S., Lozano, B., Korte, K. J., Foa, E. B., & Brady, K. T. (2019). Concurrent treatment of substance use disorders and PTSD using prolonged exposure: A randomized clinical trial in military veterans. *Addictive Behaviors, 90*, 369–377. https://doi.org/10.1016/j.addbeh.2018.11.032

Blanco, C., Wall, M. M., Okuda, M., Wang, S., Iza, M., & Olfson, M. (2016). Pain as a predictor of opioid use disorder in a nationally representative sample. *The American Journal of Psychiatry, 173*(12), 1189–1195. https://doi.org/10.1176/appi.ajp.2016.15091179

Carroll, K. M. (1998). *A cognitive-behavioral approach: Treating cocaine addiction. (NIH Publication Number 98-4308)*. National Institute on Drug Abuse.

Cochran, B. N., Flentje, A., Heck, N. C., Van Den Bos, J., Perlman, D., Torres, J., Valuck, R., & Carter, J. (2014). Factors predicting development of opioid use disorders among individuals who receive an initial opioid prescription: Mathematical modeling using a database of commercially-insured individuals. *Drug and Alcohol Dependence, 138*, 202–208. https://doi.org/10.1016/j.drugalcdep.2014.02.701

Committee on Medication-Assisted Treatment for Opioid Use Disorder. (2019). *Medications for opioid use disorder save lives*. T. N. A. Press.

Conway, K. P., Compton, W., Stinson, F. S., & Grant, B. F. (2006). Lifetime comorbidity of DSM-IV mood and anxiety disorders and specific drug use disorders: Results from the National Epidemiologic Survey on Alcohol and Related Conditions. *The Journal of Clinical Psychiatry, 67*(2), 247–257.

Davis, M. A., Lin, L. A., Liu, H., & Sites, B. D. (2017). Prescription opioid use among adults with mental health disorders in the United States. *Journal of American Board of Family Medicine, 30*(4), 407–417. https://doi.org/10.3122/jabfm.2017.04.170112

Demyttenaere, K., Bruffaerts, R., Lee, S., Posada-Villa, J., Kovess, V., Angermeyer, M. C., Levinson, D., de Girolamo, G., Nakane, H., Mneimneh, Z., Lara, C., de Graaf, R., Scott, K. M., Gureje, O., Stein, D. J., Haro, J. M., Bromet, E. J., Kessler, R. C., Alonso, J., & Von Korff, M. (2007). Mental disorders among persons with chronic back or neck pain: Results from the World Mental Health Surveys. *Pain, 129*(3), 332–342. https://doi.org/10.1016/j.pain.2007.01.022

Dindo, L., Zimmerman, M. B., Hadlandsmyth, K., StMarie, B., Embree, J., Marchman, J., Tripp-Reimer, T., & Rakel, B. (2018). Acceptance and commitment therapy for prevention of chronic postsurgical pain and opioid use in at-risk veterans: A pilot randomized controlled study. *The Journal of Pain, 19*(10), 1211–1221. https://doi.org/10.1016/j.jpain.2018.04.016

Dixon, K. E., Keefe, F. J., Scipio, C. D., Perri, L. M., & Abernethy, A. P. (2007). Psychological interventions for arthritis pain management in adults: A meta-analysis. *Health Psychology, 26*(3), 241–250. https://doi.org/10.1037/0278-6133.26.3.241

Dreifuss, J. A., Griffin, M. L., Frost, K., Fitzmaurice, G. M., Potter, J. S., Fiellin, D. A., Selzer, J., Hatch-Maillette, M., Sonne, S. C., & Weiss, R. D. (2013). Patient characteristics associated with buprenorphine/naloxone treatment outcome for prescription opioid dependence: Results from a multisite study. *Drug and Alcohol Dependence, 131*(1–2), 112–118. https://doi.org/10.1016/j.drugalcdep.2012.12.010

DuPont, R. L. (2017). Should patients with substance use disorders be prescribed benzodiazepines? No. *Journal of Addiction Medicine, 11*(2), 84–86. https://doi.org/10.1097/adm.0000000000000291

Han, B., Compton, W. M., Blanco, C., Crane, E., Lee, J., & Jones, C. M. (2017). Prescription opioid use, misuse, and use disorders in U.S. adults: 2015 National Survey on Drug Use and Health. *Annals of Internal Medicine*. https://doi.org/10.7326/m17-0865

Hassan, A. N., Le Foll, B., Imtiaz, S., & Rehm, J. (2017). The effect of post-traumatic stress disorder on the risk of developing prescription opioid use disorder: Results from the National Epidemiologic Survey on Alcohol and Related Conditions III. *Drug and Alcohol Dependence, 179*, 260–266. https://doi.org/10.1016/j.drugalcdep.2017.07.012

Hoffman, B. M., Papas, R. K., Chatkoff, D. K., & Kerns, R. D. (2007). Meta-analysis of psychological interventions for chronic low back pain. *Health Psychology, 26*(1), 1–9. https://doi.org/10.1037/0278-6133.26.1.1

Hofmann, S. G., & Smits, J. A. (2008). Cognitive-behavioral therapy for adult anxiety disorders: A meta-analysis of randomized placebo-controlled trials. *The Journal of Clinical Psychiatry, 69*(4), 621–632.

Hser, Y. I., Mooney, L. J., Saxon, A. J., Miotto, K., Bell, D. S., & Huang, D. (2017). Chronic pain among patients with opioid use disorder: Results from electronic health records data. *Journal of Substance Abuse Treatment, 77*, 26–30. https://doi.org/10.1016/j.jsat.2017.03.006

Ilgen, M. A., Trafton, J. A., & Humphreys, K. (2006). Response to methadone maintenance treatment of opiate dependent patients with and without significant pain. *Drug and Alcohol Dependence, 82*(3), 187–193. https://doi.org/10.1016/j.drugalcdep.2005.09.005

Katz, C., El-Gabalawy, R., Keyes, K. M., Martins, S. S., & Sareen, J. (2013). Risk factors for incident nonmedical prescription opioid use and abuse and dependence: Results from a longitudinal nationally representative sample. *Drug and Alcohol Dependence, 132*(1–2), 107–113. https://doi.org/10.1016/j.drugalcdep.2013.01.010

Lee, E. B., An, W., Levin, M. E., & Twohig, M. P. (2015). An initial meta-analysis of acceptance and commitment therapy for treating substance use disorders. *Drug and Alcohol Dependence, 155*, 1–7. https://doi.org/10.1016/j.drugalcdep.2015.08.004

Luoma, J. B., Kohlenberg, B. S., Hayes, S. C., & Fletcher, L. (2012). Slow and steady wins the race: A randomized clinical trial of acceptance and commitment therapy targeting shame in substance use disorders. *Journal of Consulting and Clinical Psychology, 80*(1), 43–53. https://doi.org/10.1037/a0026070

Magill, M., Ray, L., Kiluk, B., Hoadley, A., Bernstein, M., Tonigan, J. S., & Carroll, K. (2019). A meta-analysis of cognitive-behavioral therapy for alcohol or other drug use disorders: Treatment efficacy by contrast condition. *Journal of Consulting and Clinical Psychology, 87*(12), 1093–1105. https://doi.org/10.1037/ccp0000447

Marker, I., & Norton, P. J. (2018). The efficacy of incorporating motivational interviewing to cognitive behavior therapy for anxiety disorders: A review and meta-analysis. *Clinical Psychology Review, 62*, 1–10. https://doi.org/10.1016/j.cpr.2018.04.004

Marmot, M., & Allen, J. J. (2014). Social determinants of health equity. *American Journal of Public Health, 104 Suppl 4*(Suppl 4), S517–S519. https://doi.org/10.2105/ajph.2014.302200

Martel, M. O., Dolman, A. J., Edwards, R. R., Jamison, R. N., & Wasan, A. D. (2014). The association between negative affect and prescription opioid misuse in patients with chronic pain: The mediating role of opioid craving. *The Journal of Pain, 15*(1), 90–100. https://doi.org/10.1016/j.jpain.2013.09.014

Martel, M. O., Edwards, R. R., & Jamison, R. N. (2020). The relative contribution of pain and psychological factors to opioid misuse: A 6-month observational study. *The American Psychologist, 75*(6), 772–783. https://doi.org/10.1037/amp0000632

Martins, S. S., Fenton, M. C., Keyes, K. M., Blanco, C., Zhu, H., & Storr, C. L. (2012). Mood and anxiety disorders and their association with non-medical prescription opioid use and prescription opioid-use disorder: Longitudinal evidence from the National Epidemiologic Study on Alcohol and Related Conditions. *Psychological Medicine, 42*(6), 1261–1272. https://doi.org/10.1017/s0033291711002145

McGowan, S. K., & Behar, E. (2013). A preliminary investigation of stimulus control training for worry: Effects on anxiety and insomnia. *Behavior Modification, 37*(1), 90–112. https://doi.org/10.1177/0145445512455661

McHugh, R. K., Edwards, R. R., Ross, E. L., & Jamison, R. N. (2019). Does bedtime matter among patients with chronic pain? A longitudinal comparison study. *Pain Reports, 4*(3), e747. https://doi.org/10.1097/pr9.0000000000000747

McHugh, R. K., Hilton, B. T., Chase, A. M., Griffin, M. L., & Weiss, R. D. (2021). Do people with opioid use disorder and posttraumatic stress disorder benefit from dding individual opioid Drug Counseling to buprenorphine? *Drug and Alcohol Dependence, 228*, 109084. https://doi.org/10.1016/j.drugalcdep.2021.109084

Miller, W. R., & Rollnik, S. (2012). *Motivational interviewing: Helping people change* (3rd ed.). Guilford Press.

Mills, K. L., Teesson, M., Back, S. E., Brady, K. T., Baker, A. L., Hopwood, S., Sannibale, C., Barrett, E. L., Merz, S., Rosenfeld, J., & Ewer, P. L. (2012). Integrated exposure-based therapy for co-occurring posttraumatic stress disorder and substance dependence: A randomized controlled trial. *JAMA, 308*(7), 690–699. https://doi.org/10.1001/jama.2012.9071

Park, T. W. (2017). Debate: Are benzodiazepines appropriate treatments for patients with substance use disorders? Yes. *Journal of Addiction Medicine, 11*(2), 87–89. https://doi.org/10.1097/adm.0000000000000292

Rikard, S. M., Strahan, A. E., Schmit, K. M., & Guy, G. P., Jr. (2023). Chronic pain among adults - United States, 2019-2021. *MMWR. Morbidity and Mortality Weekly Report, 72*(15), 379–385. https://doi.org/10.15585/mmwr.mm7215a1

Robichaud, M., & Dugas, M. J. (2015). *The generalized anxiety disorder workbook: A comprehensive CBT guide for coping with uncertainty, worry, and fear*. New Harbinger Publications.

Rogers, A. H., Shepherd, J. M., Orr, M. F., Bakhshaie, J., McHugh, R. K., & Zvolensky, M. J. (2019). Exploring anxiety sensitivity in the relationship between pain intensity and opioid misuse among opioid-using adults with chronic pain. *Journal of Psychiatric Research, 111*, 154–159. https://doi.org/10.1016/j.jpsychires.2019.02.004

Saitz, R. (2017). Should benzodiazepines be used to treat anxiety in people with substance use disorders? Contentious debate with similar conclusions. *Journal of Addiction Medicine, 11*(2), 83. https://doi.org/10.1097/adm.0000000000000293

Sullivan, M. D., Edlund, M. J., Zhang, L., Unützer, J., & Wells, K. B. (2006). Association between mental health disorders, problem drug use, and regular prescription opioid use. *Archives of Internal Medicine, 166*(19), 2087–2093. https://doi.org/10.1001/archinte.166.19.2087

Taghian, N. R., McHugh, R. K., Griffin, M. L., Chase, A. R., Greenfield, S. F., & Weiss, R. D. (2021). Associations between childhood abuse and chronic pain in adults with substance use disorders. *Substance Use & Misuse, 56*(1), 87–92. https://doi.org/10.1080/10826084.2020.1840590

Tripp, J. C., Haller, M., Trim, R. S., Straus, E., Bryan, C. J., Davis, B. C., Lyons, R., Hamblen, J. L., & Norman, S. B. (2020). Does exposure exacerbate symptoms in veterans with PTSD and alcohol use disorder? *Psychological Trauma*. https://doi.org/10.1037/tra0000634

Weiss, R. D., Potter, J. S., Griffin, M. L., McHugh, R. K., Haller, D., Jacobs, P., Gardin, J., 2nd, Fischer, D., & Rosen, K. D. (2014). Reasons for opioid use among patients with dependence on prescription opioids: The role of chronic pain. *Journal of Substance Abuse Treatment, 47*(2), 140–145. https://doi.org/10.1016/j.jsat.2014.03.004

WHO Commission on Social Determinants of Health, & World Health Organization. (2008). *Closing the gap in a generation: Health quity through action n the social determinants of health: Commission on Social Determinants of Health final report*. W. H. Organization.

Chapter 10
Cognitive-Behavioral Therapy Targeted to the Successful Discontinuation of Benzodiazepine Medication

Laura J. Long, E. Marie Parsons, and Michael W. Otto

This chapter provides a review of the current status of cognitive-behavioral strategies for aiding the discontinuation of benzodiazepine (BZ) medication. The majority of empirical work within this domain has focused on patients with panic disorder—the disorder with particularly high rates of BZ taper failures as well as high post-discontinuation distress. To address these issues, cognitive-behavioral therapy (CBT) interventions have been utilized to treat the fear of anxiety sensations and the development of skills to tolerate BZ withdrawal sensations, while also targeting the larger issue of managing the anxiety disorders/difficulties for which BZs were originally prescribed. The development and validation of this approach to BZ discontinuation is described below as well as changes in prescribing practices and recognition of unique harms that makes issues of BZ discontinuation particularly important at the current time.

Benzodiazepine Treatment and Discontinuation Difficulties

BZ treatment has demonstrated efficacy for anxiety disorders (Offidani et al., 2013; Shinfuku et al. 2019). However, the benefits associated with BZ treatment are attenuated by the potential for concerning adverse effects including sedation, fatigue, ataxia, memory impairment, as well as the emergence of dependence and difficulties discontinuing BZ medications (American Psychiatric Association, 2009; Bandelow et al., 2012; Katzman et al., 2014). More specifically, extended periods of regular use, even at therapeutic doses, are associated with a greater likelihood of

L. J. Long · E. M. Parsons · M. W. Otto (✉)
Department of Psychological and Brain Sciences, Boston University, Boston, MA, USA
e-mail: mwotto@bu.edu

K. Wolitzky-Taylor (ed.), *Treating Comorbid Substance Use and Emotional Disorders*, CBT: Science Into Practice, https://doi.org/10.1007/978-3-031-62971-6_10

developing dependence (Winstock, 2012). Physiological dependence, defined as clinically significant discontinuation symptoms after abrupt withdrawal, is a natural consequence of changes at the BZ receptor site from chronic use, and can develop to therapeutic doses by 4–6 weeks (Konopka et al., 2016; Salzman, 1998). The reinforcing effects of BZ as an anxiolytic and sedative-hypnotic drug also carry the potential for misuse, and there is evidence that those with conditions for which this drug is typically indicated (e.g., anxiety and insomnia) are more sensitive to these reinforcing effects (Helmus et al., 2005; Votaw et al., 2019). These issues with BZ treatment have led BZs to be generally recommended for short-term rather than longer-term care of anxiety-related disorders (American Psychiatric Association, 2009; Bandelow et al., 2012; Katzman et al., 2014). Nonetheless, long-term treatment with BZs is common in clinical practice and BZs continue to be recommended by prescribers (Dubovsky & Marshall, 2022; Bruce et al., 2003; Vasile et al., 2005).

After weeks to months of regular use, abrupt withdrawal of BZ treatment is associated with moderate to severe symptoms of anxiety (Fontaine et al., 1984; Murphy et al., 1989), and a substantial number of patients still experience withdrawal, rebound anxiety, and/or relapse despite gradual tapering (Mellman & Uhde, 1986; Pecknold et al., 1988; Schweizer et al., 1991). For instance, within a study of controlled BZ discontinuation for panic disorder patients, relapse rates exceeded 70% following cessation of BZ and 60% of patients endorsed anxiety symptoms equivalent to or exceeding pre-treatment levels (Noyes et al., 1991). Whereas more gradual tapering can mitigate withdrawal and anxiety symptoms, they may not be fully eliminated (see Michelini et al., 1996; Salzman, 1993 for a review). Thus, many patients will end their attempt at discontinuation even when gradual tapering is used (Baillargeon et al., 2003; Fyer et al., 1987; Gosselin et al., 2006; Noyes et al., 1991), and there is evidence that only a minority achieve long-term abstinence with routine care or gradual dose reduction alone (see Parr et al., 2009).

BZ withdrawal symptoms tend to mirror the anxiety symptoms that initially prompted pharmacological intervention (Roy-Byrne & Hommer, 1988; Tyrer et al., 1990). The re-emergence of anxiety symptoms during tapering can interfere with discontinuation and may test the limits of patients' coping abilities. Those who are particularly fearful of experiencing anxiety and have catastrophic interpretations of their symptoms are more likely to experience difficulties. These fears define anxiety sensitivity, the fear of anxiety symptoms due to perceived catastrophic consequences (Smits et al., 2018), which is routinely measured using the Anxiety Sensitivity Index (ASI; Reiss et al., 1986; Taylor et al., 2007). Patients with panic disorder and PTSD tend to show particularly high anxiety sensitivity scores, though elevated scores are also common among individuals with social anxiety disorder, generalized anxiety disorder, OCD, and major depressive disorder (Naragon-Gainey, 2010; Olatunji & Wolitzky-Taylor, 2009). Though BZ may reduce symptoms of anxiety, catastrophic interpretations of anxiety-related sensations underlying panic disorder may persist, leaving these patients more vulnerable to relapse. In fact, BZ users with panic disorder show selective attention to threatening physical sensations (Stewart et al., 2000), which may be reinforced over time by prn (i.e., "as needed") use. Upon BZ discontinuation, patients with panic disorder are likely highly aware of bodily arousal due to concerns that their symptoms may intensify. Thus, discontinuing BZ may actually elicit the same symptoms that patient with panic find most distressing during a period when they are particularly wary of their re-emergence (Otto et al., 1992). As a result, targeting fear and distress associated with physical sensations—whether stemming from BZ withdrawal, an anxiety disorder, or some other source—can be useful for both aiding successful BZ discontinuation and addressing core underlying psychopathology.

In summary, while BZs have shown efficacy as a treatment for anxiety disorders, their possible adverse effects warrant caution against long-term use. The potential for significant symptoms of withdrawal, rebound anxiety, and relapse complicates BZ discontinuation, even when gradual tapering is used. Moreover, BZ users, particularly those with panic disorder, tend to have elevated anxiety sensitivity and are likely to be concerned about symptom reemergence during discontinuation, which can make long-term abstinence difficult to achieve. Given these problems, CBT interventions that provide training in effective management of withdrawal and anxiety symptoms are needed. Exposure-based CBT approaches to BZ discontinuation have the potential to address underlying fears and catastrophic interpretations of anxiety symptoms that are characteristic of panic disorder, as well as other anxiety-related disorders more broadly (Table 10.1).

Table 10.1 Symptoms associated with benzodiazepine discontinuation

Mood	Anxiety Irritability Depression/Sadness
Somatic	Sensitivity to light, sound, or touch Perceptual distortions Eye soreness Numbness or tingling sensations Headache Sweating Dizziness
Cognitive	Difficulty concentrating Memory problems Derealization or depersonalization
Sleep	Insomnia Nightmares
Motor, cardiovascular, & gastrointestinal	Muscle tension Tremors, shakiness Palpitations Chest tightness Nausea, low appetite, diarrhea Clumsiness

Interventions to Aid BZ Discontinuation

Cognitive-behavioral strategies have demonstrated efficacy for facilitating BZ discontinuation, providing additive benefits when paired with gradual tapering. An initial randomized controlled trial (RCT) examined the efficacy of adjunctive cognitive-behavioral therapy during tapering versus supportive tapering alone (Otto et al., 1993). The sample included 33 treatment-seeking outpatients with panic disorder who had been prescribed high-potency agents (either alprazolam or clonazepam) for 6 months or more and were attempting to discontinue BZ. The components of this 10-session CBT treatment were based on interventions addressing the core patterns of psychopathology underlying panic disorder, which would likely be exacerbated as withdrawal emerged during tapering (see Fig. 10.1).

These components included: (1) psychoeducation to illustrate the cycle of symptoms and avoidance characteristic of panic disorder and provide an overarching model for the treatment; (2) cognitive restructuring to address catastrophic interpretations of the meaning and potential outcomes of somatic symptoms due to anxiety, panic, and withdrawal; (3) exposure to feared internal sensations associated with autonomic arousal (i.e., interoceptive exposure) to promote habituation and extinction of these fears, with special attention to sensations likely to arise during BZ discontinuation; (4) when relevant, addressing agoraphobic avoidance with situational exposures to break the cycle of symptom-amplifying responses to both internal and external cues; and (5) targeted application of arousal management techniques such as muscle-relaxation techniques and diaphragmatic-breathing to specifically address withdrawal symptoms and bring them to a manageable level. Study results indicated that there were pronounced differences in outcomes between the two

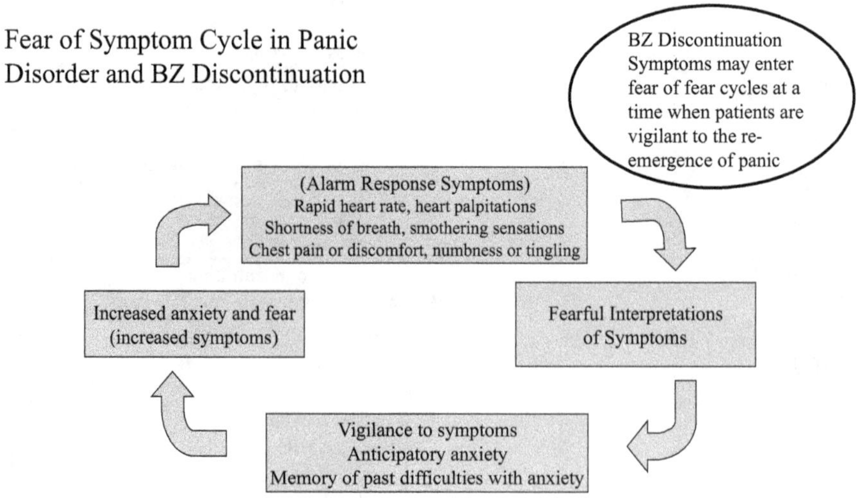

Fig. 10.1 Cognitive-behavioral model of panic disorder. (Figure adapted from Otto & Pollack, 2009a, 2009b)

treatment conditions, with 76% of patients in the exposure-based CBT group successfully discontinuing BZ compared to only 25% within the group that received slow-taper alone. In addition, patients who were able to discontinue BZ reported less distress following treatment than prior to tapering, suggesting that the intervention targeted underlying symptoms of panic disorder in addition to challenges associated with discontinuation.

To provide a more rigorous test of this approach, a subsequent RCT was conducted to control for the effects of therapist contact and support by including another treatment condition that provided the same degree of therapy contact as the supplemental exposure-based CBT but provided only relaxation training to address symptoms of anxiety and withdrawal as opposed to exposure-based strategies for extinguishing fears (Otto et al., 2010). Specifically, for this study of 47 patients with panic disorder seeking to discontinue their BZ medication, an exposure-based CBT group was compared to a control group that received taper-alone and another group that received both taper and training in relaxation. Including a relaxation condition provided the opportunity to differentiate the benefits of support and relaxation training from the presumed core effects of modifying emotional responses to internal cues (i.e., physical sensations associated with anxiety), which is believed to be the key element of CBT that equips patients to withstand withdrawal symptoms during BZ tapering (Otto et al., 2004). Consistent with this hypothesis, findings indicated that adjunctive CBT was associated with higher rates of successful BZ discontinuation than both gradual tapering alone and tapering supplemented with relaxation, with consistently medium and large effect sizes during the follow-up period that reached statistical significance by the final 6-month timepoint. These results indicate that exposure-based CBT targeting feared somatic sensations (for protocol, see Otto & Pollack, 2009a, 2009b) demonstrates specific efficacy for BZ discontinuation, even when accounting for therapist contact and training in relaxation strategies.

The results from several similar studies are consistent with these findings. During an open trial, 22 patients with panic disorder received time-limited alprazolam treatment to provide fast-acting relief from panic attacks, along with 12 weeks of CBT (Panic Control Treatment; Barlow & Craske, 1989) to address panic symptoms and facilitate discontinuation following short-term BZ treatment (Hegel et al., 1994). CBT incorporated psychoeducation, cognitive restructuring, interoceptive exposure, relaxation, and alprazolam taper began following the fourth therapy session. One year after treatment concluded, 76% of patients had abstained from using alprazolam and 85% denied experiencing panic attacks during the past 2 weeks. In addition, an RCT compared the effect of CBT combined with slow tapering to that of tapering alone within a sample of 22 outpatients seeking to discontinue alprazolam after successful treatment for panic disorder (Spiegel et al., 1994). While there were no significant differences in immediate rates of BZ discontinuation at post-treatment between conditions (80% discontinuation with taper alone compared to 90% with taper plus CBT), patients in the CBT group showed higher rates of continued abstinence from BZ throughout the 6-month follow-up period compared to patients in the group that received slow tapering alone, who were 13.5 times more likely to be using medication during follow-up. Furthermore, a long-term follow-up study with this sample and another sample of panic disorder patients who received adjunctive CBT for BZ discontinuation found that more than 75% of patients who successfully discontinued alprazolam were able to abstain from BZ use 2–5 years afterwards without requiring any additional interventions for panic disorder, and that patients who experienced greater reductions in anxiety sensitivity during treatment were less likely to experience relapse of panic disorder (Bruce et al., 1999).

The successes of these exposure-based CBT approaches to BZ discontinuation stand in contrast to the limited success reported for pharmacologic strategies to aid BZ discontinuation (see Oude Voshaar et al., 2006; Parr et al., 2009). As such, CBT featuring exposure appears to provide additive benefits above gradual tapering and other anxiety management techniques to assist patients in becoming BZ free. By directly targeting fear of somatic sensations, exposure-based CBT equips patients to persist with BZ discontinuation even in the presence of withdrawal symptoms, thus supporting abstinence in the long-term. Although much of the research examining the efficacy of adjunctive exposure-based CBT for BZ discontinuation has focused on panic disorder patients, this treatment approach is applicable to patients with other anxiety-related conditions and there has been initial evidence of its efficacy for GAD patients (Gosselin et al., 2006).

Core Treatment Procedures

Two key features of CBT for BZ discontinuation that are vital to its success are: (1) interoceptive exposure trainings targeting fears of anxiety-related symptoms regardless of their source, whether it be stress, an anxiety disorder, or BZ withdrawal symptoms; and (2) providing a framework for coping with these symptoms, given that the course of withdrawal may be persistent compared to the more discrete episodes of anxiety or panic that they typically experience. While somatic sensations associated with anxiety are generally context dependent and relatively brief, withdrawal symptoms are more persistent, lasting hours or days while homeostasis is restored within the body.

There is significant variation in terms of which withdrawal symptoms will appear and when they will appear during the process of tapering. It is important to remember that medications with a longer half-life take more time to leave the body, which means that symptoms of withdrawal will likely emerge relatively later in the tapering period. For instance, alprazolam has a briefer half-life (approximately 12–15 hours) than clonazepam, a more potent, long-lasting agent (half-life approximately 15–50 hours). Thus, withdrawal symptoms tend to emerge earlier during the tapering period for patients taking alprazolam than for those taking clonazepam. In fact, while alprazolam users commonly face a weekly surge of symptoms after each reduction in their dose, some patients taking clonazepam might reach the end of tapering having experienced minimal withdrawal symptoms, only to experience a barrage of symptoms several days after their final dose. No matter how their unique trajectories of withdrawal unfold, patients can benefit from pretraining to help them endure uncomfortable symptoms during tapering and beyond.

A variety of interoceptive exposure exercises can be used during pretraining to help patients learn to relax in the presence of these sensations and achieve relative comfort (Otto & Pollack, 2009a, 2009b). A list of common procedures and the sensations they generate can be found in Table 10.2. With therapist support, patients can shift from an amplifying response fueled by catastrophic interpretations of symptoms to an acceptance response by "doing nothing" with the sensations (see Fig. 10.2). Patients should begin interceptive exposure several weeks before tapering to allow sufficient time to practice this response before withdrawal symptoms start to emerge.

The metaphor of fear as the body's alarm system can be used to illustrate how uncomfortable physical sensations motivate avoidance and interfere with safety learning. Clinicians may begin by explaining the function of fear, as follows:

> The role of fear is to alert us to a danger. However, people with panic disorder tend to have more sensitive alarm systems that are prone to sounding false alarms in the absence of a true threat. Fear and anxiety are associated with a range of physical sensations that are uncomfortable and difficult to ignore. This is by design, because an alarm system needs to grab your attention and direct it to a potential threat. The alarm response also motivates you to remove yourself from danger so that these uncomfortable feelings subside – this is why we tend to avoid or escape situations that provoke fear or anxiety. This is also why symptoms like panic attacks can be so confusing – your body is sounding the alarm telling you that something is off, even in situations where logic would indicate you are safe. Learning to withstand false alarms can also make it easier to face situations that feel dangerous, but pose no real threat. We can treat our fear as a signal to pay attention; This emotion is simply a source of information that can be used to inform what you do next. When we allow the false alarm to pass without trying to escape it, we give ourselves the opportunity to learn through experience that what we're experiencing is actually safe.

During interoceptive exposure, the patient can be directed to notice and describe what they are feeling in their body, while also recognizing any urges to distract themselves or dampen these feelings. Their attention can also be drawn to the role of their thinking, including what they are telling themselves about the meaning of these sensations, their ability to handle them, and whether something terrible might happen next. The patient can also be primed to recognize the role of anxious behaviors in reinforcing their sense of danger, for example, through noticing how their experience changes if they adopt a more relaxed posture, such as leaning back in their chair and resting their feet on the coffee table. In this way, the patient can be coached to adopt non-anxiogenic behavioral responses, with the stated goal of "treating the situation like it's not dangerous" by reacting how they would if they weren't feeling anxious.

Continuing with interoceptive exposure during tapering allows the clinician to monitor the patient's symptoms, tailor interoceptive exercises to their unique withdrawal profile, and provide ongoing coaching as they face physical sensations at greater levels of intensity and difficulty. In this way, patients can address symptoms of withdrawal within an exposure framework and practice (a) allowing their symptoms to be exactly as they are, without trying to control or change them, and (b)

Table 10.2 Typical interoceptive exposure exercises

Exposure exercise	Generated sensations/ emotions
Head rolling: Repeatedly turning the head around in a circle (from midline, around with chin to chest, and then on around to midline) while sitting with eyes closed	Dizziness, disorientation, and very mild derealization
Hyperventilation: Rapid deep breathing (with a forceful exhale) at a rate of 1 breath per second for 60 seconds	Dizziness, numbness and tingling (face, scalp, arms), hot flushes, dry mouth
Straw breathing: Breathing in and out of a thin coffee straw/ stirrer with nose plugged for 60 seconds	Breathlessness, smothering feelings
Running: Jogging in place with high knees or running up stairs	Rapid heartbeat, pounding heart, dyspnea, heavy legs
Chair spinning: Spinning around in a swivel chair with eyes closed	Dizziness, disorientation, nausea
Breath gulps: Clasping the hands behind the head (so that the arms make a triangle), fully expanding the lungs and holding the breath, then slowly taking three additional gulps of air (while continuing to hold breath) before finally exhaling	Chest tightness
Breath holding: Hold breath for as long as possible (30–90 seconds)	Pressure to breathe, dizziness, lightheadedness, burning sensation in the lungs
Full-body tension: While seated, tensing forehead and jaw, clenching hands and bringing them tightly to the shoulders, pulling in the stomach, and pushing heals into the floor while clenching the toes. Hold for 60 seconds	Trembling, numbness/ tingling sensations
Pillow squeeze: Tightly squeeze a firm couch pillow to the chest and solar plexus with arms for 50 seconds	Chest pressure, sinking feeling in the stomach
Rapid swallowing: Repeatedly swallowing (around six swallows) while mouth is empty	Throat tightness, dry mouth
Hand staring: Staring intently into the palm for 60 seconds (without allowing the eyes to move to trigger distortions in peripheral vision (e.g., seeing a finger disappear or an extra finger to appear) *Optical illusions:* Staring intently at venetian blinds or any other array of strips alternative between dark and light (e.g., office ventilation grate) without moving the eyes for 60 seconds (alternatively, staring at stripped visual illusions available on the Internet)	Visual distortions, derealization
Rapidly raising head from below knees: Leaning forward while seated and placing the head below the knees for 60 seconds, then rising up rapidly from that position (while remaining seated)	Flushed face; facial pressure
Stomach restriction: Wearing a tight belt or pants with a full stomach (e.g., after drinking a lot of water)	Nausea

(continued)

Table 10.2 (continued)

Exposure exercise	Generated sensations/ emotions
Chocolate-covered coffee beans: Depending on the patient's typical caffeine intake, eating a half dozen beans (or rapidly drinking a large coffee) at the beginning of the session can generate diffuse symptoms of arousal symptoms that can last for hours	Diffuse over-arousal: Rapid heart rate, sweaty palms, trembling, anxiety
Hand pinch: Utilizing the nerve sensitivity within the "triangle" between the thumb, wrist, and index finger, pinching the tendon in this area to produce mild pain and discomfort while "relaxing with the sensation"	Pain-related discomfort

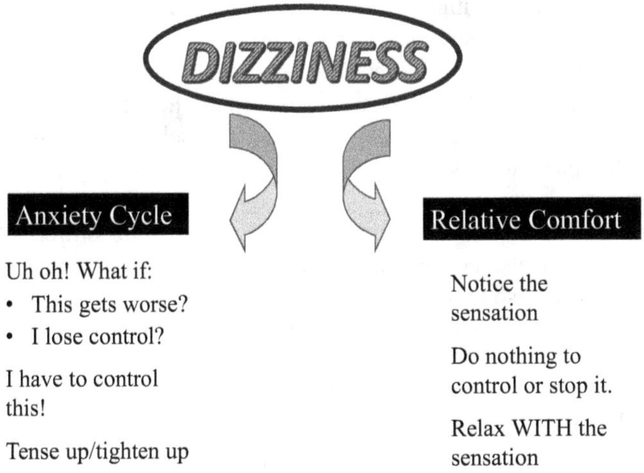

Fig. 10.2 Training in non-anxiogenic responses to symptoms using interoceptive exposure. (Figure adapted from Otto & Pollack, 2009a, 2009b)

viewing them through the lens of the "benzodiazepine flu" (see below). Ultimately, this equips patients to respond to rebound anxiety and withdrawal effectively as they transition from pharmacotherapy to psychotherapy.

The "benzodiazepine flu" metaphor also provides a useful framework for patients to understand and manage their withdrawal symptoms (Otto & Pollack, 2009a, 2009b). Likening withdrawal to flu symptoms provides a sense of safety and familiarity around somatic sensations that may arise during this vulnerable transition period. This frame of reference also helps patients draw on existing coping skills for addressing physical discomfort during common illnesses, which are also applicable to BZ tapering. During a benign illness such as the flu or the common cold, most patients can cope with their symptoms and nurse themselves back to health while maintaining some level of functioning. Though they may not necessarily enjoy the experience and may even face significant discomfort during their recovery, they are able to endure their symptoms without fearing the worst.

The clinician may begin with Socratic questioning to help the patient recognize their usual symptoms when they have the flu or a particularly nasty cold, making a mental note of which are similar to BZ withdrawal. Afterwards, the clinician may explore how the patient coped with the illness and managed their symptoms, for example, inquiring about whether they called out sick from work or skipped their appointments to probe how well they were able to fulfill their role obligations. Finally, the clinician may ask if they were frightened by their symptoms. The purpose of this conversation is to help the patient articulate their ways of coping with somatic sensations and discomfort without letting go of their responsibilities (e.g., I still had to get my children ready for school even though it was a really difficult; I still had to meet a deadline at work and that was a challenge) and their willingness to self-soothe and prioritize their recovery when possible (e.g., I let myself take a break and watch a movie) without worrying about the consequences. Marvel at how the patient (1) experienced significant uncomfortable symptoms (particularly those that mirror symptoms of BZ withdrawal); (2) but was able maintain some of their responsibilities (e.g., related to childcare, work, school, household chores, or activities of daily living); (3) while also taking care of themselves and self-soothing; (4) and waiting for them to pass without viewing them as dangerous of cause for concern.

This response can be framed as a skill for coping with uncomfortable somatic sensations, which can also be applied to withdrawal symptoms. Note how BZ withdrawal symptoms are also time-limited and follow a predictable course before eventually clearing up. As noted above, patients are encouraged to consider their withdrawal symptoms as case of the "benzodiazepine flu" and treat themselves like they would during any common illness. Although they may not find the experience to be enjoyable, they can tolerate it during a limited period of tapering. In fact, being able to tolerate withdrawal symptoms is applicable to managing symptoms of their anxiety disorder—whether their symptoms are attributable to anticipatory anxiety, stress, panic, withdrawal or any other scenario, including and illness or physical exertion during exercise.

Development of the BZ taper program falls to the patient's prescriber, who, in consultation with the clinician, will choose an appropriate pace based on the patient's clinical presentation and goals for BZ discontinuation. The objective is to achieve a rate of taper that is safe, manageable, and mitigates the most intense symptoms of withdrawal. The role of the clinician is to train patients in non-anxiogenic responding to their symptoms and provide coaching as they rehearse this strategy during structured interoceptive exposure.

Attending to Context

In most cases, the meaning we ascribe to somatic sensations and emotions depends on the situation. Experiencing breathlessness and elevated heart rate during vigorous exercise would have different implications than if this suddenly occurred during a casual stroll down the street. Similarly, crying in front of a long-term romantic partner after a hard day would be viewed differently than crying on a first date. The broader context of the situation impacts the availability of escape, avoidance, assistance, or embarrassment, thus influencing the perceived catastrophic outcomes of symptoms.

Clinical experience working with patients with panic disorder provides a sense of the unique ways that concerns about somatic sensations contribute to distinct patterns of avoidance for each individual. For one patient, experiencing symptoms in a crowded place where escape might be difficult, such as a concert venue or movie theater, may feel particularly threatening. Another may be more concerned about experiencing symptoms while driving due to fear of losing control and putting themselves and other drivers in danger—and then what if their children are in the car?

The clinician's office provides the initial context for interoceptive exposure. Here, the process of explanation, induction, and processing symptom meanings and their outcomes is typically repeated several times for each target symptom (typically at least 3–5 trials). The main objective of in-session exposure is for the patient to practice non-anxiogenic responding by "leaning in" to the anxiety and resisting the urge to engage in safety behaviors, so that extinction can occur. Between sessions, patients have opportunities to practice exposure in a wider variety of contexts. Patients may benefit from practicing a final trial of exposure alone in the therapy room without the clinician present to prepare for home practice. Prior to introducing the homework, the clinician may provide the following explanation:

> Now that you have some initial practice under your belt, the next step is to continue practicing this exposure at home, enough times that you eventually "get bored" by the sensations you feel. I would suggest practicing three exposures every day this week to help you get comfortable with the symptoms while gradually working your way up to greater intensities. You have a sense of what these exposures will be like based on our practice today, but your experience may be different when you practice them on your own while I'm not there. To prepare you for this, I'm going to have you induce the same symptoms here one more time, while I step out of the room (or turning off the clinician's camera and microphone during telehealth sessions). I want you to pay attention to whether your internal monologue changes, or if you have more of an urge to push away the symptoms while I'm not here with you. Remember, the goal is to do nothing with the sensations and relax alongside them.

It is important to remember that the context for exposure includes internal factors in addition to external ones. Engaging in interoceptive exposure after a good night's rest feels different than after a night of fitful sleep. Similarly, engaging in exposure with family support feels different than it would after an argument with a loved one. Of course, the patient's patterns of thinking also influence how these sensations are experienced and the meaning that is assigned to them. For example, engaging in interoceptive exposure while thinking "I can't handle this, it feels like it's never going to end" feels different than when thinking "I've done this before and it won't last forever."

Practicing interoceptive exposure in a variety of contexts helps develop an unconditional sense of safety around feared sensations. Patients may habituate to autonomic arousal in the therapist's office, but certain "what if" thoughts may remain—what if I start feeling panicky while I'm driving on the highway 200 miles away from home? What if this happens while I'm climbing up the stairs and I lose control and fall when there is nobody around to help me? Incorporating relevant contextual factors into interoceptive exposure practice provides more opportunities to violate patient's expectations about catastrophic outcomes of symptoms and create new safety memories (e.g., I can still climb the stairs while hyperventilating and feeling lightheaded without falling, even if my hands are shaking I can still maintain my grasp on the steering wheel). While the patient's past experiences cannot be erased, the more competing safety memories the patient creates, the more likely the association with safety will dominate the next time the cue is encountered. Over time, being able to tolerate physical sensations in the therapist's office will no longer be considered a "special case" as a more global sense of safety surrounding autonomic arousal is developed in a variety of contexts. This can be discussed with the patient as follows:

Therapist Now that you have a lot of practice with straw breathing and running in place, let's talk about how we can build a broader sense of safety around the feeling of labored breathing that we've been targeting with these exercises. I remember you mentioning that this sensation feels more alarming while you're climbing the stairs, is that right?

Patient Yes, I started to feel that way last month when I was taking the stairs up to my office to grab my coat at the end of the day. I was worried I might have a panic attack and I could lose my footing and fall down the stairs. Then I started thinking how that nobody would find me until the next morning since there aren't many people in the office that late.

Therapist What did you do next?

Patient I got off at the next floor and took the elevator the rest of the way up. Come to think of it, it's been a while since I've taken the stairs up to my office.

Therapist What about now, while you're sitting here relaxed in your chair—how likely does it seem that you would start panicking an lose you footing if were to take the stairs up to your office tomorrow?

Patient It doesn't seem as likely. I've taken the stairs a million times in the past, but it's another story when I'm feeling panicky.

Therapist And yet, you've experienced labored breathing many times now while practicing straw breathing and high knees running, including down the hallway. Have you ever lost control of your body and fell over?

Patient No *[laughs]*

Therapist I'd like us to try taking the stairs at the clinic today. We can start slow at first and then build up to running. Let's think of this as an opportunity to prove to yourself that you can tolerate the feeling of labored breathing, even while climbing the stairs. We can treat this like an experiment and test out whether you suddenly lose your footing. It's one thing to recognize that logically, there's a low chance this would happen, and another to learn that its safe through experience. How would you feel about that?

Patient: It still sounds a bit intimidating, but I'm willing to give it a try. I would really like to be able to take the stairs again at work because I'm trying to get more steps in.

Therapist: That's great! Later on, I would like you to practice climbing up the stairs to your office. Eventually, we can work up to taking the stairs later in the evening when there will be less people around. That way you can really prove to yourself that feeling breathless while taking the stairs is safe, no matter the circumstances.

Considering the Prototypical Session and Intervention

In general, the structure of each interoceptive exposure session targeting fear of emotions and associated somatic sensations includes: (1) preparing patients for the sensations they will experience, with pre-rehearsal of doing nothing to manage these sensations (i.e., to relax alongside the sensations, not necessarily relax away the sensations); (2) generating the feared sensations; (3) paying attention to the sensations and the way they are experienced while practicing acceptance and non-anxiogenic responding; (4) processing what was learned from interoceptive exposure; (6) repeating these steps several times during the session; and (7) assigning home practice, ensuring that in-session exposures provided a sufficient foundation for the patient to complete assigned exposures on their own.

The specific exposure exercises are tailored to the patient's case formulation, selecting the type, intensity, and context that will best target the core elements of their fear. Clinicians should approach each session with a specific learning objective in mind ("By the end of today's session, I want the patient to learn..."), though the plan for the session is always developed collaboratively with the patient. Head rolling is particularly suited for introducing interoceptive exposure, whereas hyperventilation or straw breathing are broadly effective for extending treatment gains in later sessions.

Each session follows this general format, with earlier sessions focusing on safety learning with lower order fear cues and ensuring that the patient can engage in non-anxiogenic responding. Subsequent sessions may incorporate a broader variety of interoceptive cues at increasing levels of intensity and difficulty during exposure. Once a sense of safety is developed in the presence of these cues, the focus may shift to expanding the context in which these cues are perceived as safe. This involves fading safety behaviors and varying contextual factors associated with threat (e.g., feared situations, internal states such as fatigue or heightened stress, interpersonal threat, varying times of day, specific distressing thoughts). The final phase of treatment may focus on more naturalistic exposure procedures and transition towards value-based exposures that promote emotional acceptance more broadly. In this way, the clinician can support the patient not only in reducing their symptoms, but enhancing their well-being by addressing a broader range of emotional and situational cues that may be considered challenging for most people.

Case Example: BZ Discontinuation for a Patient with Panic Disorder

Case Introduction: Mira is a 32-year-old, married woman referred for help discontinuing her benzodiazepine medication prescribed by her psychiatrist. She has been taking this medication (clonazepam) for 6 years, since the onset of her panic disorder. In addition to the panic, Mira describes herself as having difficulties with anxiety ever since childhood, reporting a pattern of worry and anxiety symptoms consistent with an early diagnosis of overanxious disorder and continuing on to an adulthood diagnosis of generalized anxiety disorder. She describes her distress in relation to these symptoms as mild to moderate and she did not seek treatment other than a few sessions with a High School counsellor around test anxiety. She explains that she assumed her chronic anxiety and worry was a trait and that she should probably just make do minimizing it. But when panic attacks emerged at age 26, she immediately sought attention in the emergency department for her prominent symptoms of chest pain, derealization, and dizziness. Despite medical reassurance, Mira quickly began to fear that her symptoms were either a sign of a pending heart attack, or that these symptoms might mean she was going crazy or losing control of her mental faculties.

Mira experienced in the range of 5–10 panic attacks a week until finally being referred to a psychiatrist, who prescribed the clonazepam. She noted fairly immediate relief from her daily dose of clonazepam (0.5 mg in the AM and 0.5 mg in the PM) but reported she experienced less control of her panic over time. Within a year, she was taking 0.5 mg three times a day. At this dose, she reported her panic was mostly controlled, although she continued a pattern of anticipatory anxiety and agoraphobic avoidance around a variety of situations where she felt most at risk for panic: crowded stores, driving distances from the house (especially at night), air or boat travel, and elevators (other than 1–2 floors).

Aside from her medication treatment, Mira met with a mental health counsellor who focused on her longstanding patterns of worry, including a review of childhood events that may have made her feel at risk. She describes her counsellor as a really nice woman who makes her feel safe and is good to talk to; Mira did not describe any significant change in symptoms arising from this psychotherapy.

Mira states her reason for seeking out specialty CBT for the purpose of discontinuing her benzodiazepine medication as twofold. First, she notes that she never felt fully comfortable being on the clonazepam (with encouragement from her mother to try getting off the medication). Second, and more importantly, her reason to finally pursue discontinuation was due to her desire to get pregnant in the next year. Her psychiatrist discussed the risk-benefit ratio of staying on benzodiazepine medications, but agreed to facilitate a referral for a discontinuation attempt. Mira's mental health counsellor was supportive of this referral.

Initial Elements of Treatment

Upon initiation of treatment, Mira's CBT therapist reviewed her motivation for discontinuing her clonazepam, the profile of common benzodiazepine discontinuation symptoms, and the plan to "get ahead" of these symptoms with a program of interoceptive exposure designed to change her relationship with these sensations (learn to relax with them) and to apply this skill to the treatment of her panic disorder and generalized anxiety disorder. The initiation of the benzodiazepine taper was set for after 3 sessions of treatment. Mira and her CBT therapist had a preliminary discussion of the rate of taper (a start somewhere between 10% and 25% reduction per week) and then Mira discussed and confirmed the following rate of week-by-week taper with her psychopharmacologist: 1.5 mg, 1.25 mg, 1.0 mg, 0.75 mg, 0.5 mg, 0.25 mg, to 0 mg. The 0.25 mg dosage reductions were to take place sequentially across the midday, evening, then morning dosages (i.e., 0.5 mg in the morning, 0.25 mg midday, and 0.5 mg in the evening for the first week of taper, and then 0.5 mg morning, 0.25 mg midday, and 0.25 mg evening dose for the second week of taper). All providers agreed that a temporary slowing of the taper when the lowest doses are reached is a reasonable alternative and denotes nothing about the likelihood of ultimate success. Mira's CBT therapist thus contracted for an initial 12 sessions of treatment: 3 sessions after the diagnostic intake session to provide initial skills, 6 weekly sessions during the planned taper, and then at least 2 weekly sessions after taper to help her further her skill attainment and further apply them to her anxiety conditions. Booster sessions can then be scheduled for monthly or bimonthly to allow further consolidation of treatment gains.

During initial interoceptive exposure (the induction of dizziness with head rolling; see Table 10.2), Mira showed strong bracing responses—grabbing the arms of her chair upon completion of the head rolling. Her therapist then began instruction in relaxing with the induced sensations.

Therapist	Mira, I noticed you grabbed the sides of your chair just now; what were you thinking and feeling?
Mira	I just felt so dizzy and I needed to make it stop.
Therapist	You wanted the dizziness to stop, why did that seem important? What felt so bad about the dizziness?
Mira	I don't know; I just hate it. I don't want it to get worse.
Therapist	What do you think might happen if it got worse?
Mira	I don't really know. I just don't want to lose control.
Therapist	Tell you what, let's have you head roll again, and while you head roll, I would like you to pay attention to what the dizziness actually feels like and ask yourself, "what is so bad about this feeling? Can I let myself just feel this for a while and see how I do?" Does that sound ok?
Mira	It doesn't sound good, but I guess I am willing to at least try it again.

Head rolling is repeated, with the therapist reminding Mira to notice what the sensations of dizziness feel like while doing nothing to try to control the sensations. Upon completion of the 20-second trial, the therapist queries her reactions

Therapist Ok, tell me all you can about what you are feeling right now?

Mira It feels weird. I feel off-center. I am not too dizzy, it is more feeling weird.

Therapist Ok, while you are feeling weird, would you lean back in your chair and just embrace the feelings of weirdness? And instead of gripping the arms of your chair, lean back and let your hands relax in your lap. Get comfortable in the chair and let yourself continue to feel weird. I want you to have the experience of weird and relaxed instead of feeling weird and tensing and bracing. What is that like for you?

Mira I still feel weird.

Therapist Oh good. I want you to continue to feel weird and off-center and maybe a bit dizzy so that you can practice getting comfortable with these sensations. What do you notice now?

Mira I am not so dizzy, not so feeling weird. I feel better already.

Therapist I am glad you feel better; that comes from relaxing with the sensations from head rolling. Take a moment and see if you can still find ways you may feel a bit dizzy, and I want you to sit back and just relax with those sensations. Remember, we are not hurrying any sensations away. Instead, we are inviting them to stay and getting comfortable with the sensations.

The therapist then completes another head rolling experience, this time preparing Mira for an alternative interpretive frame coming from the memory of having enjoyed getting dizzy from rolling down a hill with her friends.

Therapist Mira, this time when you opened your eyes from head rolling you did not brace at all. In fact, I think you smiled a little.

Mira Oh my gosh. It was so different. I was dizzy, but I remembered that I used to love rolling down a hill trying to get dizzy with my friend Amanda. It is not like I liked feeling weird just now, but it was harder to fear it while remembering I actually used to like this sensation.

Therapist That is amazing. Mira, you are noticing that your comfort with the bodily sensations you induced depends on how you interpret them. In just three exposures here today, you went from bracing and fearing sensations from head rolling to being able to sit comfortably and actually smile at the very same sensations. This really is the essence of the treatment we are doing. If we can help you feel more comfortable with a wide range of bodily sensations, then you will be able to do well with the natural sensations of withdrawal that can happen when you taper your dose of benzodiazepine medication. Also, if we can help you continue to relax with sensations of anxiety, we can help end the escalating patterns of vigilance, worry, and anxious responding to these sensations that is at the heart of many anxiety disorders, panic disorder in particular. Our next step is to send you home to practice head rolling at least twice daily, to help you get really bored with these sensations so that they have no power in making you feel anxious.

Mid-Treatment Stage

Mira has completed most of the interoceptive exposure procedures and targets in Table 10.2. In terms of assessment measures, this progress should be reflected by decreased anxiety sensitivity scores relative to her baseline. This should occur despite some increases in general distress due to the ongoing taper. The time course and type of symptoms to be experienced cannot be known with certainty, but by mid-treatment, most patients will be experiencing several days of strong symptoms after each dose reduction. This is the case with Mira when she presents for his seventh session of treatment (4 weeks after initiation of her benzodiazepine taper).

Therapist	How are you doing today?
Mira	Ugh. I feel lousy. I have been jittery all day following my last dose reduction, and I have more of that odd metallic taste in my mouth; I hate that. My muscles are also more tense and achy than usual.
Therapist	Oh yeah. You are in the midst of the Benzodiazepine Flu. Last session we talked in some detail about applying the "flu coping" model to your medication taper symptoms. Has that been useful at all?
Mira	It really has been. I mean, I hate the symptoms, but I have not been scared of them this week. Well, mostly not scared of them. I still have that panic voice in my head, saying, "what if it all gets worse?"
Therapist	I am glad the flu model is working for you, and let's do some rehearsals to help you with that persistent panic voice (thinking pattern). Let's take a moment and have you practice relaxing with symptoms, just like we do every week with interoceptive exposure, but let's do them with the symptoms you have. I would like you to sit back and relax your shoulders and hands and go ahead and pay attention to your achy muscles and your feelings of jitteriness. You know why you have these sensations (due to the medication taper), let them be present, and let's have you relax with them the best you can. And while you are relaxing with the symptoms, let's make sure you hear that old panic voice saying, "what if the symptoms get worse" or "what if you lose control." Hear that voice and still keep sitting back in your chair comfortably while you hear those catastrophic thoughts that are so common in panic disorder.

As Mira progresses with these skills with her existing symptoms, the therapist will hone this training by adding in additional symptoms with interoceptive exposure using one of the procedures in Table 10.2. Home practice with interoceptive exposure will continue, with the therapist and treating physician monitoring the taper progress.

Final Stage of Weekly Treatment

As Mira completes her taper (either on schedule or after some pauses in her taper schedule), the task of the therapist is to make sure Mira applies her learned skills to eliminating the full panic pattern. At this point, Mira has become a relative expert at replacing anxiogenic responses to symptoms—at least those symptoms due to interoceptive exposure and benzodiazepine taper. Her task is now to apply these skills to her panic patterns and the anxiety that accompanies her worry. She already has experience noting but not attending to anxiogenic thoughts associated with her taper ("what is these symptoms get worse?"). In the last few sessions, it is her therapist's task to help her apply this skill to the "what if" thoughts that characterize generalized anxiety disorder as well as panic disorder.

In addition, the therapist can also transition from interoceptive exposure assignments to in vivo exposure: where the patient is asked to use situations to cue uncomfortable sensations but to lean into those sensations and relax with them, while also learning to enjoy the benefits of staying in once-avoided situations. Follow-up sessions will then be scheduled as "booster" sessions to continue to hone these skills for ending panic and worry patterns.

New Applications of CBT for BZ Discontinuation

The opioid crisis has heightened concerns about BZ use and highlighted the need for expanding BZ discontinuation care to additional populations. Anxiety disorders commonly co-occur with opioid use disorder (OUD; Grant et al., 2004; Compton et al., 2007) and individuals with OUD often receive BZ prescriptions to manage their symptoms (Hawkins et al., 2019; Mooney et al., 2022). Additionally, individuals with pain are often prescribed both opioids and BZs (Hawkins et al., 2019; Mooney et al., 2022). In addition to the previously discussed negative impacts of BZ use, BZ use while taking opioids confers added risks, including the potential for overdose (Yeh et al., 2011; Nielsen et al., 2007, 2015; McCance-Katz et al., 2010; Cho et al., 2020). Indeed, there is a specific relationship between BZ daily dose and risk of death (Park et al., 2015; Garg et al., 2017). From 2005 to 2009 the most common cause of polysubstance overdose death occurred due to the combination of opioids and BZs (Calcaterra et al., 2013). Moreover, there was a tenfold increase in overdose deaths involving BZs between 1999 and 2017 (Overdose Death Rates, 2020).

Despite these serious and established risks for harm with concomitant BZ and opioid use (Lembke et al., 2018; Limandri, 2018), there is a lack of effective clinical guidelines for treating BZ misuse in this population. Although clinical guidelines for BZ taper exist (e.g., AU guideline; RACGP, 2023), these guidelines are not widely distributed and are primarily based on clinical census rather than research evidence. There is also a dearth of research to inform clinical practice and many healthcare settings lack both the resources and time to address this need (Wolitzky-Taylor et al., 2023).

Modifications of the BZ Discontinuation Program for Opioid Use Disorder

To fill this gap and facilitate BZ discontinuation in adults taking opioid medications, a number of modifications have been made in the CBT BZ discontinuation program published by Otto and Pollack (2009a, 2009b). The modifications are to: (1) de-emphasize the focus on panic disorder and broaden a focus on BZ discontinuation for individuals with any number of anxiety-related conditions, (2) enhance the focus on applying lessons learned from BZ discontinuation to the management of a broader set of anxiety difficulties, (3) include applications of skills for distress management around chronic pain (given that many patients taking both BZs and opioids suffer from pain-related complaints), and (4) include more of a principle-based rather than a protocol-based approach to manualized treatment. This modified protocol is currently under study in a federally funded pilot study of the efficacy of this care delivered by telehealth to individuals taking both BZ and opioid medications (Wolitzky-Taylor et al., 2018).

Of these modifications, two deserve additional comment. First, in broadening the focus on additional anxiety disorders, the interoceptive exposure component of treatment was conceptualized as general training to provide a non-anxiogenic response to stress, worry, and anxiety, regardless of source. Interoceptive exposure can be an effective way to introduce the concept of "leaning in" to anxiety by "doing nothing" to control it, and allows patients to develop a more concrete understanding of what non-anxiogenic responding entails through experiential learning. Many patients resonate with the objective of learning to relax in the presence of physical sensations that typically arise when they are anxious, but in the absence of an actual feared situation. Even if the sensations generated by interoceptive exposure exercises are not similar to how the patient feels when anxious, interoceptive exposure can be framed as a way to build tolerance of discomfort more broadly so it is experienced as less distressing.

Patients with low distress tolerance may particularly benefit from interoceptive exposure, especially before facing more emotionally activating fear cues, such as social anxiety-inducing interactions. Beginning with interoceptive exposure can also be particularly helpful if safety behaviors are overlearned and have become a reflexive way of responding under high levels of stress. When patients have initial success with interoceptive exposure and experience habituation, this builds a sense of mastery and confidence that an exposure-based approach will work for them. It may also result in greater willingness to confront more salient feared situations and experience the anxiety this produces. The physical symptoms of anxiety that arise in these situations may also seem less intimidating and may no longer be interpreted as a sign of danger with this initial practice under their belt.

Second, extending treatment procedures to the management of chronic pain also deserves note. The focus on modifying anxious responses to symptoms—the essence of intervening for anxiety sensitivity—is highly apt for chronic pain populations. We have shown in a meta-analytic review that AS is reliably linked to the experience of pain, particularly to the fearful appraisals of pain (Ocanez et al., 2010). Importantly, AS is also linked to greater avoidance, thereby reducing functional activities and facilitating the progression from acute to chronic pain (Asmundson & Taylor, 1996; Norton & Asmundson, 2004). Indeed, in the diathesis stress model of chronic pain proposed by Turk (2002), anxiety sensitivity has a significant direct effect on fear of pain and pain catastrophizing (accounting for 75% and 73% of the variance respectively), and fear of pain had a direct effect on escape/avoidance (accounting for 65% of the variance; Asmundson & Taylor, 1996). AS also has core linkages to Fear Avoidance models of pain disability (Leeuw et al., 2007), including application to those with co-occurring pain and PTSD (Martin et al., 2010). These findings support targeting AS as a modifiable risk factor for the management of chronic pain, with additional support for this model coming from clinical trial data (Fitzgerald et al., 2021).

Accordingly, in our current protocol (Wolitzky-Taylor et al., 2023) non-anxiogenic responses to symptoms are rehearsed in the context of discomfort exposures (interoceptive exposure to mildly painful stimuli), with rehearsal of the application of this skill to ongoing pain complaints. As such, interoceptive exposure broadly facilitates habituation and non-anxiogenic responding to somatic sensations, anxiety, pain, and distress. By targeting anxiety sensitivity and related avoidance, our protocol addresses core processes underlying both anxiety disorders and chronic pain that are prevalent among dual BZ and opioid users and may interfere with long-term BZ discontinuation. Thus, our protocol has the potential to promote greater success in BZ discontinuation by addressing symptoms of anxiety and chronic pain that may have prompted BZ and opioids use in the first place.

Conclusion

Although BZ have utility as a short-term treatment for anxiety disorders, discontinuation can present a challenge due to the potential for withdrawal symptoms, rebound anxiety, and even relapse, making long-term abstinence difficult to achieve. Exposure-based CBT interventions for BZ discontinuation have the benefit of directly targeting fear of sensations associated with anxiety and withdrawal alike, thus serving a dual function in promoting successful BZ discontinuation while addressing anxiety-related problems that first occasioned the BZ prescription. These interventions involve repeated exposure to internal sensations that mimic both anxiety and withdrawal symptoms while encouraging patients to engage in non-anxiogenic responding (e.g., "relaxing with" the anxiety and "doing nothing" to change it). Withdrawal symptoms are also framed as a case of the "benzodiazepine flu," which can be endured using the same strategy. When used in combination with gradual tapering, exposure-based CBT is associated with higher rates of successful BZ discontinuation among panic disorder patients compared to either gradual dose reduction alone or when paired with other arousal management techniques like relaxation training. These interventions also show promise for BZ users with a broader range of anxiety disorders and comorbidities including opioid use disorder and chronic pain.

References

American Psychiatric Association. (2009). *Practice guidelines for the treatment of patients with panic disorder.* https://psychiatryonline.org/pb/assets/raw/sitewide/practice_guidelines/guidelines/panicdisorder.pdf

Asmundson, G. J., & Taylor, S. (1996). Role of anxiety sensitivity in pain-related fear and avoidance. *Journal of Behavioral Medicine, 19*(6), 577–586. https://doi.org/10.1007/BF01904905

Baillargeon, L., Landreville, P., Verreault, R., Beauchemin, J.-P., Grégoire, J.-P., & Morin, C. M. (2003). Discontinuation of benzodiazepines among older insomniac adults treated with cognitive-behavioural therapy combined with gradual tapering: A randomized trial. *Canadian Medical Association Journal, 169*(10), 1015–1020.

Bandelow, B., Sher, L., Bunevicius, R., Hollander, E., Kasper, S., Zohar, J., & Möller, H.-J. (2012). Guidelines for the pharmacological treatment of anxiety disorders, obsessive–compulsive disorder and posttraumatic stress disorder in primary care. *International Journal of Psychiatry in Clinical Practice, 16*(2), 77–84. https://doi.org/10.3109/13651501.2012.667114

Barlow, D. H., & Craske, M. G. (1989). *Mastery of your anxiety and panic (MAP).* Graywind.

Bruce, T. J., Spiegel, D. A., & Hegel, M. T. (1999). Cognitive–behavioral therapy helps prevent relapse and recurrence of panic disorder following alprazolam discontinuation: A long-term follow-up of the Peoria and Dartmouth studies. *Journal of Consulting and Clinical Psychology, 67*(1), 151–156. https://doi.org/10.1037/0022-006X.67.1.151

Bruce, S. E., Vasile, R. G., Goisman, R. M., Salzman, C., Spencer, M., Machan, J. T., & Keller, M. B. (2003). Are benzodiazepines still the medication of choice for patients with panic disorder with or without agoraphobia? *The American Journal of Psychiatry, 160*(8), 1432–1438. https://doi.org/10.1176/appi.ajp.160.8.1432

Calcaterra, S., Glanz, J., & Binswanger, I. A. (2013). National trends in pharmaceutical opioid related overdose deaths compared to other substance related overdose deaths: 1999–2009. *Drug and Alcohol Dependence, 131*(3), 263–270. https://doi.org/10.1016/j.drugalcdep.2012.11.018

Cho, J., Spence, M. M., Niu, F., Hui, R. L., Gray, P., & Steinberg, S. (2020). Risk of overdose with exposure to prescription opioids, benzodiazepines, and non-benzodiazepine sedative-hypnotics in adults: A retrospective cohort study. *Journal of General Internal Medicine, 35*(3), 696–703. https://doi.org/10.1007/s11606-019-05545-y

Compton, W. M., Thomas, Y. F., Stinson, F. S., & Grant, B. F. (2007). Prevalence, correlates, disability, and comorbidity of DSM-IV drug abuse and dependence in the United States: Results from the National Epidemiologic Survey on Alcohol and Related Conditions. *Archives of General Psychiatry, 64*(5), 566–576. https://doi.org/10.1001/archpsyc.64.5.566

Dubovsky, S. L., & Marshall, D. (2022). Benzodiazepines remain important therapeutic options in psychiatric practice. *Psychotherapy and Psychosomatics, 91*(5), 307–334. https://doi.org/10.1159/000524400

Fitzgerald, H. E., Hoyt, D. L., Kredlow, M. A., Smits, J. A. J., Schmidt, N. B., Edmondson, D., & Otto, M. W. (2021). Anxiety sensitivity as a malleable mechanistic target for prevention interventions: A meta-analysis of the efficacy of brief treatment interventions. *Clinical Psychology: Science and Practice, 28*(4), 323–337. https://doi.org/10.1037/cps0000038

Fontaine, R., Chouinard, G., & Annable, L. (1984). Rebound anxiety in anxious patients after abrupt withdrawal of benzodiazepine treatment. *The American Journal of Psychiatry, 141*(7), 848–852. https://doi.org/10.1176/ajp.141.7.848

Fyer, A. J., Liebowitz, M. R., Gorman, J. M., Campeas, R., Levin, A., Davies, S. O., Goetz, D., & Klein, D. F. (1987). Discontinuation of alprazolam treatment in panic patients. *The American Journal of Psychiatry, 144*(3), 303–308. https://doi.org/10.1176/ajp.144.3.303

Garg, R. K., Fulton-Kehoe, D., & Franklin, G. M. (2017). Patterns of opioid use and risk of opioid overdose death among Medicaid patients. *Medical Care, 55*(7), 661–668. https://doi.org/10.1097/MLR.0000000000000738

Gosselin, P., Ladouceur, R., Morin, C. M., Dugas, M. J., & Baillargeon, L. (2006). Benzodiazepine discontinuation among adults with GAD: A randomized trial of cognitive-behavioral therapy. *Journal of Consulting and Clinical Psychology, 74*(5), 908–919. https://doi.org/10.1037/0022-006X.74.5.908

Grant, B. F., Stinson, F. S., Dawson, D. A., Chou, P., Dufour, M. C., Compton, W., Pickering, R. P., & Kaplan, K. (2004). Prevalence and co-occurrence of substance use disorders and independent mood and anxiety disorders: Results from the National Epidemiologic Survey on Alcohol and Related Conditions. *Archives of General Psychiatry, 61*(8), 807–816. https://doi.org/10.1001/archpsyc.61.8.807

Hawkins, E. J., Goldberg, S. B., Malte, C. A., & Saxon, A. J. (2019). New coprescription of opioids and benzodiazepines and mortality among veterans affairs patients with posttraumatic stress disorder. *The Journal of Clinical Psychiatry, 80*(4), 18m12689. https://doi.org/10.4088/JCP.18m12689

Hegel, M. T., Ravaris, C. L., & Ahles, T. A. (1994). Combined cognitive-behavioral and time-limited alprazolam treatment of panic disorder. *Behavior Therapy, 25*, 183–195.

Helmus, T. C., Tancer, M., & Johanson, C. E. (2005). Reinforcing effects of diazepam under anxiogenic conditions in individuals with social anxiety. *Experimental and Clinical Psychopharmacology, 13*(4), 348–356. https://doi.org/10.1037/1064-1297.13.4.348

Katzman, M. A., Bleau, P., Blier, P., Chokka, P., Kjernisted, K., & Van Ameringen, M. (2014). Canadian clinical practice guidelines for the management of anxiety, posttraumatic stress and obsessive-compulsive disorders. *BMC Psychiatry, 14*(Suppl 1). https://doi.org/10.1186/1471-244X-14-S1-S1

Konopka, A., Pełka Wysiecka, J., & Samochowiec, J. (2016). Chapter 32—Benzodiazepine misuse and addiction. Risk factors and adverse behavioral aspects. In V. R. Preedy (Ed.), *Neuropathology of drug addictions and substance misuse* (pp. 327–333). Academic Press. https://doi.org/10.1016/B978-0-12-800634-4.00032-9

Leeuw, M., Goossens, M. E. J. B., Linton, S. J., Crombez, G., Boersma, K., & Vlaeyen, J. W. S. (2007). The fear-avoidance model of musculoskeletal pain: Current state of scientific evidence. *Journal of Behavioral Medicine, 30*(1), 77–94. https://doi.org/10.1007/s10865-006-9085-0

Lembke, A., Papac, J., & Humphreys, K. (2018). Our other prescription drug problem. *New England Journal of Medicine, 378*, 693–695. https://doi.org/10.1056/NEJMp1715050

Limandri, B. J. (2018). Benzodiazepine use: The underbelly of the opioid epidemic. *Journal of Psychosocial Nursing and Mental Health Services, 56*, 11–15. https://doi.org/10.3928/02793695-20180521-03

Martin, A. L., Halket, E., Asmundson, G. J. G., Flora, D. B., & Katz, J. (2010). Posttraumatic stress symptoms and the diathesis-stress model of chronic pain and disability in patients undergoing major surgery. *The Clinical Journal of Pain, 26*(6), 518–527. https://doi.org/10.1097/AJP.0b013e3181e15b98

McCance-Katz, E. F., Sullivan, L. E., & Nallani, S. (2010). Drug interactions of clinical importance among the opioids, methadone, and buprenorphine, and other frequently prescribed medications: A review. *The American Journal on Addictions, 19*(1), 4–16. https://doi.org/10.1111/j.1521-0391.2009.00005.x

Mellman, T. A., & Uhde, T. W. (1986). Withdrawal syndrome with gradual tapering of alprazolam. *The American Journal of Psychiatry, 143*(11), 1464–1466. https://doi.org/10.1176/ajp.143.11.1464

Michelini, S., Cassano, G. B., Frare, F., & Perugi, G. (1996). Long-term use of benzodiazepines: Tolerance, dependence and clinical problems in anxiety and mood disorders. *Pharmacopsychiatry, 29*(4), 127–134. https://doi.org/10.1055/s-2007-979558

Mooney, L. J., Zhu, Y., Yoo, C. K., Wolitzky-Taylor, K., & Hser, Y. I. (2022). Association between benzodiazepine and opioid prescription and mortality among patients in a large healthcare system. *Journal of Addiction Medicine, 16*(1), 65–71. https://doi.org/10.1097/ADM.0000000000000828

Murphy, S. M., Owen, R., & Tyrer, P. (1989). Comparative assessment of efficacy and withdrawal symptoms after 6 and 12 weeks' treatment with diazepam or buspirone. *The British Journal of Psychiatry, 154*, 529–534. https://doi.org/10.1192/bjp.154.4.529

Naragon-Gainey, K. (2010). Meta-analysis of the relations of anxiety sensitivity to the depressive and anxiety disorders. *Psychological Bulletin, 136*(1), 128–150. https://doi.org/10.1037/a0018055

Nielsen, S., Dietze, P., Lee, N., Dunlop, A., & Taylor, D. (2007). Concurrent buprenorphine and benzodiazepines use and self-reported opioid toxicity in opioid substitution treatment. *Addiction, 102*(4), 616–622. https://doi.org/10.1111/j.1360-0443.2006.01731.x

Nielsen, S., Lintzeris, N., Bruno, R., Campbell, G., Larance, B., Hall, W., Hoban, B., Cohen, M. L., & Degenhardt, L. (2015). Benzodiazepine use among chronic pain patients prescribed opioids: Associations with pain, physical and mental health, and health service utilization. *Pain Medicine, 16*(2), 356–366. https://doi.org/10.1111/pme.12594

Norton, P. J., & Asmundson, G. J. G. (2004). Anxiety sensitivity, fear, and avoidance behavior in headache pain. *Pain, 111*(1–2), 218–223. https://doi.org/10.1016/j.pain.2004.06.018

Noyes, R., Garvey, M. J., Cook, B., & Suelzer, M. (1991). Controlled discontinuation of benzodiazepine treatment for patients with panic disorder. *American Journal of Psychiatry, 148*, 517–523.

Ocañez, K. L. S., McHugh, R. K., & Otto, M. W. (2010). A meta-analytic review of the association between anxiety sensitivity and pain. *Depression and Anxiety, 27*(8), 760–767. https://doi.org/10.1002/da.20681

Offidani, E., Guidi, J., Tomba, E., & Fava, G. A. (2013). Efficacy and tolerability of benzodiazepines versus antidepressants in anxiety disorders: A systematic review and meta-analysis. *Psychotherapy and Psychosomatics, 82*(6), 355–362. https://doi.org/10.1159/000353198

Olatunji, B. O., & Wolitzky-Taylor, K. B. (2009). Anxiety sensitivity and the anxiety disorders: A meta-analytic review and synthesis. *Psychological Bulletin, 135*(6), 974–999. https://doi.org/10.1037/a0017428

Otto, M. W., & Pollack, M. H. (2009a). *Stopping anxiety medication (Therapist guide, 2nd ed.)*. Oxford University Press.

Otto, M. W., & Pollack, M. H. (2009b). *Stopping anxiety medication (Patient Workbook, 2nd Ed.)*. Oxford University Press.

Otto, M. W., Pollack, M. D., Meltzer-Brody, S., & Rosenbaum, J. F. (1992). Cognitive-behavioral therapy for benzodiazepine discontinuation in panic disorder patient. *Psychopharmacology Bulletin, 28*, 123–130.

Otto, M. W., Pollack, M. H., Sachs, G. S., Reiter, S. R., Meltzer-Brody, S., & Rosenbaum, J. F. (1993). Discontinuation of benzodiazepine treatment: Efficacy of cognitive-behavior therapy for patients with panic disorder. *American Journal of Psychiatry, 150*, 1485–1490.

Otto, M. W., Safren, S. A., & Pollack, M. H. (2004). Internal cue exposure and the treatment of substance use disorders: Lessons from the treatment of panic disorder. *Journal of Anxiety Disorders, 18*(1), 69–87. https://doi.org/10.1016/j.janxdis.2003.07.007

Otto, M. W., McHugh, R. K., Simon, N. M., Farach, F. J., Worthington, J. J., & Pollack, M. H. (2010). Efficacy of CBT for benzodiazepine discontinuation in patients with panic disorder: Further evaluation. *Behaviour Research and Therapy, 48*(8), 720–727. https://doi.org/10.1016/j.brat.2010.04.002

Oude Voshaar, R. C., Couveé, J. E., Van Balkom, A. J. L. M., Mulder, P. G. H., & Zitman, F. G. (2006). Strategies for discontinuing long-term benzodiazepine use: Meta-analysis. *The British Journal of Psychiatry, 189*(3), 213–220. https://doi.org/10.1192/bjp.189.3.213

Overdose Death Rates. (2020, Revised March). https://www.drugabuse.gov/related-topics/trends-statistics/overdose-death-rates

Park, T. W., Saitz, R., Ganoczy, D., Ilgen, M. A., & Bohnert, A. S. (2015). Benzodiazepine prescribing patterns and deaths from drug overdose among US veterans receiving opioid analgesics: Case-cohort study. *BMJ, 350*, h2698. https://doi.org/10.1136/bmj.h2698

Parr, J. M., Kavanagh, D. J., Cahill, L., Mitchell, G., & Young, R. M. (2009). Effectiveness of current treatment approaches for benzodiazepine discontinuation: A meta-analysis. *Addiction, 104*(1), 13–24. https://doi.org/10.1111/j.1360-0443.2008.02364.x

Pecknold, J. C., Swinson, R. P., Kuch, K., & Lewis, C. P. (1988). Alprazolam in panic disorder and agoraphobia: Results from a multicenter trial: III Discontinuation effects. *Archives of General Psychiatry, 45*(5), 429–436. https://doi.org/10.1001/archpsyc.1988.01800290043006

Reiss, S., Peterson, R. A., Gursky, D. M., & McNally, R. J. (1986). Anxiety sensitivity, anxiety frequency and the predictions of fearfulness. *Behaviour Research and Therapy, 24*(1), 1–8. https://doi.org/10.1016/0005-7967(86)90143-9

Roy-Byrne, P. P., & Hommer, D. (1988). Benzodiazepine withdrawal: Overview and implications for the treatment of anxiety. *American Journal of Medicine, 84*, 1041–1052.

Salzman, C. (1993). Benzodiazepine treatment of panic and agoraphobic symptoms: Use, dependence, toxicity, abuse. *Journal of Psychiatric Research, 27*, 97–110.

Salzman, C. (1998). Addiction to Benzodiazepines. *Psychiatric Quarterly, 69*(4), 251–261. https://doi.org/10.1023/A:1022125929946

Schweizer, E., Rickels, K., Case, W. G., & Greenblatt, D. J. (1991). Carbamazepine treatment in patients discontinuing long-term benzodiazepine therapy: Effects on withdrawal severity and outcome. *Archives of General Psychiatry, 48*(5), 448–452. https://doi.org/10.1001/archpsyc.1991.01810290060012

Shinfuku, M., Kishimoto, T., Uchida, H., Suzuki, T., Mimura, M., & Kikuchi, T. (2019). Effectiveness and safety of long-term benzodiazepine use in anxiety disorders: A systematic review and meta-analysis. *International Clinical Psychopharmacology, 34*(5), 211–221. https://doi.org/10.1097/YIC.0000000000000276

Smits, J. A. J., Otto, M. W., Powers, M. B., & Baird, S. O. (Eds.). (2018). *Anxiety sensitivity: A clinical guide to assessment and treatment*. Academic Press.

Spiegel, D. A., Bruce, T. J., Gregg, S. F., & Nuzzarello, A. (1994). Does cognitive behavior therapy assist slow-taper alprazolam discontinuation in panic disorder. *American Journal of Psychiatry, 151*, 876–881.

Stewart, S. H., Westra, H. A., Thompson, C. E., & Conrad, B. E. (2000). Effects of naturalistic benzodiazepine use on selective attention to threat cues among anxiety disorder patients. *Cognitive Therapy and Research, 24*(1), 67–85. https://doi.org/10.1023/A:1005403025084

Taylor, S., Zvolensky, M. J., Cox, B. J., Deacon, B., Heimberg, R. G., Ledley, D. R., Abramowitz, J. S., Holaway, R. M., Sandin, B., Stewart, S. H., Coles, M., Eng, W., Daly, E. S., Arrindell, W. A., Bouvard, M., & Cardenas, S. J. (2007). Robust dimensions of anxiety sensitivity: Development and initial validation of the Anxiety Sensitivity Index-3. *Psychological Assessment, 19*(2), 176–188. https://doi.org/10.1037/1040-3590.19.2.176

The Royal Australian College of General Practitioners. (2023). *Discontinuing benzodiazepines*. https://www.racgp.org.au/clinical-resources/clinical-guidelines/key-racgp-guidelines/view-all-racgp-guidelines/drugs-of-dependence/part-b/discontinuing-benzodiazepines

Turk, D. C. (2002). A diathesis-stress model of chronic pain and disability following traumatic injury. *Pain Research and Management, 7*(1), 9–19. https://doi.org/10.1155/2002/252904

Tyrer, P., Murphy, S., & Riley, P. (1990). The benzodiazepine withdrawal symptom questionnaire. *Journal of Affective Disorders, 19*(1), 53–61. https://doi.org/10.1016/0165-0327(90)90009-W

Vasile, R. G., Bruce, S. E., Goisman, R. M., Pagano, M., & Keller, M. B. (2005). Results of a naturalistic longitudinal study of benzodiazepine and SSRI use in the treatment of generalized anxiety disorder and social phobia. *Depression and Anxiety, 22*(2), 59–67. https://doi.org/10.1002/da.20089

Votaw, V. R., Geyer, R., Rieselbach, M. M., & McHugh, R. K. (2019) The epidemiology of benzodiazepine misuse: A systematic review Drug and Alcohol Dependence, 200, 95–114. https://doi.org/10.1016/j.drugalcdep.2019.02.033

Yeh, H. H., Chen, C. Y., Fang, S. Y., Chang, I. S., Wu, E. C., & Lin, K. M. (2011). Five-year trajectories of long-term benzodiazepine use by adolescents: Patient, provider, and medication factors. Psychiatric Services (Washington, D.C.), 62(8), 900–907. https://doi.org/10.1176/ps.62.8.pss6208_0900

Winstock, A. R. (2012). 29—Psychoactive drug misuse. In P. Wright, J. Stern, & M. Phelan (Eds.), *Core psychiatry (third edition)* (pp. 439–462). W.B. Saunders. https://doi.org/10.1016/B978-0-7020-3397-1.00029-X

Wolitzky-Taylor, K., Krull, J., Rawson, R., Roy-Byrne, P., Ries, R., & Craske, M. G. (2018). Randomized clinical trial evaluating the preliminary effectiveness of an integrated anxiety disorder treatment in substance use disorder specialty clinics. *Journal of Consulting and Clinical Psychology, 86*(1), 81–88. https://doi.org/10.1037/ccp0000276

Wolitzky-Taylor, K., Mooney, L. J., Otto, M. W., Metts, A., Parsons, E. M., Hanano, M., & Ram, R. (2023). Augmenting the efficacy of benzodiazepine taper with telehealth-delivered cognitive behavioral therapy for anxiety disorders in patients using prescription opioids: A pilot randomized controlled trial. *Contemporary Clinical Trials, 133*, 107334. https://doi.org/10.1016/j.cct.2023.107334

Index

K. Wolitzky-Taylor (ed.), *Treating Comorbid Substance Use and Emotional Disorders*, CBT: Science Into Practice, https://doi.org/10.1007/978-3-031-62971-6

Printed in the USA
CPSIA information can be obtained
at www.ICGtesting.com
CBHW071922200924
14722CB00003B/132

9 783031 629709